Lung function testing is a vital part of the clinical assessment and evaluation of patients with respiratory dysfunction and disease. It provides a basis for diagnosis and can allow the disease process to be monitored and the efficacy of treatment to be assessed. However, the usefulness of the tests depends on the rigorous application of theoretical and practical knowledge. The clinician must know which tests to apply, how to interpret the results and how to recognise the limitations of the methods used.

This book provides a clear and comprehensive introduction to the use and interpretation of lung function tests in clinical practice. Early chapters consider the various tests which are available and review the basic physiological concepts of lung function necessary to understand their application and interpretation. The book then goes on to describe and discuss the use of breathing tests in a variety of clinical situations, providing helpful guidance and explanation of which test to apply and how to assess the results.

As a practical handbook and source of reference, *Pulmonary Function* will be of the utmost value to clinicians entering the field of respiratory medicine, as well as to all scientists and technical staff working with patients in the pulmonary function laboratory.

D1479718

# PULMONARY FUNCTION

# PULMONARY FUNCTION
## A GUIDE FOR CLINICIANS

Gabriel Laszlo

*Consultant Physician, Bristol Royal Infirmary,
and Clinical Lecturer in Medicine, University of Bristol*

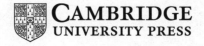

CAMBRIDGE
UNIVERSITY PRESS

Published by the Press Syndicate of the University of Cambridge
The Pitt Building, Trumpington Street, Cambridge CB2 1RP
40 West 20th Street, New York, NY 10011-4211, USA
10 Stamford Road, Oakleigh, Melbourne 3166, Australia

© Cambridge University Press 1994

First published 1994

Printed in Great Britain at the University Press, Cambridge

*A catalogue record for this book is available from the British Library*

*Library of Congress cataloguing in publication data*

Laszlo, Gabriel.
Pulmonary function : a guide for clinicians / Gabriel Laszlo.
p.  cm.
Includes index.
ISBN 0 521 43050 X (hardback). – ISBN 0 521 44679 1 (pbk.)
1. Pulmonary function tests.    I. Title.
[DNLM: 1. Respiratory Function Tests.    2. Lung Diseases –
physiopathology.    3. Respiration – physiology.    WF 600 L349p 1994]
RC734.P84L38    1994
616.2'4075 – dc20
DNLM/DLC
for Library of Congress    93-25546    CIP

ISBN 0 521 43050 X hardback
ISBN 0 521 44679 1 paperback

For Olwen

# CONTENTS

# PREFACE

This book has been written to provide a detailed insight into the application of clinical physiology to the investigation and treatment of respiratory disease. I have tried to fulfil two purposes: to place respiratory physiology into a clinical context and to discuss it rigorously in sufficient detail to provide the reader with the theoretical basis needed to evaluate and keep abreast with the literature in this field.

I have assumed a knowledge of general internal medicine at a standard expected of house staff, and the elementary knowledge of the basic physiology of respiration and acid–base balance expected of medical students, which is similar to that required for students working for degrees or diplomas in physiology, physiotherapy, nursing and physiological measurement. The book starts with a reminder of the way in which lung function tests can often explain the difficulties experienced with breathing by patients with lung disease. A systematic description of the investigation of lung mechanics and gas exchange follows. The next chapters place breathing tests into their clinical context. Chapters 10 to 12 describe my approach to the management of respiratory failure in the medical wards and the investigation of breathlessness. Chapter 13 is a critical account of exercise testing in the respiratory laboratory. Chapter 14 consists of a collection of essays on the theoretical aspects of oxygen and carbon dioxide exchange and on the control of ventilation. The book ends with a personal view of the rapidly changing field of sleep-related disorders of breathing. The technology of physiological measurement and details of epidemiological standards and reference values are mentioned only briefly as they are well covered elsewhere.

## Acknowledgments

Many colleagues, senior, contemporary and more recent have contributed to my understanding of respiratory physiology and will recognise their ideas in these pages. I have been fortunate in my teachers. Moran Campbell, Charles Fletcher and Dick Riley introduced me to the study of respiration; Frank Scadding and Stephen Semple encouraged me to show how it can be applied in daily clinical practice in a general medical setting.

Sheila Willatts kindly commented on sections of this work. Rob Ellis made the drawings. Janice Cooper's skill has made the production of the final drafts as painless as possible. I am very grateful to Jim Catterall who reviewed the whole work from beginning to end, as it is meant to be read, and suggested numerous improvements. Finally I would like to thank all those at Cambridge University Press who have been such a continual source of encouragement and for their excellent work on this text.

Any errors, obscurities and omissions that remain are mine. I hope the originators of any ideas which are not acknowledged in the references will be flattered. Some unconscious plagiarism is inevitable and if this book is quoted from memory once in a while, I shall be very pleased.

*Gabriel Laszlo*

*Bristol, July 1993*

# SYMBOLS IN RESPIRATORY PHYSIOLOGY

| Description | Symbol | Example |
|---|---|---|
| *Gas phase* | | |
| Flow | $\dot{V}$ | $\dot{V}_A$ Alveolar ventilation |
| Volume | $V$ | $V_A$ Alveolar volume |
| Inspired | Subscript I | $V_I$ Inspired volume |
| | | $\dot{V}_I$ max    Maximal inspiratory flow |
| Expired | Subscript E | $\dot{V}_E$ Expired ventilation |
| Alveolar | Subscript A | $\dot{V}_A$ Alveolar ventilation |
| Dead space | Subscript D | $V_D$ |
| Tidal | Subscript T | $V_T$ Tidal volume |
| *Blood phase* | | |
| Volume | $Q$ | $Q_C$ Pulmonary capillary volume |
| Flow | $\dot{Q}$ | $\dot{V}_A/\dot{Q}$    Ventilation – perfusion ratio |
| | | $\dot{Q}_S/\dot{Q}_{tot}$    Shunt fraction |
| Arterial | Subscript a | $P_aO_2$ |
| Mixed venous | Subscript $\bar{v}$ | $P_{\bar{v}}CO_2$    Partial pressure of carbon dioxide in mixed venous blood |
| Capillary | Subscript c | $P_cO_2$ |
| End-capillary | Subscript c' | $P_{c'}O_2$ |
| *Gases* | | |
| Oxygen | $O_2$ | $\dot{V}O_2$ Oxygen intake |
| Carbon dioxide | $CO_2$ | $\dot{V}CO_2$ Carbon dioxide output |
| Nitrogen | $N_2$ | $F_IN_2$ Fractional inspired concentration of nitrogen |
| Water vapour | $H_2O$ | |
| Helium | He | $F_I$HE |
| Carbon monoxide | CO | |
| Sulphur hexafluoride | $SF_6$ | |
| Partial pressure | P | $P_aCO_2$ |
| Fractional concentration | F | $F_IO_2$ |
| Blood content | C | $C_aO_2$ |
| Haemoglobin saturation | S | $S_aO_2$ |
| Barometric pressure | PBAR | |

*Tests*

| | |
|---|---|
| PEF | Peak expiratory flow |
| $MEF_{25}$ | Maximal expiratory flow when 25% of vital capacity remains to be exhaled* |
| $MIF_{50}$ | Maximal inspiratory flow at 50% of vital capacity* |
| $FEV_1$ | Forced expired volume (in the first second of forced expiration) |
| FVC | Forced vital capacity |
| VC | Slow vital capacity |
| EVC | Slow vital capacity (from full to empty) |
| IVC | Slow vital capacity (from empty to full) |
| TLC | Total lung capacity |
| FRC | Functional residual capacity |
| RV | Residual volume |
| ERV | Expiratory reserve volume |
| IC | Inspiratory capacity |
| $R_{AW}$ | Airway resistance |
| $G_{AW}$ | Airway conductance |
| $C_L$ | Lung compliance |
| $R_{OS}$ | Resistance, by oscillometric method |
| $TL_{CO}$ | Transfer factor for carbon monoxide |
| DL | Diffusing capacity |
| R | Respiratory exchange ratio $\dot{V}_{CO_2}/\dot{V}_{O_2}$ |
| RQ | Respiratory quotient |
| $f_b$ | Frequency of breathing |
| $f_c$ | Heart rate |

*Sometimes 25%, 50% of total lung capacity.

# 1 Introduction. Tests of lung function: how and why they are measured, how they are interpreted

Breathing is the only bodily function which, though continuing automatically throughout life, is performed by voluntary muscles and can be controlled at will. Cortical impulses can, consciously or unconsciously, override or augment the neural and chemosensitive control systems which regulate the cyclical actions of the respiratory muscles.

The purpose of breathing is to transfer oxygen from the inspired air to the circulating blood. The most logical way of testing the integrity of the lungs would be to analyse the arterial blood and the expired air (the end product and waste product of pulmonary ventilation), and the rate, depth and force of breathing. This can be done at rest or under stress. In practice, this is not easy, because the use of mouthpieces and arterial cannulation upsets the delicate adjustment of the rate and depth of breathing.

The most useful basic lung function tests involve standardised respiratory manoeuvres such as the forced vital capacity which are not part of the normal breathing process but which give information about the integrity of the lungs. In either case, the patient performs the test with the help of the operator. In this respect, the investigation of pulmonary function is like that of locomotor and psychological testing and unlike the investigation of the circulation or the endocrine glands. In the process, patients learn something about their disorder in a language shared with the investigator, because both cooperate in the measurement of performance in relation to effort.

The diagnostic acumen of the clinician improves rapidly as a result of performing investigations into the clinical physiology of respiratory disorders. The tests which are most easy to interpret are those which are elicited personally.

Breathing tests measure one or more of the three aspects of respiratory function: ventilatory mechanics, ventilatory control and gas exchange. Tests are selected to answer specific questions that may be posed:

1. Is the respiratory system damaged?
2. Why is the patient abnormally breathless?
3. How severe is the patient's bronchopulmonary disease?
4. Can anything be learned about the mechanism whereby disease causes disability?

Sometimes, patterns of physiological abnormality are seen which can be used to make deductions about the presence of structural abnormalities in the lungs, such as obstruction to the airways or diffuse lung fibrosis. These are often very useful, but breathing tests can only point towards broad diagnostic groupings or, occasionally, suggest that a provisional diagnosis may be incorrect.

## The need to breathe and the ability to breathe

The lungs are ventilated with air to provide oxygen and to remove carbon dioxide. The latter is present in inspired air at a concentration of only 0.3%. Thus it is easiest to consider first the elimination of carbon dioxide by pulmonary ventilation, and to treat the lungs as a single large gas exchanger connected to the outside by a tracheal dead space, so named because no measurable gas

Single gas exchanger (alveolus)

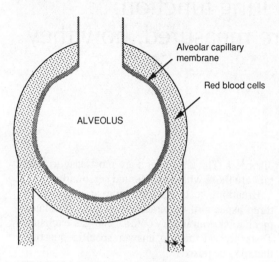

Fig. 1.1. Gas exchange in a single alveolus.

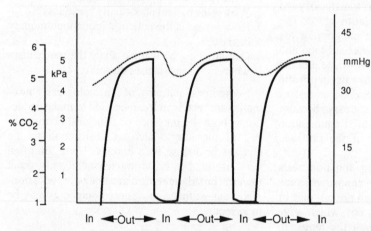

In ◄—Out—► In ◄—Out—► In ◄—Out—► In

and this blood returns to the lungs at a higher $P_{CO_2}$. The $CO_2$ diffuses from the venous blood into the alveoli, until the partial pressure in the alveolar gas is the same as in the blood in the pulmonary capillary. If the breath is held, alveolar partial pressure gradually reaches that in the blood returning to the lungs. Alveolar gas is renewed regularly by a tidal breath which dilutes the alveolar gas with room air. The partial pressures of alveolar gas oscillate with each tidal breath, and to a lesser extent as each heart beat sends another pulse of blood to the lungs (Fig. 1.2). In the following discussion these pulsations will be averaged, which introduces little error when considering events occurring over several respiratory cycles and when analysing blood and expired air over similar long periods. Thus, if arterial $P_{CO_2}$ is to remain at 42 mmHg (5.5 kPa), the average concentration of $CO_2$ in the alveoli must be 42/703, that is, 6% of the total gas pressure, less the water vapour pressure, at sea level.

Fig. 1.3 shows how $CO_2$ output and oxygen

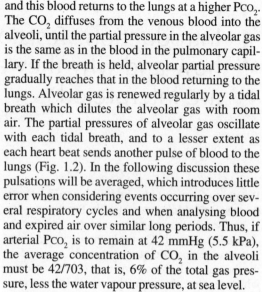

Fig. 1.2. Oscillations of $P_{CO_2}$. Continuous line, analysis of tidal $CO_2$ concentrations at the mouth; interrupted line, calculated mean alveolar $CO_2$ concentration.

exchange takes place there (Fig. 1.1). It is assumed that the alveolar temperature is constant at 37 °C (a close approximation) and the partial pressure of water vapour constant at 47 mmHg (6.25 kPa) in the saturated alveolar gas. The $CO_2$ in the air is ignored. The partial pressures of the other alveolar gases add up to 713 mmHg (95 kPa) when atmospheric pressure is 760 mmHg (101.2 kPa).

In health, ventilatory control mechanisms set arterial $P_{CO_2}$, sensed in the chemoreceptors of the brain, within close limits, usually 36–44 mmHg (5–6 kPa). $CO_2$ is added to the blood in the tissues

consumption may be measured. Expired gas is collected over several breaths in a bag or reservoir and analysed. Ventilation is expressed in litres per minute. The fractional concentration of $CO_2$ in the expired gas is measured by analysis and $CO_2$ output is calculated:

$CO_2$ output l/min = expired ventilation l/min ×
expired $CO_2$ concentration fraction   (1.1)

If the lung is represented as in Fig. 1.1, all the $CO_2$ is produced in the alveoli, but only part of the expired ventilation comes from the alveoli, the

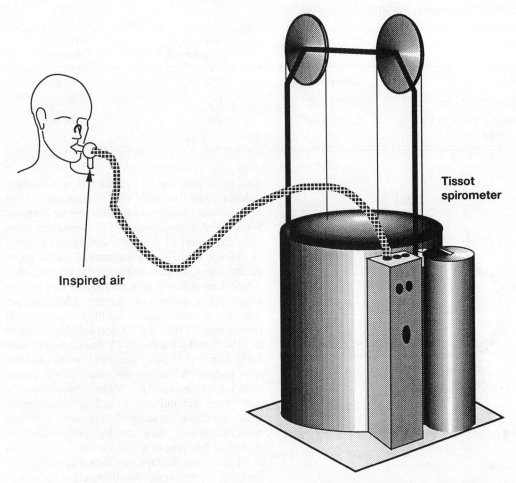

**Tissot spirometer**

**Inspired air**

Fig 1.3. Experimental determination of expired ventilation and expired gas concentrations.

rest coming from the dead space and containing no carbon dioxide. Thus:

$$CO_2 \text{ output} = \text{'alveolar ventilation'} \times \text{mean alveolar } CO_2 \text{ concentration} \quad (1.2)$$

This can be rearranged to express the principle underlying this equation:

$$\text{Alveolar } CO_2 \text{ concentration} = CO_2 \text{ output} \times \text{alveolar ventilation} \quad (1.3)$$

In other words, if alveolar $CO_2$ concentration is to remain constant (and thus arterial $PCO_2$), alveolar ventilation must be regulated to change pro-

portionally with the amount of $CO_2$ being added to the venous blood by metabolism. This varies considerably according to the amount of exertion, as shown in Table 1.1

Under normal circumstances, the actual amount of air breathed in is greater than in 'alveolar ventilation' by a factor of 10% to 20%, because of the ventilation 'wasted' in the trachea, bronchi and those few alveoli where no $CO_2$ exchange takes place (Fig. 1.4).

### Maximum ventilation: classical test of maximal breathing capacity

The total amount of air that can be moved in and out of the lungs varies with age and height, the

Table 1.1. *The regulation of alveolar ventilation*

| Effort | $CO_2$ production | = | Alveolar $CO_2$ concentration | × | Alveolar ventilation |
|---|---|---|---|---|---|
| At rest | $0.240 \; l\cdot min^{-1}$ | | 6% | of | $4 \; l\cdot min^{-1}$ |
| Walking on the level | $0.960 \; l\cdot min^{-1}$ | | 6% | of | $16 \; l\cdot min^{-1}$ |
| Walking at 3 mph (5 km·h⁻¹) up a slope | $2.400 \; l\cdot min^{-1}$ | | 6% | of | $40 \; l\cdot min^{-1}$ |

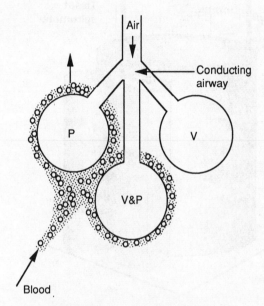

Fig. 1.4. Uneven distribution of ventilation and perfusion. V&P, ventilated and perfused alveoli: site of normal gas exchange. V, ventilated but not perfused alveoli: 'alveolar dead space'. P, perfused and poorly ventilated alveoli: 'physiological shunt'. 'V' and 'P' cause inefficient oxygen and $CO_2$ exchange because pulmonary ventilation and blood flow are wasted in these regions of the lung.

major determinants of lung volumes and mechanics in people of the same sex and race. Experimentally, a healthy young man of average height, breathing in and out of a spirometer as fast as he can for about 15 seconds, can achieve about 35 litres of ventilation or 140 litres per minute.

This procedure, the 15 second test of maximum voluntary ventilation (MVV), was the earliest test of ventilatory ability, low results being obtained when there is weakness of the respiratory muscles, alterations of the distensibility of the lungs or thoracic cage, loss of the normal elastic recoil of the lungs, or narrowing of the air passages. About four fifths of this ventilation can be sustained for 4 minutes or longer; 120 litres per minute in the same healthy young man (Freedman, 1970). The 15 second (Matthews *et al.*, 1989) and 4 minute MVV correlate well with maximum ventilation measured when patients with various pulmonary diseases perform heavy exercise (Clark *et al.*, 1969). Most healthy individuals are unlikely to achieve their maximum breathing capacity during even vigorous exercise, unless their cardiac performance is trained to the limit (Table 1.1). The 4 minute test of maximum voluntary ventilation is difficult to perform, so maximum breathing capacity is usually derived from single breath tests of forced expiration.

## Timed forced vital capacity: a test of ventilatory function

The timed forced vital capacity is the most widely used test of breathing, from which many clinical deductions may be made about the size of the lungs, the extent of lung damage and whether the airways are patent or narrowed. The patient takes a full breath in and breathes out as fast as possible into a spirometer arranged to draw a graph of expired volume against time (Fig. 1.5). Timed forced vital capacity was introduced as a simple method of assessing the maximum breathing

Table 1.2. *Mean values of FEV$_1$ and MVV for populations of European descent*

| Height (m) | Man aged 20 | | Man aged 60 | | Woman aged 20 | | Woman aged 60 | |
|---|---|---|---|---|---|---|---|---|
| | FEV$_1$ | MVV | FEV$_1$ | MVV | FEV$_1$ | MVV | FEV$_1$ | MVV |
| 1.6 | 3.6 | 108 | 2.4 | 72 | 3.2 | 93 | 2.1 | 63 |
| 1.7 | 4.0 | 120 | 2.7 | 81 | | | | |
| 1.8 | 4.4 | 132 | 3.0 | 90 | | | | |

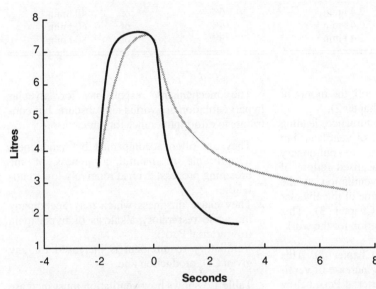

Fig. 1.5. Forced inspiration and expiration recorded on a kymograph connected to a spirometer. Bold line, young normal subject. Eighty per cent of the breath is expelled in 1 second and 100% in 3 seconds during a maximal expiratory effort starting with full lungs. Feint line, mild chronic airflow obstruction. Less than 70% is expelled in the initial second of forced expiration, which is prolonged. Forced expiratory flow rate is reduced at all lung volumes.

capacity (Tiffeneau and Pirelli, 1947). The expired volume in the first second of a maximum forced expiration (FEV$_1$) is approximately one thirtieth of the 4 minute maximum voluntary ventilation (Freedman, 1970). This is easy to understand if one allows a second for inspiration and for expiration at a respiratory rate of 30 breaths each minute, although even in heavy exercise, few healthy subjects and only some patients with lung disease breathe in this way. The early literature refers to several published formulae relating FEV$_1$ and FEV$_{0.75}$ to maximum voluntary ventilation which are valid for normal subjects, but are unfortunately misleading in disease states (Pineda *et al.*, 1984). Nevertheless, FEV$_1$ predicts maximum exercise capacity fairly well. With additional information about the power of the diaphragm and the gas exchange capacity of the

lung it is possible to predict maximum exercise capacity with some confidence (Dillard *et al.*, 1989).

Mean values of FEV$_1$ (litres) and estimated 4 minute MVV for populations of European descent are given in Table 1.2.

## Shortness of breath, ventilation and gas exchange

Shortness of breath normally occurs when ventilation exceeds about 50% of maximum (Hyatt, 1965). Three types of damage may interfere with a normal sensation of ventilation in exercise, caused by disturbances of lung mechanics, gas exchange or control of breathing:

1. Reduced ventilatory capacity: because of dis-

Table 1.3. *The increase in alveolor ventilation necessary if $P_{CO_2}$ falls to 28 mmHg (3.8 kPa)*

|  | CO$_2$ production | = | Alveolar CO$_2$ concentration | × | Alveolar ventilation |
|---|---|---|---|---|---|
| At rest | 0.24 l·min$^{-1}$ |  | 6% | of | 4 l·min$^{-1}$ |
|  | 0.24 l·min$^{-1}$ |  | 4% | of | 6 l·min$^{-1}$ |
| Walking on the level | 0.96 l·min$^{-1}$ |  | 6% | of | 16 l·min$^{-1}$ |
|  | 0.96 l·min$^{-1}$ |  | 4% | of | 24 l·min$^{-1}$ |
| Cycling up an incline | 2.4 l·min$^{-1}$ |  | 6% | of | 40 l·min$^{-1}$ |
|  | 2.4 l·min$^{-1}$ |  | 4% | of | 60 l·min$^{-1}$ |
|  | 2.4 l·min$^{-1}$ |  | 3% | of | 80 l·min$^{-1}$ |

eases of the airways, the alveoli, the thorax or the muscles of respiration (Chapter 2).

2. Pulmonary gas exchange disturbance, leading to an increase in the volume of ventilated but unperfused alveoli. Damage to pulmonary blood vessels may cause localised failure of pulmonary blood supply; ventilation to the zones is wasted and the volume of the alveolar dead space is increased (Chapter 3). This results in an excessive ventilation for the workload.

3. Alveolar hyperventilation (Chapter 3). This phrase is used to describe an increase of ventilation resulting in a fall of arterial $P_{CO_2}$ below the normal range. This occurs when the normal control mechanism is overridden. Sometimes this may readily be explained by increased chemoreceptor activity because of arterial hypoxaemia, metabolic acidosis or adrenal medullary stimulation. Interruption of cortical inhibitory pathways may result in central neurogenic hyperventilation, which is occasionally seen in central nervous system disease. Psychologically-induced hyperventilation is a feature of arousal, due to anxiety or occasionally hysteria (Brashear, 1983). Some diseases of the heart, lungs and pulmonary circulation cause alveolar hyperventilation in exercise or occasionally at rest. This is sometimes attributed to abnormal stimulation of receptors adjacent to pulmonary vessels, but there is no direct evidence for this.

The mechanisms responsible for alveolar hyperventilation are varied and obscure, but contribute to effort intolerance for three reasons:

1. They are often accompanied by heightened, disagreeable or painful awareness of the breathing process, even at relatively low ventilation.
2. They cause dizziness which may accompany the acute respiratory alkalosis of hypocapnia (low arterial $P_{CO_2}$).
3. Ventilatory requirement is increased for any given CO$_2$ production rate.

Table 1.3 shows how ventilation must increase if alveolar $P_{CO_2}$ falls to 28 mmHg (3.8 kPa) (4% alveolar concentration). The increase from 4 l·min$^{-1}$ to 6 l·min$^{-1}$ at rest is trivial and usually not noticed by the patient or the observer, in contrast to what happens during exercise when even a modest degree of hyperventilation is a major cause of dyspnoea. Fig. 1.6 illustrates this relationship graphically.

Table 1.4 illustrates how physical working capacity is lost by the effects of only moderate abnormalities of all the three components of respiratory function: ventilatory capacity, gas exchange and control of ventilation. The patient is trying to walk at 3 miles per hour up a 10% incline. In the example given, the metabolic requirement for exercise is identical in the normal subject and the patient, but the ventilatory requirement is calculated, on the basis of the

Table 1.4. *Loss of physical working capacity as a result of abnormalities in respiratory function*

| How obtained | Test | Normal | Patient |
|---|---|---|---|
| Assumed | $CO_2$ output | 2.4 | 2.4 $l\cdot min^{-1}$ |
| Measured | $FEV_1$ | 4.0 | 2.5 $l\cdot min^{-1}$ |
| Calculated | Sustainable ventilation | 120 | 75 $l\cdot min^{-1}$ |
| Assumed | Arterial $Pco_2$ | 42 | 35 mmHg |
| | | 5.6 | 4.7 kPa |
| Calculated | Alveolar $CO_2$ concentration | 6% | 5% |
| Calculated | Alveolar ventilation | 40 | 48 $l\cdot min^{-1}$ |
| Assumed | Wasted ventilation | 9% | 25% |
| Calculated | Total ventilation | 44 | 64 $l\cdot min^{-1}$ |
| Calculated | Total/maximal ventilation | 37% (44/120) | 85% (64/75) |

The tests were done when both the normal subject and the patient were trying to walk at 3 mph (5 $km\cdot h^{-1}$) up a 10% incline.

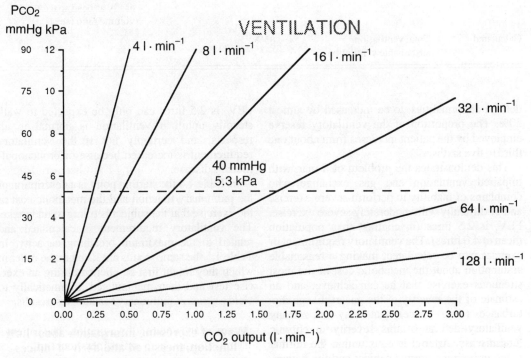

Fig. 1.6. Relationship between alveolar $Pco_2$, $CO_2$ output and total ventilation (isopleths).

Table 1.5. *The results from Table 1.4 manipulated to yield a series of pulmonary function test results*

| How obtained | Test | Result | Units | How calculated |
|---|---|---|---|---|
| Measured | $FEV_1$ | 2.5 | l | |
| Calculated | Sustainable ventilation | 75 | $l \cdot min^{-1}$ | $FEV_1 \times 30$ |
| Measured | Total ventilation | 64 | $l \cdot min^{-1}$ | |
| Measured | Expired $CO_2$ concentration | 3.75% | | |
| Calculated | $CO_2$ output | 2.4 | $l \cdot min^{-1}$ | Ventilation $\times$ expired $CO_2$ |
| Measured | Arterial $P_{CO_2}$ | 35.6 / 4.7 | mmHg / kPa | |
| Conceptual | Alveolar $CO_2$ concentration | 5% | | Arterial $CO_2$ partial pressure (barometric pressure – water vapour pressure) |
| Conceptual | Alveolar ventilation | 48 | $l \cdot min^{-1}$ | $CO_2$ output alveolar $CO_2$ concentration |
| Conceptual | Wasted ventilation | 16 | $l \cdot min^{-1}$ | Total – alveolar ventilation |
| Conceptual | Wasted/total ventilation | 25% | | This may be derived more easily as dead space/tidal volume ratio (see text) |
| Calculated | Total ventilation/ sustainable ventilation | 85% | | |

defined abnormalities, to be increased by almost 50%. The proportion of the ventilatory reserve employed by the patient increases from about one third to five sixths.

This demonstrates the problem of a man with impaired ventilation and gas exchange who complains of inability to perform severe exercise and of difficulty with moderately severe exercise. $FEV_1$ is 2.5 litres (in contrast to a population mean of 4.0 litres). The ventilatory requirement of exercise can be calculated, making a reasonable assumption about the metabolic cost of the most strenuous exercise that he can achieve, and an estimate of the severity of the gas exchange disturbance (dead space) that may accompany ventilatory defects of this severity in chronic lung disease. Arterial $P_{CO_2}$ is within the normal range in both the normal subject and the patient, but the slight increase of alveolar ventilation in this patient contributes to his ventilatory limitation. The conclusion is that a man whose $FEV_1$ is 2.5 litres can only be expected to walk steadily uphill if ventilation is normal in all respects, and certainly not if the ventilatory requirement is increased because of bronchopulmonary disease.

In Table 1.4 the starting point is a description of the pulmonary function and the metabolic cost of the exercise that the subject is trying to undertake. The ventilatory requirement is calculated and related to the maximum breathing capacity. In Table 1.5 the same results are listed in the order in which they might first be elicited during an exercise test and then manipulated arithmetically to yield a series of pulmonary function test results.

## Ways of expressing information about lung function: measured and derived indices

The tests listed in Table 1.4 illustrate some of the different ways used to describe the function of the breathing apparatus

- *FEV₁* is a measurement made while the patient performs a standard procedure unrelated to normal breathing. With the vital capacity, it gives information about the state of the lung and provides an indirect measurement of the maximum air flow rate that can be achieved. This is an important limiting factor for exercise in patients with respiratory disease (Chapter 2). $FEV_1$ is reproducible to within 5% in patients whose condition is stable. If allowance is made for height, age, sex and racial origin it can be used to indicate a degree of probability that lung damage is present, because it is distributed normally in groups of healthy individuals. One standard deviation is approximately 10–15% of the average 'predicted normal'. In the example in Table 1.4, $FEV_1$ is 4 residual standard deviations below the population mean value which means that the patient is most unlikely to be normal. Normal values do not exclude disease, but abnormal values are unlikely to be associated with health.
- *Ventilation at submaximal exercise.* This is a simple, direct measurement. By analogy with a factory, the system is being tested under normal operating conditions to identify maximum performance without stress.
- *Expired $CO_2$ concentration.* This is required for the calculation of metabolic rate, and may be used as an index of ventilation in relation to metabolic demand (Chapter 3).
- *$CO_2$ output.* With oxygen consumption, this identifies the size of the stress on the external respiratory system.

## Partial pressure of $CO_2$ in arterial blood

Generating normal arterial blood gases under all conditions is the main purpose of breathing. The measurement of partial pressures of gases in the arterial blood under conditions of increased metabolic demand shows whether the lungs are performing their ventilatory and gas exchanging function appropriately.

### Alveolar carbon dioxide concentration and alveolar ventilation

Alveolar $CO_2$ concentration and alveolar ventilation are conceptual figures because they are derived by employing a 'model' of the lung. A

physiological model is a simplified way of looking at the function of a system or organ, so that its total effectiveness can be described in orderly mathematical terms. Real lungs consist of millions of alveoli all exchanging oxygen and $CO_2$ at their own rate. When the glomerular filtration of the kidney is derived from creatinine clearance, no account is taken of the differing behaviour of each nephron. Similarly, in the 'model' of the lung shown in Fig. 1.1, gas exchange is considered to take place in a volume of uniformly ventilated alveoli, each claiming the same share of the pulmonary blood flow and allowing equilibrium to be achieved between the gas leaving the alveolus and the blood leaving the lung (Riley and Cournand, 1951). Thus $CO_2$ concentration in this model alveolus is defined by the arterial $P_{CO_2}$; the expired ventilation theoretically emanating from the model alveolus may be calculated from this and from the $CO_2$ output, because it is assumed that all the $CO_2$ excreted comes from there. If the alveolar ventilation is subtracted from the total ventilation, the remainder is wasted, so far as $CO_2$ exchange is concerned. If the volume wasted is greater than may be accounted for by the volume of the trachea and bronchi, there must be alveoli present which are contributing expired gas to the total ventilation but not excreting $CO_2$ into it: a form of inefficiency (Fig. 1.3).

This model of the lung is used very widely and needs to be examined critically (Chapter 3). There are many ways in which 17 million different alveoli can fail to arterialise the venous blood with the smallest amount of wasted effort. Even if every alveolus is taking part in gas exchange, the need to ventilate the trachea and bronchi results in small differences between arterial and expired gas pressures. The importance of this type of analysis is that it helps to identify minor degrees of abnormality; values of arterial $P_{CO_2}$ and $P_{O_2}$ which are individually within normal limits may be abnormal when taken in combination, because they differ too much from $P_{CO_2}$ and $P_{O_2}$ in the expired air.

## References

Brashear, R.E. (1983). Hyperventilation syndrome. *Lung*, **161**, 257–273.

Clark, T.J.H., Freedman, S., Campbell, E.J.M. & Winn. R.R. (1969). The ventilatory capacity of patients with chronic airways obstruction. *Clinical Science*, **36**, 307–316.

Dillard, T.A., Pantadosi, S. & Rajagopal, K.R. (1989). Determinants of maximum exercise capacity in patients with chronic airflow obstruction. *Chest*, **96**, 267–271.

Dubois, A.B., Britt, A.G. & Fenn, W.O. (1952). Alveolar $CO_2$ during the respiratory cycle. *Journal of Applied Physiology*, **4**, 535–548.

Freedman, S. (1970). Sustained maximum voluntary ventilation. *Respiration Physiology*, **8**, 230–44.

Hyatt, R.K. (1965). Dynamic lung volumes. In *Handbook of Physiology*, section 3, vol. II, ed. W. Fenn & H. Rahn, p. 1395. Washington, D.C.: APS.

Matthews, J.I., Bush, B.A. & Ewald. F.W. (1989). Exercise responses during incremental and high intensity and low intensity steady state exercise in patients with obstructive lung diseases and normal control subjects. *Chest*, **96**, 11–17.

McFadden, E.R., Pichurko, B.M., Bowman H.F., Ingenito, E., Burns, S., Dowling, V. & Solway, J. (1985). Thermal mapping of the airways in humans. *Journal of Applied Physiology*, **58**, 564–570.

Pineda, H., Haas, F. & Axen, K. *et al.* (1984). Accuracy of pulmonary function tests in predicting exercise tolerance in chronic obstructive pulmonary disease. *Chest*, **86**, 564–567.

Riley, R.L. & Cournand, A. (1951). Analysis of factors affecting partial pressure of oxygen and carbon dioxide in gas and blood of lungs: theory. *Journal of Applied Physiology*, **4**, 77–101.

Tiffeneau, R. & Pirelli, A. (1947). Air circulant et air captif dans l'exploration de la function ventilatrice pulmonaire. *Paris Médicale*, **133**, 624–628.

# 2 Testing the mechanics of breathing

In health, ventilation of the lungs varies between about 4 litres per minute in repose and 40–80 litres per minute in heavy exercise. Considerable work has to be performed by the inspiratory muscles when ventilation increases above basal levels (Fig. 2.1). The work of inspiration has to overcome mainly:

1. The resistance of the air passages to the flow of air (viscous resistance).
2. The elastic recoil of the lungs.
3. The inertia of the tissues of the lung and chest wall (tissue resistance).
4. The elastic recoil of the chest wall. The resting position of the thorax is near full inspiration which has to be overcome to reach full expansion.

Many lung diseases affect the mechanical properties of the lungs and thorax and cause an increase in the work of breathing. At the same time, they may cause alterations in the size and shape of the chest and in the pattern of ventilation.

In clinical practice, direct measurement of the resistance to inspiratory air flow and of the elastic properties of the lungs is more complex and until recently was subject to more experimental error than measurement of the lung volumes and ventilation. Therefore, investigation of the mechanics of breathing usually starts with measurement of the static lung volumes and with measurement of the largest breath than can be taken, the maximum inspiratory and expiratory flow that can be achieved and the maximum force that can be generated by the respiratory muscles.

## Static lung volumes

Lung volumes are usually expressed in litres, BTPS. These need careful definition (Fig. 2.2):

- *Total lung capacity (TLC)*. The volume of air in the lungs at full inspiration. This is a reproducible measurement.
- *Vital capacity (VC)*. VC is defined as the volume change of air at the mouth between the positions of full inspiration and full expiration. The measurement may be made in several ways, which under certain circumstances need to be distinguished.
  *Expired vital capacity*, measured from total lung capacity without force (EVC). This was the first test of lung function measured (made by Hutchinson in 1844).
  *Inspired vital capacity*, measured after the delivery of a full expiration (IVC).
  *Forced (expired) vital capacity (FVC)*. This is the maximum volume that can be expired during a maximal forced expiration (terminated by convention after 14 seconds or when expiratory flow falls to less than 0.05 litres per second (Quanjer, 1993). FVC generally exceeds or equals the other measurements in healthy normal individuals and patients without airflow obstruction. In these subjects, the measurement is reproducible to within 5%. Patients with airflow obstruction empty the lungs more fully if a breath is not first taken and if airway closure is not enhanced by undue force.
- *Residual volume (RV)*. The volume of air remaining in the lungs after full expiration. With practice, this is reproducible in normal subjects.

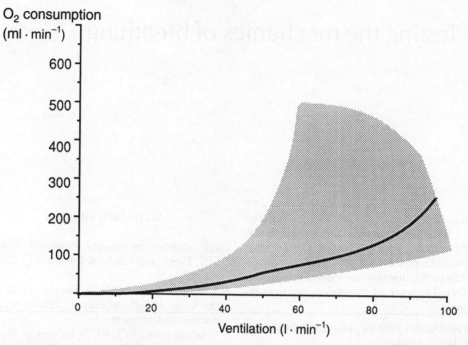

Fig 2.1. Estimates of the oxygen cost of breathing. The thick line is the generally accepted best estimate (Bartlett, Brubach & Specht, 1958). In a recent study, Aaron et al. (1992*a, b*) showed that in normal subjects breathing maximally, the cost of ventilation rose to 3 ml oxygen per litre of additional ventilation. (Oxygen uptake increases by approximately 40 ml per litre of ventilation.)

- *Functional residual capacity (FRC)*. The volume of air in the chest at the end of a quiet breath, when the respiratory muscles are at their lowest activity.
- *Expiratory and inspiratory reserve volumes (ERV, IRV)*. The volumes that may be expired or inspired from FRC to TLC and RV respectively.

## Determinants and interpretation of the static lung volumes

### Functional residual capacity

FRC is the lung volume at the end of expiration. It is determined by the tendency of the rib cage to spring open which is opposed by the elastic recoil of the lung. FRC is mainly determined by the elastic recoil of the lungs, being increased when recoil is reduced, and low when the lungs are 'stiff'. Lying down reduces FRC because the weight of the abdominal viscera pushes the diaphragm up.

A true reading of resting lung volume cannot always be obtained. Patients with severe acute airways obstruction caused by bronchial asthma cannot empty their lungs to a sufficiently low volume to reach the point where the elastic recoils cancel; electromyographs show that there is activity even at the point of maximum tidal expiration (Muller, Bryan & Zamel, 1981). Similarly, patients with expiratory muscle paralysis due to cervical cord section, who would be expected to be unable to breathe out below FRC, maintain an end-expiratory volume by continued inspiratory muscle activity.

### Vital capacity

VC was the first pulmonary measurement to be applied in clinical practice (Hutchinson, 1844). Normal values (3–6 litres) depend on sex, age and height. The test is reproducible to 5% from day to day. Results from healthy individuals are distributed normally about the mean, 2 standard devia-

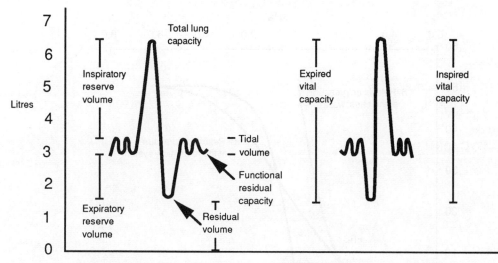

Fig 2.2. Static lung volumes. For definitions, see text.

tions being about 1 litre or 20% of the predicted value. Inspiration is limited by the distensibility of the lungs, as described later. In young adults expiration ceases when the ribs are lying against each other (Leith & Mead, 1967). In elderly subjects and patients with bronchial diseases, expiration ceases when airways are compressed by the pressure generated by the expiratory muscles (LeBlanc, Ruff & Milic-Emili, 1970).

Vital capacity may be reduced by:

1. Loss of inspiratory reserve (lung fibrosis, obliteration of alveoli, rigidity of the chest wall, respiratory muscle weakness).
2. Increased volume of residual air (trapped by closure of obstructed airways).

These may be distinguished by obtaining an estimate of total lung capacity. Vital capacity is a very useful measurement which correlates with disability and with the degree of disturbance of pulmonary gas exchange.

### Residual volume

The residual volume is the amount of air left in the lung after a full expiration. As explained above, it replaces the lower portion of the vital capacity as age advances. Residual volume should not exceed 37% of the total lung capacity.

High values of RV/TLC are generally caused by airflow obstruction or, occasionally, by expiratory muscle weakness.

### Expiratory reserve volume

Low volumes (less than 0.5 litres in adults) are found in pregnancy and obesity. Again, expiratory muscle weakness can reduce ERV.

### Total lung capacity

Inspiration is limited (at total lung capacity) because the lungs are almost fully stretched at TLC (Fig. 2.3). The maximum inspiratory pressure depends on the strength of the muscles. Full inspiration occurs normally only in sighing, yawning, sneezing and coughing.

## Measurement of static lung volumes

Measurement of lung volumes is straightforward in normal subjects, but poses a number of problems in patients which influence the reliability of reports of pulmonary function tests.

There are three different measurements of resting lung volume:

1. The volume of accessible air which exchanges with the atmosphere.
2. The thoracic gas volume, which includes alveoli not directly in contact with patent bronchi.
3. The volume of the thoracic cage.

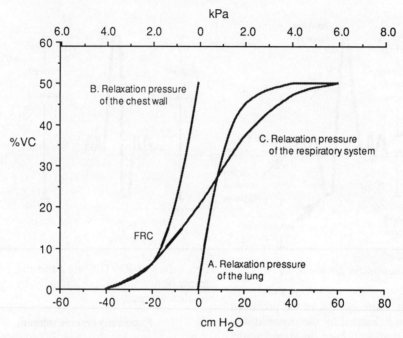

Fig 2.3. Static properties of the respiratory system. Relaxation pressures of the lung and chest wall are shown throughout the full range of vital capacity. The lung (line A) tends to empty by its own elastic recoil at all volumes above zero. The thoracic cage (line B) is at rest at about half way between TLC and RV. Line C is the sum of (A) and (B) and represents the whole respiratory system. At FRC the tendency of the lungs to empty is exactly counteracted by the expansile tendency of the thorax; the sum of their elastic recoil pressures is zero. FRC is the volume of air in the thorax when the respiratory muscles are at rest. The slopes of the volume–pressure curves (A, B and C) are the compliances of the lung (A), the chest wall (B) and the thorax (C) respectively. (After Rahn, Otis, Chadwick & Fenn, 1946.)

### Closed circuit spirometry

Accessible lung volume at FRC is measured by the dilution of an insoluble gas during closed circuit spirometry (McMichael, 1939). This produces an accurate measurement of FRC in normal subjects in whom the gas mixes with the air in the lungs in under 5 minutes, though accuracy is less in individuals whose lungs are small in relation to the size of the rebreathing circuit. Gases diffuse slowly into and out of regions affected by

bronchial obstruction. In patients with bronchial disease gas dilution tends to underestimate FRC and an end point is difficult to define (Ferris, 1978). When there are sizable poorly ventilated regions, leaks in the circuit and swallowing of air by the subject can affect the measurement because equilibration takes a long time to complete and these inaccuracies, normally unimportant, affect the measurement of the true lung volume.

### Body plethysmography

Lung volume can be measured in a variable pressure body plethysmograph shown in Fig. 2.4 (Dubois, Botelho & Comroe, 1956). This is a closed leak-proof booth of 60 litres capacity in which the subject sits. The subject makes inspiratory and expiratory efforts through a mouthpiece against a closed shutter and the oscillations of pressure are recorded at the mouth and in the plethysmograph. The change of volume of the thoracic contents caused by compression and rarefaction during these efforts is accompanied by fluctuations of volume and pressure which can be measured inside the body plethysmograph. These

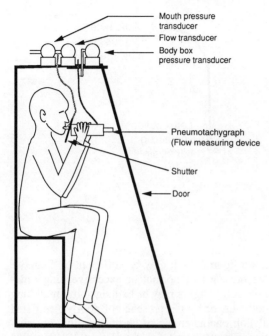

Mouth pressure transducer

Flow transducer

Body box pressure transducer

Pneumotachygraph (Flow measuring device)

Shutter

Door

Fig. 2.4. Measurement of lung volume and airway resistance by body plethysmography. The relationship between volume and pressure in the body plethysmograph depend on Boyle's Law: at constant temperature the product of volume and pressure in a closed system is constant: P1V1 = P2V2. The oscillations of volume and pressure are recorded in the plethysmograph as the subject attempts to breathe against a closed shutter. This compresses and rarefies the air in the thorax (Palv) and in the box. Thus:

Atmospheric pressure × thoracic gas volume = (atmospheric pressure × ± δ Palv) × (thoracic gas volume + δVthor)

The change in volume in the thorax (Vthor) is obtained by measuring the oscillations of volume in the closed box. In a variable volume device a rapidly responding spirometer records these oscillations directly. The variable pressure box has to be calibrated by pumping a known volume of air in and out of the box with the subject inside and measuring the oscillations of box pressure that result. This equation is expanded and solved for thoracic gas volume, ignoring the term δPalv x δPbox which is very small. To measure airways resistance, the subject breathes through the pneumotachygraph with the shutter open. The flow signal is displayed on the y axis of an oscilloscope and the pressure signal on the x axis. The slope Flow/Pbox is measured. The shutter is then closed while the subject attempts to breathe against it, which, in the absence of flow yields

are determined by the ratio of the volumes of the gas in the box outside the chest and the intrathoracic gas volume. This approach assumes that pressure swings in the intrathoracic gas are reflected accurately by the pressure recorded at the mouth. This is only true when all the airways are in continuity with the alveoli. In patients with severe airflow obstruction, discontinuity between the alveoli and the mouth results in pressure transients which do not reflect the swings of alveolar pressure in the whole thorax, but measure only the properties of the ventilated zones and the conducting airways (Brown, Scharf & Ingram, 1980; Rodenstein & Stanescu, 1982; Shore et al., 1983; Piquet et al., 1984).

Compression and rarefaction of the abdominal gas can also result in errors. The amount depends on whether panting is achieved by downward descent of the diaphragm (which results in an underestimate of thoracic gas volume) or, as is more common, by the splinting of the diaphragm with predominant activity of the muscles of the upper thorax (which includes abdominal gas in the estimate of gas volume). The errors due to abdominal gas are small, generally not more than 0.2 litres and in the direction of an overestimate (Habib & Engel, 1978; Brown et al., 1978). These problems are minimised by adopting a slow breathing frequency near TLC which has the effect of opening as many airways as possible, allowing those with slow ventilation to take part and reducing the proportion of the gas which is in the abdomen. Studies of lung volume in airflow obstruction published before 1982 employed a

an estimate of pressure within the airways and the alveoli. The slope Palv/Pbox gives a figure which allows changes in alveolar pressure to be calculated from changes in the pressure inside the plethysmograph. Since resistance is the flow generated by a change in pressure,

Airway resistance   = (Alveolar pressure/Flow)
                = (δPalv/δPbox)/(δFlow/
                    δPbox)

Panting is sometimes recommended to adduct the larynx and to minimise fluctuations of temperature, but good estimates of lung volumes and airways resistance may be obtained during quiet breathing if the inspired air is warmed and humidified.

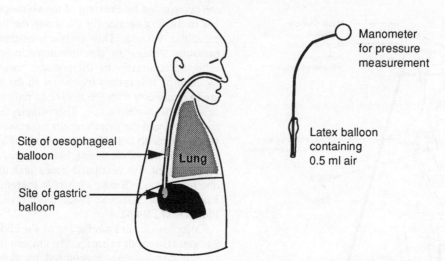

Manometer
for pressure
measurement

Site of oesophageal
balloon

Lung

Site of gastric
balloon

Latex balloon
containing
0.5 ml air

Fig. 2.5. Use of oesophageal and gastric balloons for the measurement of intrathoracic and abdominal pressure. Changes in trans-diaphragmatic pressure are used to measure the power of the diaphragm.

panting method at a rapid respiratory rate and have to be evaluated in the light of these observations.

### Radiographic measurement of lung volumes

Lung volumes can be assessed from postero-anterior and lateral chest radiographs taken in full inspiration. Formulae employing hand calculation (Loyd, String & Dubois, 1966; Harris, Pratt & Kilburn, 1971) and digitisation techniques on computers are available (Pierce *et al.*, 1979). The results agree well with plethysmographic estimates in normal subjects and exceed those obtained by helium dilution by approximately 0.4 litres. The method depends on the assumption of normal values of lung tissue volume which are subtracted from the volume occupied by the lungs, normally around 0.7 litres. This approximation introduces an unknown error in estimates in patients with emphysema or pulmonary fibrosis. Various forms of X-ray, CT and isotope densitometry are available, but none are sufficiently accessible to solve this problem.

For clinical evaluation body plethysmography yields the best results. A technically satisfactory estimate of helium dilution volume yields a mini-

mum figure which may be sufficient to diagnose the presence of normal or excessive lung inflation. A low figure may be explained by small lung volumes, or by the presence of poorly ventilated alveoli characteristic of chronic airflow obstruction. Slowly ventilated alveoli may be identified by measuring the difference between thoracic gas volume and accessible lung volume, or demonstrated by radioisotope studies of ventilation. Slow wash-in or wash-out of foreign gases also provides indirect evidence of the presence of poorly ventilated alveoli.

### Static lung compliance

The lungs resist inflation and recoil when inflated because of elastin, collagen and surface tension. The elastin fibres unwind during inspiration while the collagen fibres probably are important in limiting full inspiration (Setnikar & Meschia, 1986; Hoppin *et al.*, 1986).

The static lung volumes depend on the mechanical properties of the lungs and chest wall (Fig. 2.2). Static compliance is the name given to the measurement of distensibility of the lungs or chest wall. The units are litres of distension per unit increase of distending pressure ($l \cdot cm\ H_2O^{-1}$ or $l \cdot kPa^{-1}$). Lung compliance is usually described as if the lungs are removed from the chest and inflated directly from a syringe as shown in Fig. 2.6. Increased volume results in increased elastic

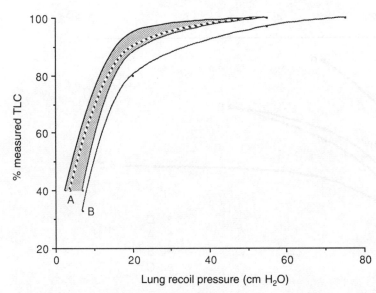

Fig. 2.6. Compliance curve of the lung, with volume expressed as a percentage of the total lung capacity. This allows for the size of the lung and the number of alveoli. The stippled area represents the normal range. Patients with reduced TLC are able to distend their lungs more forcibly and achieve higher pressures, because the inspiratory muscles are less fully contracted. Patient A (broken line), who has a reduced TLC, has normal alveolar distensibility and a high distending pressure. Patient B (continuous line) has reduced alveolar distensibility. (After Gibson & Pride 1976.)

recoil pressure, which is the total pressure in the system when air is not flowing.

During normal respiration the lung is inflated because inspiratory muscle activity makes the pressure around the lungs more negative. The pressure inside the oesophagus, about two thirds of the distance between the mouth and the diaphragm, gives an approximate estimate of the average pressure in the thorax. With some care, this may be measured by means of a balloon swallowed and connected to a manometer, but the method does not work with the patient lying flat (Fig. 2.5) (Milic-Emili *et al.*, 1964).

The capacity of a lung to expand under pressure depends on its size. The lungs of small animals and children are less compliant than those of adult humans because the alveoli are smaller and less numerous.

Static lung compliance is reported in various ways. The volume–pressure relationship may be expressed as if it is linear over the tidal range. The elasticity of the lung at or near full inflation may be expressed as the volume at a given recoil pressure or as the recoil pressure at a given lung volume. The most elaborate method consists of fitting an exponential function to the pressure–volume curve (Gibson *et al.*, 1979; Colebatch, Greaves & Ng, 1979). Both the last two methods are applicable to post-mortem stud-

ies of the pathophysiology of the lung. If volume changes are expressed as a fraction of TLC, the results are to some extent 'normalised' for lung size.

Disease may reduce static lung compliance (Fig. 2.6) by:

1. Obliteration of alveoli.
2. Increasing alveolar stiffness.
3. Increasing the thickness of the alveolar walls.
4. Reducing the secretion of surfactant material.

Increased static compliance is a feature of pulmonary emphysema and bronchial asthma when elastic recoil is reduced. In emphysematous lungs there is loss of alveolar walls and increased lung size (Fig. 2.7). The variable compliance in bronchial asthma is unexplained (Chapter 6).

### Chest wall compliance

The chest wall has a tendency to spring open until its volume is about 1 litre less than total lung capacity. Muscular effort is needed to expand it further.

### Total thoracic compliance

The measurement of total thoracic compliance is a useful guide to lung function during assisted ventilation in anaesthetised or unconscious patients. The respiratory muscles must be relaxed.

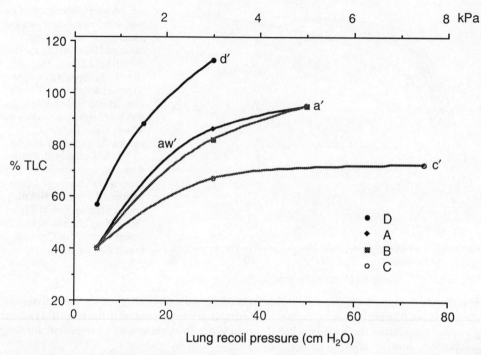

Fig. 2.7. Compliance curve of the lung, with lung volume expressed as a percentage of the expected lung volume (predicted on the basis of age, sex and height). Static lung recoil pressure (Ppl) is plotted against lung volume. A, Normal Caucasian adult male, expiratory curve (standard compliance curve). B, Same subject, inspiratory curve. Greater pressure is required to open closed airways and to overcome alveolar volume hysteresis caused by surface and elastic forces. C, A similar male with lung fibrosis causing reduced compliance. D, A patient with pulmonary emphysema causing increased distensibility. a', maximal pressure at TLC under normal circumstances; aw', weakness of respiratory muscles can limit maximal recoil and TLC. c', d', the respiratory muscles are more efficient at lower lung volumes and less so at high lung inflation, so maximal Ppl is high in alveolar disease and low in emphysema.

Alveolar pressure is measured at various levels of lung inflation. Mouth pressure is equal to alveolar pressure when there is no air flow and the glottis is open. A few patients (about one in three) can be trained to relax against a closed tap when conscious.

Total compliance at FRC has been estimated by adding weights to the bell of a water-filled spirometer and measuring change of FRC and change of mouth pressure (Heaf & Prime, 1956). Little clinical information has emerged from this.

### Work of breathing

The inspiratory muscles act to overcome:

1. The elastic recoil of the lungs, and, if a large breath is taken, the elastic recoil of the chest wall.
2. The resistance to flow offered by the air passages (airways resistance).
3. The inertia of the system (less important).

Under normal circumstances, expiration is passive, the expiratory pressure being provided by the elastic recoil of the stretched lung. When breathing is laboured, the abdominal muscles contract and push the abdominal contents against the lower surface of the diaphragm, reducing the end-expiratory volume: this assists expiration.

## Resistance to the flow of air in the airways

Resistance of a tube to airflow is defined by the pressure that is required to generate a certain flow down it:

$$\text{Resistance} = \frac{\text{Pressure}}{\text{Flow}} \qquad (2.1)$$

The units are cm $H_2O$/litre per second (kilopascals/litre per second).

### Methods of measuring airways resistance

The total resistance of the airways was first estimated by measuring the changes of intrathoracic (balloon) pressure and airflow during tidal breathing (Mead & Whittenberger, 1953) (Fig. 2.8). Whole body plethysmography (Dubois, Botelho & Comroe, 1956) is now generally employed (Fig. 2.4).

The calculation of airways resistance requires an estimate of the difference between alveolar and mouth pressure (driving pressure) and the flow of air during panting or tidal breathing. First, airflow ($\dot{V}$) is measured and the fluctuations of pressure within the box are recorded as the patient breathes the air enclosed in the box. If there were no resistance, there would be no compression or decompression of the air in the thorax during tidal breathing. Thus, changes of pressure as the patient breathes inside the closed box reflect the specific airways resistance (resistance/lung volume). Lung volume is measured as described earlier, providing an estimate of airways resistance.

Quite minor technical problems cause abnormal traces. The analysis is very dependent on obtaining linear relationships between flow, box pressure and mouth pressure. Humidity and temperature have to be stabilised and the box made almost completely leakproof. Pressure gauges must have equal response times. Patients with airflow obstruction have regions of lung which equilibrate more slowly than others, resulting in difficulties in interpretation (Fig. 2.9).

The physiological meaning of total airways resistance is obscured by the complexity of the branching system of airways. As the bronchi branch towards the periphery, each daughter pair

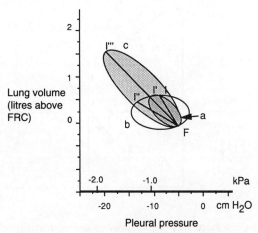

Fig. 2.8. The work of breathing. Relationship between pleural pressure and lung volume during quiet breathing (a), during rapid forced shallow breathing (b), and with increased tidal volume (c). The work required to overcome the static recoil and inertia of the lung in moving from F to I' is the elastic work. To this is added the resistive work needed to overcome the resistance of the airway to the movement of gas. Thus the pressure–volume curve of the lung is different at high (a) and low (b) flow rates. The slope of the line FI is the static compliance. FI', FI'' and FI''' are the dynamic compliances at different frequency and tidal volume. The relationship between pressure change and work of breathing depends on the pattern of tidal respiration and is complex (Roussos & Campbell, 1986). In a fluid system, work is the change in pressure multiplied by the change in volume; this is represented by the area of the diagram of pressure/lung volume.

has a total diameter greater than the parent by a factor of about 1.3:1. It follows that the resistance to airflow, and for the same reason its velocity, is greatest in the narrowest part of the larynx, which accounts for half of the airways resistance. The trachea and major bronchi are thought to account for some 30%, only 20% normally being sited in airways smaller than 2 mm in diameter (Macklem & Mead, 1967). These early estimates may be too low (Hoppin, Green & Morgan, 1978), but it is known that peripheral resistance is much higher in patients with chronic airflow obstruction (Hogg, Macklem & Thurlbeck (1968). Airways resistance, measured in the body plethysomo-

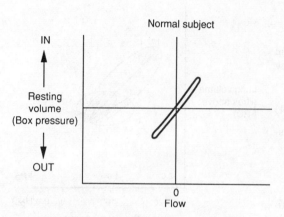

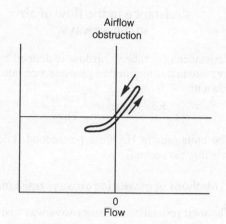

Fig. 2.9. Relationship between air flow and thoracic volume (measured by body plethysmography during panting at FRC) in a normal subject and a patient with airflow obstruction.

graph, is therefore very sensitive to changes of calibre in the larynx and proximal airways.

### Oscillometric measurement of airways resistance

The mechanics of the respiratory system can be studied during quiet breathing into and out of a tube. An oscillation of flow is superimposed at various frequencies by means of a loudspeaker. These oscillations generate variations of pressure which are subjected to Fourier analysis in a computer. The theoretical analysis depends on the simple idea that if pressure is applied to a system of tubes, the flow of air into it depends on the resistance to flow and the elasticity of the system. Elastic forces limit flow at all frequencies, but narrowing of the tube has a greater effect when the pressure is applied rapidly at high frequency. The physiological analysis of this phenomenon is forbidding (Peslin, 1986), but commercially made equipment is now available and has the advantage of generating values for airways resistance during quiet breathing by means of an experiment which is quite simple for the subject. The values are not strictly comparable to those obtained by other methods and the model employed provides a different approximation to airways resistance from that used in body plethysmography.

## Dynamic spirometry to detect airflow obstruction

In clinical practice, airflow obstruction is usually identified by measurements of airflow during forced inspiration and expiration. We now explore these tests and their applications.

### Timed forced expiration: forced expired volume–time curve

The forced expiratory volume–time curve is sometimes known as the 'spirogram'. Simply, if a patient exhales forcibly to RV after a full inspiration to TLC, any airflow obstruction present will reduce the speed at which the lungs can be emptied. $FEV_1$, the volume expired in the first 1 second interval of forced expiration, should be greater than 75% of the forced vital capacity. It is normally greater than 80% of VC in women and men under 30, 90% in most teenagers and 70% in elderly men (Fig. 2.10).

$FEV_1$, FVC and VC are important indicators of ventilatory capacity. The ratio $FEV_1$/VC is an indicator of the presence of airways obstruction.

Occasionally, patients with severe obstruction are unable to exhale for more than 2 seconds, so ratios of greater than 75% may be misleading under these conditions. It follows that improvement may be accompanied at first by a fall of the ratio $FEV_1$/VC, because vital capacity improves faster than $FEV_1$ (Fig. 2.10).

*Peak flow rate* is the maximum flow rate (sus-

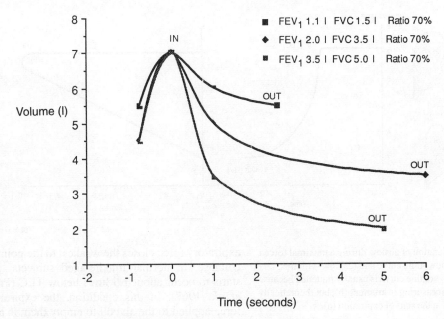

Fig. 2.10. FEV1, forced vital capacity and their ratio: (top) during an acute attack of airflow obstruction, (middle) during recovery, and (bottom) after recovery.

tained for 10 milliseconds) that can be achieved during a brief forced expiration from TLC. A portable meter may be used to measure expiration of flow at TLC after maximal effort. The normal range (380–700 l·min⁻¹) is wide, but the test is useful for measuring changes with treatment or during the course of one individual's illness and for detecting moderate or severe reduction of airflow rates. Readings of less than 100 l·min⁻¹ after bronchodilator drugs indicate a substantial risk of ventilatory failure during acute illnesses.

### The shape of the forced expired flow–time trace (Hyatt, 1983)

Dynamic spirometry is the starting point in the investigation of pulmonary function and may be all that is required because it readily detects airflow obstruction. Measurements of maximal expiratory flow are highly reproducible and widely used. Their physiological significance is worth exploring.

### Determinants of maximal expiratory flow rate

Airways are kept open by their own intrinsic anatomical rigidity and by their attachments to surrounding structures. Airways outside the thorax tend to collapse in inspiration (like a weak tube when sucked). Like alveoli, intrathoracic airways widen in inspiration and narrow in expiration. They collapse during forced expiration because of the rise of pleural pressure around the lung.

Forced expiratory flow decelerates (Fig. 2.11). This is because the elastic recoil diminishes and the airways narrow progressively when pleural pressure is increased by the effort of expiration. Maximal expiratory efforts

- *aid* expiration by adding to elastic recoil pressure around the alveoli but
- *hinder* expiration by obstructing the intrathoracic airways.

This is 'dynamic airways compression'. The interpretation of measurements of airflow in forced expiration depends on whether the airways are compressed to the point of obstruction.

When a normal subject breathes in fully to TLC and exhales forcibly, the airways are fully open.

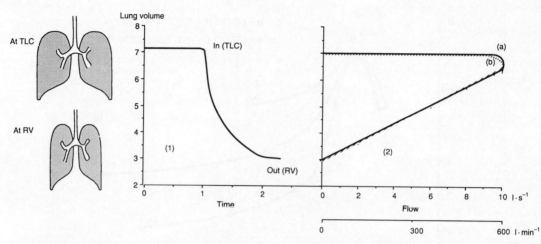

Fig. 2.11. Deceleration of airflow during a maximal forced expiration: (1) flow–time curve and (2) flow–volume curve. The flow–volume curve is usually flattened because of inertia in the measuring instrument (b), but theoretically flow is maximal at the start of expiration (a).

Peak flow depends on

1. The effort employed.
2. The elastic recoil of the lung.
3. The conductivity of the whole airway.

Arithmetically

$$\text{Flow} = \frac{(\text{alveolar pressure - atmospheric pressure})}{\text{airways resistance}}$$

= (alveolar pressure - atmospheric pressure) × airway conductance

or

$$V = \text{Palv} - \text{PBAR}/\text{Raw} \qquad (2.2)$$

When

Alveolar pressure = (pleural pressure caused by expiratory effort) + (elastic recoil pressure of lungs)

i.e.

$$\text{Palv} = \text{Ppl} + \text{Pel} \qquad (2.3)$$

The relationship between flow and effort alters when the airways are on the point of compression. As expiration proceeds, the airways narrow progressively as the lung becomes less distended. The pressure holding them open diminishes and

expiratory force closes the weakest to the point of collapse. In normal middle-aged subjects, this starts to occur about 1.5 litres below TLC (Pride *et al.*, 1967). In this condition, the expiratory force applied to the alveoli to empty them is also transmitted to the airways to obstruct airflow. When expiratory pressure overcomes the intrinsic rigidity of the bronchial walls and collapses the airways, further effort causes no further increase of expiratory flow, which now depends on the elastic recoil pressure of the lungs and the conductivity of the airways between the alveoli and the collapsed segment of airway.

The airway collapses when pleural pressure exceeds the transmural pressure. At this time the force of expiration overcomes the intrinsic rigidity of the airway plus the splinting effect of the air flowing out of the lung. Intrinsic rigidity cannot be measured. If it is ignored and the airway treated as a floppy tube, then it can be shown that flow should be independent of the expiratory effort applied, and depends entirely on the elastic recoil of the lung and the degree of obstruction caused by the bronchi between the alveoli and the collapsed segment.

Pressure aiding expiration    = Pleural pressure and elastic recoil pressure
                              = Ppl + Pel
Pressure obstructing expiration = Ppl    (2.4)

Resistance to airflow is equal to the resistance of the airways between the alveoli and the collapsed

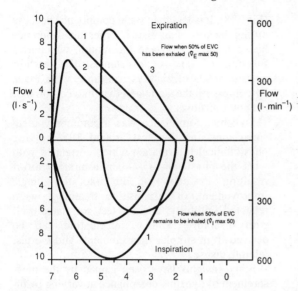

Fig. 2.12. Flow–volume curves: normal curve (1) and airflow obstruction (2). Maximal flow is reduced at all lung volumes but proportionally more near residual volume, resulting in a downward convexity of the curve. In fibrosing alveolitis (3) the lung volumes are reduced, with relatively high values of airflow rate if allowance is made for total lung capacity.

bronchial segment (Rp), because the airways downstream from the site of compression offer no effective resistance. Therefore

$$\text{Flow} = \frac{Ppl + Pel - Ppl}{Rp}$$

$$= \frac{Pel}{Rp} \qquad (2.5)$$

This equation explains how pulmonary emphysema causes airflow obstruction even when the bronchi are not demonstrably abnormal because the loss of elastic recoil causes reduction of airflow even if peripheral airways resistance is normal. Conversely, high flow rates are seen, as expected, in forced expiratory tests in some patients with fibrosing alveolitis in whom elastic recoil is increased proportionally more than the resistance of the peripheral airways (Fig. 2.12).

This analysis shows that if the airways are very easily collapsible, expiratory flow is virtually independent of expiratory effort once the intrinsic rigidity of the airways is overcome by the force of expiration.

Bronchography shows that in normal subjects, the first or second generation of bronchi collapse during forced expiration about 1–1.5 litres below

TLC (Macklem, Fraser & Bates, 1965). Patients with chronic airways obstruction show evidence of collapse of airways in forced expiration even at TLC and the site of the collapse is more distal (Macklem, Fraser & Brown, 1965). Thus, in normal subjects, achievement of maximal readings of peak flow and the first portion of the FEV/time curve, depends on maximal effort, while the lower portions of the FEV/time curve require only moderate expiratory force to achieve maximum readings (Fig. 2.13). Patients with moderately severe airways obstruction collapse their airways on forced expiration, even at full inspiration. In such subjects the FEV curve and peak flow are very reproducible, depending only on full inspiration and reasonable effort.

This explanation of the effort-independence of forced expiratory tests is satisfying, but there probably is another mechanism, related to the distensibility of the bronchi. The velocity of airflow through a non-rigid tube cannot exceed the velocity of the propagation of a wave down its substance (Dawson & Elliott, 1977). Intuitively, this means that when air is forced into a non-rigid bronchus, the velocity of forward flow down the tube is reduced by the extent to which the tube bulges. This mechanism of flow limitation (called the 'choke point') probably also operates in inspiration.

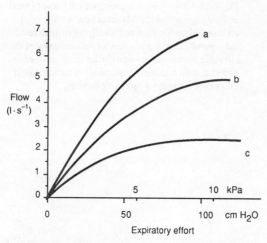

Fig. 2.13. Isovolume pressure–flow curves: relationship between expiratory flow achieved ($y$ axis) and expiratory effort (pleural pressure: $x$ axis). In this example, a normal subject, maximal expiratory flow rate (a; peak flow) depends on the strength of the respiratory muscles, but becomes less dependent on effort as the lung volume diminishes. Curve b was obtained at 60% of TLC when flow-limitation is usually detectable in normal adults. Curve c was obtained at 30% TLC. The tangent of the upslope yields an estimate of airways resistance at the volume under study, and demonstrates progressive airway narrowing during expiration.

### Flow volume plots

The familiar FEV curve shows volume plotted against time. Plotting flow against volume (Fig. 2.11) uses the same information, but illustrates certain aspects of airway function more clearly.

Maximum inspiratory and expiratory flow are about equally reduced by diffuse intrathoracic airways obstruction. Effort is generally thought to be the main determinant of inspiratory flow, although airway distensibility may play a part (Denison *et al.*, 1982). Many subjects find the measurement of forced inspiratory flow difficult to perform and it has, therefore, been neglected, except in the study of narrowing of the larynx and trachea (Chapter 6).

### Dynamic compliance

Dynamic compliance is the change of intra-thoracic pressure with volume during breathing (Fig. 2.8). It is less than static compliance because during the flow of air there is a pressure difference between the alveoli and the mouth, which is a function of airways resistance. The earliest measurements of airways resistance were made by comparing the static and dynamic compliance at known airflows.

Dynamic compliance was a commonly measured lung function test around 1955, giving physiological information which correlated with what the physician saw – an inspiratory effort resulting in entry of air into the lungs. Improvement, or response to treatment, were reflected faithfully, and the test correlated well with disability. Similar information can be derived from simpler measurements and the test fell into disuse.

Some insights have been gained by the measurement of dynamic compliance at varying respiratory frequency, as an indicator of occlusion of the small airways (Fig. 2.8). The interpretation of this depends on the concept of time constants (Otis *et al.*, 1956). By analogy with electronic circuits, if a pressure is applied to a lung unit consisting of airway and alveolus, it fills more rapidly if it has a low compliance or low resistance; less rapidly if it has a high compliance or high resistance.

$$\text{Time constant} = \text{resistance}^{-1} \times \text{compliance}^{-1}$$

If respiratory frequency is very rapid, there is insufficient time to fill the alveoli with long time constants, and pressure is not equalised throughout the lung, so a small volume change is obtained for a given inspiratory effort than at lower rates. A fall of dynamic compliance with increasing frequency of breathing ('frequency dependence of compliance') was shown to occur in smokers and others who might be supposed to have early disease of small airways (Woolcock, Vincent & Macklem, 1969), and the validity of the analysis was confirmed by inducing small airways obstruction in experimental animals, but the test is not very reproducible (Guyatt *et al.*, 1975) and has been abandoned as an epidemiological test of narrowing of small airways. The phenomenon is responsible for the variation of the results of airway resistance measurements with breathing frequency when measured in the body plethysmograph, as pointed out earlier.

## Functional anatomy of the respiratory muscles (Roussos, 1985; Green & Moxham, 1985)

### The diaphragm

The diaphragm is a more or less cylindrical tube of muscle, partly in contact with the lower rib cage, with a fibrous dome at the top (Fig. 2.14). The main action of the diaphragm is to pull down the dome, thus enlarging the thorax and sucking air into the lungs. Contraction of the diaphragm reduces the pressure within the thorax, and increases it in the abdomen. Exactly what happens is determined by the position of the subject, and by the extent to which the abdominal muscles are allowed to relax. If they relax completely, contraction of the diaphragm causes very little outward movement of the lower rib cage. If the abdominal muscles are held rigid, or the abdomen is swollen and cannot distend further, the positive pressure of the abdomen pushes out the ribs with which it is in contact. Since these are hinged so as to move outwards and upwards in the normal expiratory position, contraction of the diaphragm may raise and evert the lower ribs.

Near total lung capacity, the diaphragm assumes a horizontal position and its fibres are shortened. It therefore becomes more inefficient. A very hard pull may, paradoxically, pull the lower ribs inwards. Although acutely shortened muscles are inefficient, a slowly progressive chronic increase in lung volume probably results in resetting of the length–tension relationship of respiratory muscles (Farkas & Roussos, 1983; Arora & Rochester, 1987).

### Other muscles of inspiration

The sterno-mastoid muscle pulls the sternum upwards and the scalenus anterior exerts upward traction on the first rib. The external intercostals are inspiratory, maintaining the integrity of the chest wall and enabling it to move together. The parasternal muscles are also inspiratory but the interosseous parts of the internal intercostals are expiratory, and these have the action of apposing the lower ribs.

The scalenus anterior muscles are not palpably involved in quiet respiration in the semi-recum-

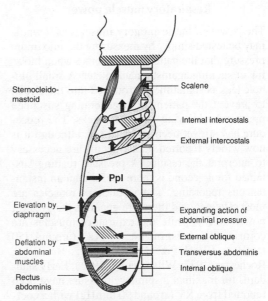

Fig. 2.14. Diagrammatic representation of the function of the respiratory muscles (redrawn from Roussos, 1985). By pressing downwards and increasing abdominal pressure (Pab), the diaphragm uses the abdominal contents as a lever to push the sternum forwards and the lower ribs outwards, thus expanding the thorax.

bent position with the trunk at rest, as in clinical examination, but needle electrode studies show some activity during quiet breathing under almost all conditions. They probably help to hold the upper chest in position during expiration. Their power and importance may in part be due to the fact that they shorten very little between full expiration and full inspiration.

The sterno-mastoid muscles elevate the first rib and sternum and are active during sniffing, during heavy exercise and in respiratory distress and when breathing near total lung capacity.

### The abdominal muscles

The external oblique, the internal oblique, the transversus abdominis and rectus abdominis muscles have important respiratory functions. They can increase intra-abdominal pressure and force the diaphragm upwards. They can contract to pull down the lowest ribs, increasing rib cage deflation.

## Respiratory muscle power

The power of the respiratory muscles as a whole may be tested simply by measuring the maximum pressure that the patient can generate when blowing or sucking against a manometer. A small pinhole leak is sometimes introduced into the circuit to prevent the patient from generating sustained pressure by blowing with the cheeks. The procedure has not yet been standardised, although it is now widely reported. Exact details are necessary to interpret the results. A pressure reading sustained for 1 second is more useful than an instantaneous recording. The inspiratory muscles are most efficient, and therefore generate the greatest power at RV while the expiratory muscles are correspondingly strongest at TLC (around 150 mmHg) (Black & Hyatt, 1969; Braun & Rochester, 1977; Wilson et al., 1981). Early standards for maximal inspiratory pressure have been reported from RV (around 90 mmHg) with a coefficient of repeatability of about 10%, but the test is better performed at FRC, because at RV there is some tendency for the chest wall to spring back to FRC. This means that there is a positive result even in the absence of any inspiratory effort, producing an important error in the presence of weakness. Sniffing produces higher pressures (Koulouris et al., 1989), but the measurements do not accurately reflect pleural pressure in patients with airflow obstruction because of slow time constants in some parts of the lung (Mulvey et al., 1991).

Maximal pressures are reduced early in the course of progressive neuromuscular disease, though not reliably. The measurement of VC and $Pco_2$ are the most useful indicators of the severity of progressive muscular weakness. Severe weakness also reduces lung compliance, because of the lack of frequent distension by yawning or sighing (Gibson et al., 1977).

### Assessing the function of the diaphragm

Contraction of the diaphragm results in inspiration by downward (caudad) movement of the dome and by upward (cephalad) traction on the lower ribs. As a result, there is overall downward movement of the diaphragm. The pressure gradient between the thorax and the abdomen increases during inspiration when the diaphragm is functioning, intrathoracic pressure becoming more negative and abdominal pressure more positive. When there is paralysis of the diaphragm, the gradient does not change during inspiration. Weakness results in a lower than normal change. Diaphragmatic power may be measured most accurately by balloon manometry (Mier et al., 1988). Balloons are passed into the oesophagus and stomach (Fig. 2.5). At FRC, when the diaphragm is relaxed, there is a slight positive pressure in the stomach due to gastric tone, and a slight negative pressure in the thorax due to elastic recoil. There is no pressure generated by the diaphragm (Pdi = 0), but there is a balloon pressure difference of about 8 cm $H_2O$ (8 kPa). If both hemi-diaphragms are paralysed, the pressure difference does not increase. Pdi increases to a lower limit of 5 during tidal breathing and should exceed 25 during maximal inspiration. Sniffing produces a maximal effort, normally greater than 80 cm $H_2O$ at FRC. When other inspiratory muscles are intact they can generate negative intrathoracic pressure, but if the diaphragm is paralysed the abdominal wall is sucked paradoxically upwards and inwards, and the abdominal pressure becomes more negative by an equal amount. Transdiaphragmatic pressure provides a quantitative assessment of the strength of diaphragmatic contraction, especially if a sniff is used. The integrity of the phrenic nerves can be tested separately by measurement of the transdiaphragmatic pressure during stimulation, preferably by surface electrodes (Mier & Brophy, 1991).

During assessment, diaphragm paralysis may be suspected if there is respiratory weakness and reduction of VC in recumbency. Bilateral diaphragmatic paralysis causes reduction of vital capacity, usually of more than 50%, with a further deterioration of more than the normal 25% on lying down (Allen, Hunt & Green, 1985). Residual ventilatory function may be adequate to maintain normal blood gases when awake in the upright position, with the development of dyspnoea or respiratory failure in the recumbent position or in sleep.

Unilateral phrenic paralysis may be diagnosed by demonstrating paradoxical movement of the diaphragm when respiration is observed under fluoroscopy. This is not entirely reliable in bilateral paralysis because many patients learn to breathe by active expiration below FRC, followed by relaxation of the abdominal muscles when the thorax springs back to its resting position. In these circumstances the diaphragm appears to move normally and fluoroscopists may be deceived, unless they take care to observe the pattern of breathing and to examine inspirations to TLC.

When only one hemi-diaphragm is paralysed, the reduction of VC is usually slight, amounting to no more than 20%, and VC is therefore within normal limits. Again, VC falls on lying down.

Lower cervical cord injury causes paralysis of the expiratory accessory muscles and the intercostals, with preservation of the diaphragm and cervical inspiratory muscles. VC and inspiratory power are reduced to about 50% with some capacity to improve with training.

### Respiratory muscle fatigue

The diaphragm and probably the other muscles of respiration cannot sustain more than 40% of their maximal force indefinitely without fatigue (Roussos & Macklem, 1977) though greater power can be generated for shorter periods (Tenney & Reese, 1968). Fatigue is the inability to sustain the required force with continued contractions and results in the development of submaximal power (Green & Moxham, 1985). Patients with disturbances of lung mechanics are liable to develop fatigue of the diaphragm, which may be detected clinically. The signs include inability to increase the tidal volume above resting levels, lack of downward pressure palpable in the epigastrium during inspiratory efforts, and 'respiratory alternans' which is the alternate recruitment of the diaphragm and the accessory muscles of the neck over a few respiratory cycles. The respiratory rate usually falls. The situation is worsened by

1. High lung volume, which shortens the resting length of the muscles.
2. A high inspiratory resistance, which lengthens the time needed for inspiration (McCool et al. 1986).

3. A rapid inspiratory rate (Bellemare & Grassino 1982a, b).
4. Low cardiac output, which may reduce blood flow to the diaphragm.

The need to adopt breathing strategies to avoid respiratory muscle fatigue is probably an important factor in determining whether $Pco_2$ rises above normal in patients with severe chronic respiratory disease (Bégin & Grassino, 1991).

Experimental demonstration of fatigue is not possible by direct means as there are no definite electromyographic or physiological features which can determine its presence at a single time. Central fatigue (loss of volition) may be diagnosed experimentally by stimulating the sternomastoids and demonstrating that further contraction occurs. In clinical practice, fatigue is diagnosed over a period of time by progressive failure of performance.

## Tidal breathing

Rate and depth of breathing have interested both physiologists and clinicians for many years (von Euler, Herrero & Wexler, 1970). Experimental studies in animals show that respiratory activity is stimulated by a progressive increase in the medullary output of the inspiratory neurones until these are switched off (Clark & von Euler, 1972). This occurs as a result of the increased firing of inhibitory neurones. In some animals, stress receptors in the bronchi stimulate the Hering-Breuer reflex, but this is very weak in man.

Inspiration is an active process and the need to overcome elastic, resistive and inertial forces has been discussed. In theory, expiration could proceed passively since elastic recoil of the lung should return the thorax to its resting position. In fact, this is not the case (Milic-Emili & Zin, 1986). In normal quiet breathing, expiration is slower than would occur if the lungs were allowed to deflate. This braking is caused by continued activity of the inspiratory muscles at the onset of expiration and, to some extent, by an increased resistance of the larynx and upper airway. With an increasing demand for ventilation, the expiratory brake is gradually withdrawn and active expiration is invoked, with a tendency to empty the lungs below resting FRC.

Inspiration becomes more difficult as lung volume increases and it is common observation that patients with stiff lungs adopt a shallow breathing pattern. The factors which select the most efficient inspiratory flow rate are hardly understood, but they relate to the sensation of breathing and are probably mediated by chest wall receptors.

The factors which determine the proportion of the respiratory cycle allocated to inspiration (the duty cycle) are very complex and capable of fine adjustment (Milic-Emili & Zin, 1986; Stradling, 1990). The pattern of breathing is hardly altered by quite major changes of nasal resistance, the necessary adjustment being made by altering the force of inspiration. With increasing ventilation, the proportion of time allocated to expiration falls. If expiration is slowed, because of airflow obstruction, there is a danger that the end-expiratory volume may rise uncomfortably above FRC, which in turn makes inspiration more difficult because of the increasing elastic recoil of the lung at high lung volumes. To prevent this, the time of inspiration is progressively shortened and this accounts for the ready development of inspiratory muscle fatigue during exercise in patients with chronic airflow obstruction. The factors which control the switching on and off of inspiration and expiration have been studied intensively in experimental animals, but our understanding of these processes in human disease remains quite simplistic.

The cyclical drive to breathing which is initiated in the medullary reticular formation is regulated in four ways:

1. *Metabolic*. Medullary and peripheral chemoreceptors modulate breathing to keep arterial $P_{CO_2}$ and pH within certain limits which can be defined for any set of circumstances (the constitution of ambient air, metabolic acidosis, body temperature and the like), and can be modified by drugs and disease affecting the control mechanisms. There are several important techniques which may be used experimentally to measure the sensitivity of the chemoreceptors to $CO_2$ and hypoxaemia (Chapter 14).

2. *Behavioural*. The instructions from the brain stem to perform the act of inspiration at regular intervals may be modified by non-metabolic functions of the breathing apparatus. These include coughing, sniffing and sneezing, speaking, crying or singing, and, in certain animals, thermoregulatory panting. These vary with degree of arousal.

3. *Reflex*. There are three reflexes carried by vagal afferent pathways which arise from the lungs and airways and may induce hyperventilation (Coleridge & Coleridge, 1984):
   (a) irritation of the airway causes panting or coughing;
   (b) the Hering–Breuer reflex, poorly developed in humans, causes cessation of inspiration when the airways are stretched;
   (c) C-fibre receptors, some of which are juxta-alveolar ('J' receptors), respond to increased pulmonary capillary pressures and other forms of irritation.

3. *Voluntary*. Ability to hold the breath may have survival value when diving or hiding from enemies, but it is limited by metabolic effects of hypoxia and $CO_2$ retention and by an overwhelming desire to breathe. This is satisfied by a gas mixture which does not improve the blood gases. Breath-holding and voluntary hyperventilation may both cause clouding of consciousness by hypoxia and respiratory alkalosis respectively.

### Techniques for the study of tidal breathing in health and disease

Accurate measurements of tidal volume and minute ventilation have classically been made with a mouthpiece and occasionally with a face mask and these stimulate breathing (Gilbert *et al.*, 1972; Rodenstein, Mercenier & Stanescu, 1985). Trained subjects and placid subjects soon settle down to a regular pattern of ventilation, which may be slightly deeper and more rapid than in repose. Most patients with lung disease also breathe in a regular fashion. Total ventilation must be interpreted in the light of oxygen uptake allowing for the effect of the additional dead space of the apparatus on gas exchange. A highly irregular trace or one with frequent sighs suggests that there is psychogenic hyperventilation, with or without

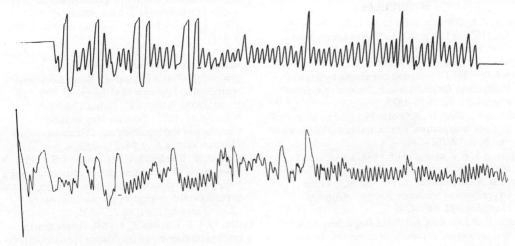

Fig. 2.15. Spirometric traces obtained from 2 patients with psychogenic hyperventilation. Note the frequent sighs and irregular breathing pattern.

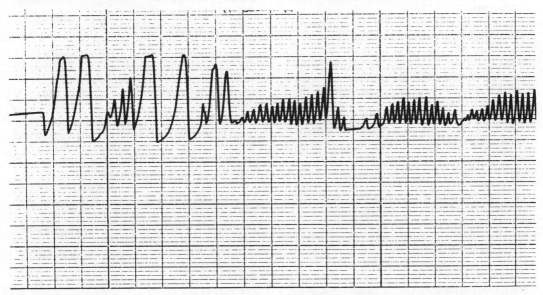

Fig. 2.16. Spirometric trace of Cheyne-Stokes respiration (from right to left).

pulmonary disease (Fig. 2.15). Periodic irregularity (Cheyne-Stokes breathing) due to heart failure, may be detected by spirometry (Fig. 2.16).

It is possible to measure rate and depth of breathing in conscious subjects without the use of mouthpieces and with correspondingly less interference. Using respiratory jackets or other devices which respond to chest wall and abdominal movement, it is clear that normal subjects breathe at a lower frequency at rest than has been supposed.

# References

Aaron, E.A., Johnson, B.D., Seow, C.K. & Dempsey, J.A. (1992a). Oxygen cost of hyperpnea: measurement. *Journal of Applied Physiology*, **72**, 1810–1817.

Aaron, E.A., Seow, C.K., Johnson, B.D. & Dempsey, J.A. (1992b). Oxygen cost of exercise hyperpnea: implications for performance. *Journal of Applied Physiology*, **72**, 1818–1825.

Allen, S.M., Hunt, B., & Green, M. (1985). Fall in vital capacity with posture. *British Journal of Diseases of the Chest*, **79**, 267–271.

Arora, N.S. & Rochester, D.F. (1987). COPD and human muscle dimensions. *Chest*, **91**, 719–724.

Bartlett, R.G., Brubach, H.F. & Specht, F. (1958). Oxygen cost of breathing. *Journal of Applied Physiology*, **12**, 413–424.

Bégin, P. & Grassino, A. (1991). Inspiratory muscle dysfunction and chronic hypercapnia in chronic obstructive pulmonary disease. *American Review of Respiratory Disease*, **143**, 905–912.

Bellemare, F. & Grassino, A. (1982a). Effect of pressure and time of contraction on human respiratory muscle fatigue. *Journal of Applied Physiology*, **53**, 1190–1195.

Bellemare, F. & Grassino, A. (1982b). Evaluation of human diaphragm fatigue. *Journal of Applied Physiology*, **53**, 1196–1206.

Black, L.F. & Hyatt, R.E. (1969). Maximal respiratory pressures: normal values and relationship to age and sex. *American Review of Respiratory Disease*, **99**, 696–702.

Braun, N.M.T. & Rochester, D.F. (1977). Respiratory muscle function in chronic obstructive pulmonary disease. *American Review of Respiratory Disease*, **115**, 91P.

Brown, R., Hoppin, F.G., Ingram, R.H., Saunders, N.A. & McFadden, E.R. (1978). Influence of abdominal gas on the Boyle's law determination of thoracic gas volume. *Journal of Applied Physiology*, **44**, 469–473.

Brown, R., Scharf, S. & Ingram, R.H. (1980). Non-homogeneous alveolar pressure swings in the presence of airway closure. *Journal of Applied Physiology*, **49**, 398–402.

Clark, F.J. & von Euler, C. (1972). On the regulation of depth and rate of breathing. *Journal of Physiology (London)*, **222**, 267–295.

Colebatch, A.J.H., Greaves, I.A. & Ng, C.K.Y. (1979). Experimental analysis of elastic recoil and ageing in healthy males and females. *Journal of Applied Physiology: Respiratory, environmental and exercise physiology*, **47**, 683–691.

Coleridge, J.C.G. & Coleridge, H.M. (1984). Afferent vagal C fibre innervation of the lungs and airways and its functional significance. *Review of Physiology, Biochemistry and Pharmacology*, **99**, 1–110.

Dawson, S.V. & Elliott, E.A. (1977). Wave speed limitation on expiratory flow: a unifying concept. *Journal of Applied Physiology*: Respiratory, environmental and exercise physiology, **43**, 498–515.

Denison, D.M., Waller, J.F., Turton, C.W.G. & Sopwith, T. (1982). Does the lung work? 5. Breathing in and breathing out. *British Journal of Diseases of the Chest*, **76**, 237–252.

Dubois, A.B., Botelho, S.Y. & Comroe, J.H. (1956). A raw method for measuring airway resistance using a body plethysmograph: values in normal subjects and in patients with respiratory disease. *Journal of Clinical Investigation*, **35**, 327–335.

Farkas, G.A. & Roussos, C. (1983). Diaphragm in emphysematous hamsters: Sarcomere adaptibility. *Journal of Applied Physiology*, **54**, 1635–1640.

Ferris, B.G. (1978). Epidemiology standardisation project. *American Review of Respiratory Disease* **6** (Suppl), 1–120.

Gibson, G.J. & Pride, N.B. (1976). Lung distensibility. The static pressure–volume curve of the lungs and its use in clinical assessment. *British Journal of Diseases of the Chest*, **70**, 143–184.

Gibson, G.J., Pride, N.B., Davis J. & Schroter, R.C. (1979). Exponential description of the static pressure–volume curve of normal and diseases lungs. *American Review of Respiratory Disease*, **120**, 799–811.

Gibson, G.J., Pride, N.B., Newsom Davis, J. & Loh, L.C. (1977). Pulmonary mechanics in patients with respiratory muscle weakness. *American Review of Respiratory Disease*, **115**, 389–395.

Gilbert, R, Auchinloss, H., Brodosky, J. & Boden, W. (1972). Changes to tidal volume, frequency and ventilation induced by their measurement. *Journal of Applied Physiology*, **33**, 252–254.

Green, M. & Moxham, J. (1985). The respiratory muscles. *Clinical Science*, **68**, 1–10.

Guyatt, A.R., Siddorn, J.A., Brash, H.M. & Flenley, D.C. (1975). Reproducibility of dynamic compliance and flow volume curves in normal man. *Journal of Applied Physiology*, **39**, 341–348.

Habib, M.P. & Engel, L.A. (1978). Influence of the panting technique on the measurement of thoracic gas volume. *Journal of Applied Physiology*, **117**, 265–271.

Harris, T.R., Pratt, P.C. & Kilburn, K.H. (1971). Total lung capacity measured by roentgenograms. *American Journal of Medicine*, **50**, 756–763.

Heaf, P.J.D. & Prime, F.J. (1956). The compliance of

the thorax in normal human subjects. *Clinical Science*, **15**, 319–327.

Hogg, J.C., Macklem, P.T. & Thurlbeck, W.M. (1968). Site and nature of airway obstruction in chronic obstructive lung disease. *New England Journal of Medicine*, **278**, 1355–1360.

Hoppin, F.G., Green, M. & Morgan, M.S. (1978). Relationship of central and peripheral airway resistance to lung volume in dogs. *Journal of Applied Physiology*, **44**, 728–737.

Hoppin, F.G., Stothert, J.C., Greaves, I.A., Lai, Y-L, & Hildebrandt J. (1986). Lung recoil: elastic and biological properties. In *Handbook of Physiology*, section 3, The respiratory system, Vol. III, Part 1, ed. P.T. Macklem & J. Mead, pp. 204–205. Bethesda: APS.

Hutchinson, J. (1844). Pneumatic apparatus for valuing the respiratory powers. *Lancet*, **i**, 390–391.

Hyatt, R.E. (1983). Expiratory flow limitation. *Journal of Applied Physiology*, **55**, 1–8.

Koulouris, N.G., Mulvey, D.A., Laroche, C.M., Sawicka, E.M., Green M. & Moxham, J. (1989). The measurement of inspiratory muscle strength by sniff oesophageal, nasopharyngeal and nasal pressures. *American Review of Respiratory Disease*, **139**, 641–646.

LeBlanc, P. Ruff, F. & Milic-Emili, J. (1970). Effects of age and body position on airway closure in man. *Journal of Applied Physiology*, **28**, 448–451.

Leith, D.E. & Mead, J. (1967). Mechanisms determining the residual volume of the lungs in normal subjects. *Journal of Applied Physiology*, **23**, 221–227.

Loyd, H.M., String, S.T. & Dubois, A.B. (1966). Radiographic and plethysmographic determination of total lung capacity. *Radiology*, **86**, 7–14.

McCool, F., McCann, D.R., Leith, D.E. & Hoppin, F.G. (1986). Pressure flow effects on endurance of the respiratory muscles. *Journal of Applied Physiology*, **60**, 299–303.

Macklem, P.T., Fraser, R.G. & Bates, D.V. (1965). Bronchial pressures and dimensions in health and obstructive airways disease. *Journal of Applied Physiology*, **18**, 699–706.

Macklem, P.T., Fraser, R.G. & Brown, W.G. (1965). Bronchial pressure measurements in emphysema and bronchitis. *Journal of Clinical Investigation*, **44**, 897–905.

Macklem, P.T. & Mead, J. (1967). Resistance of central and peripheral airways measured by a retrograde catheter. *Journal of Applied Physiology*, **22**, 395–401.

McMichael, J. (1939). A rapid method of determining lung capacity. *Clinical Science*, **4**, 167–173.

Mead, J. & Whittenberger, J.L. (1953). Physical properties of the lung measured during spontaneous respiration. *Journal of Applied Physiology*, **5**, 779–796.

Mier-Jedrzejowicz, A., Brophy, C., Moxham, J. & Green, M. (1988). Assessment of diaphragm weakness. *American Review of Respiratory Disease*, **137**, 877–883.

Mier, A. & Brophy, C. (1991). Measurement of twitch transdiaphragmatic pressure: surface versus needle electrode stimulation. *Thorax*, **46**, 669–670.

Milic-Emili, J., Mead, J., Turner, J.M. & Glauser, E.M. (1964). Improved technique for estimating pleural pressure from oesophageal balloons. *Journal of Applied Physiology*, **19**, 207–211.

Milic-Emili, J. & Zin, W.A. (1986). Relationship between neuromuscular respiratory drive and ventilatory output. In *Handbook of Physiology,* vol. III, part 2, ed. P.T. Macklem & J. Mead, p. 641. Bethesda: APS.

Muller, N., Bryan, A.C. & Zamel, N. (1981). Tonic inspiratory muscle activity as a cause of hyperinflation in asthma. *Journal of Applied Physiology*, **50**, 279–282.

Mulvey, D.A., Elliott, M.W., Koulouris, N.G., Carroll, M.P., Moxham, J. & Green, M. (1991). Sniff oesophageal and nasopharyngeal pressures and maximal relaxation rates in patients with respiratory dysfunction. *American Review of Respiratory Disease*, **43**, 950–953.

Otis, A.B., McKerrow, C.B., Bartlett, R.A., Mead, J., McIlroy, M.B., Selverstone, N.J. & Radford, E.P. (1956). Mechanical factors in distribution of pulmonary ventilation. *Journal of Applied Physiology*, **8**, 427–443.

Peslin, R. (1986). Methods for measuring total respiratory impedance by forced oscillations. *Bulletin Européen Physiopathologie Respiratoire*, **22**, 621–631.

Pierce, K.J., Brown, D.J., Holmes, M., Cumming, G. & Denison, D.M. (1979). The estimation of lung volumes from chest radiographs using shape information. *Thorax*, **34**, 726–734.

Piquet, J., Harf, A., Lorino, H., Atlan, G. & Bignon, J. (1984). Lung volume measurements in the plesythmograph in chronic obstructive pulmonary disease. Influence of the panting pattern. *Bulletin Européen Physiopathologie Respiratoire*, **20**, 31–36.

Pride, N.B., Permutt, S., Riley, R.L. & Bromberger-Barnea, B. (1967). Determinants of maximal expiratory flow from the lungs. *Journal of Applied Physiology*, **23**, 646–662.

Quanjer, Ph. H. (1993). Standardized lung function testing. *European Respiratory Journal*, **6** (Suppl. 16), 3–102.

Rahn, H., Otis, A.B., Chadwick, I.E., Fenn, W.O.

(1946). The pressure volume diagram of the thorax and lung. *American Journal of Physiology*, **146**, 161–178.

Rodenstein, D.D., Mercenier, C., Stanescu, D.C. (1985). Influence of the respiratory route on the testing breathing pattern in humans. *American Review of Respiratory Disease*, **131**, 163–165.

Rodenstein, D.D. & Stanescu, D.C. (1982). Reassessment of lung volume measurement by helium dilation and by body plesythmography in chronic airflow obstruction. *American Review of Respiratory Disease*, **126**, 1040–1044.

Roussos, C. (1985). Function and fatigue of respiratory muscles. *Chest*, **88**, 127S–132S.

Roussos, C. & Campbell, E.J.M. (1986). Respiratory muscle energetics. In *The Handbook of Physiology: The Respiratory System,* vol. III, part 2, ed. P.T. Macklem & J. Mead, pp. 493–501. Bethesda: APS.

Roussos, C.S. & Macklem, P.T. (1977). Diaphragmatic fatigue in man. *Journal of Applied Physiology*, **43**, 189–197.

Setnikar, I. & Meschia, G. (1986). Proprieta elastiche del polmone e di modelle mechanici. *Archives Fisiologica*, **52**, 288–302.

Shore, S.A., Huk, O., Mannix, S. & Martin, J.G. (1983). Effect of panting frequency on the plesythmographic determination of thoracic gas volume in chronic obstructive pulmonary disease. *American Review of Respiratory Disease*, **128**, 54–59.

Stradling, J.R. (1990). Control of breathing. In *Respiratory Medicine*, ed. R.A.L. Brewis, G.J. Gibson & D.M. Geddes, pp. 168–172. London: Baillière Tindall.

Tenney, S.M. & Reese, S.G. (1968). The ability to sustain great breathing efforts. *Respiration Physiology*, **5**, 187–201.

Von Euler, C., Herrero, F. & Wexler, I. (1970). Control mechanisms determining rate and depth of respiratory movements. *Respiration Physiology*, **10**, 93–108.

Wilson, J.H., Cookc, N.T., Edwards, R.II.T. & Spiro, S.G. (1981). Predicted normal values for maximal respiratory pressure in Caucasian adults and children. *Thorax*, **39**, 535.

Woolcock, A.J., Vincent, N.J. & Macklem, P.T. (1969). Frequency dependence of compliance as a test for obstruction in small airways. *Journal of Clinical Investigation*, **4**, 1097–1106.

# 3 Pulmonary oxygen and carbon dioxide exchange

Pulmonary gas exchange replenishes the oxygen removed in the tissues from the arterial blood, and results in the excretion of $CO_2$.

In health, $P_{CO_2}$ and the saturation of oxygen in the arterial blood are set within fairly narrow limits (40 mmHg (6 kPa) and 95% respectively). Respiratory disease usually results in some abnormality at rest or during exercise. Generally, $P_{O_2}$ is low in relation to the amount of pulmonary ventilation; $P_{CO_2}$ may be low, normal or high.

The purpose of this chapter is firstly to explain how normal blood gas levels are achieved; secondly, to explore how damage to the pulmonary gas exchanging surface results in derangement of arterial blood gases; and thirdly, to show how arterial blood gas measurements may be used as tests of the integrity of pulmonary ventilation and gas exchange.

For a discussion of pulmonary gas exchange, respiratory quotient, respiratory exchange ratio, the concept of steady state and the meaning of dissociation curves of gases in blood and other body fluids need to be defined.

### Respiratory quotient (RQ)

RQ is the ratio of $CO_2$ output to oxygen consumption applied to cellular metabolism. When carbohydrate is the only substrate, RQ is 1. Fats and fatty acids yield less $CO_2$ for each mole of oxygen, about 0.7 moles; protein yields about 0.8. In the basal state, RQ is about 0.8; this falls to 0.7 after prolonged fasting, as the proportion of fat to other metabolic substrates increases.

### Respiratory exchange ratio (R)

R is the ratio $CO_2$ output/$O_2$ consumption applied to measurements of pulmonary gas exchange.

Over short periods of time, this is affected by variations in cardiac output and pulmonary ventilation, as well as by metabolic rate.

### Steady state

In physiology generally, a steady state occurs when the *milieu intérieur* (Bernard 1865) is approximately constant. A 'steady state' of gas exchange is present when inspired and expired gas concentrations and venous and arterial blood gas contents change little over a period of time. Therefore the respiratory exchange ratio, R, measured by collection of expired gases, represents the respiratory quotient, RQ. This situation is difficult to achieve experimentally. Non-steady states are easier to define. They occur when the metabolic rate is changing in response to variations in physical work and when ventilation and cardiac output are varying. Hyperventilation and breath-holding produce rapid changes in R because the tissues of the body store more $CO_2$ than oxygen.

## Dissociation slopes for oxygen and carbon dioxide

Dissociation curves (correctly adsorption–dissociation curves) are graphs which show how partial pressures and content of gases relate in body fluids. The most familiar are those of $O_2$ and $CO_2$ in whole blood (Fig. 3.1).

Partial pressures of gases when dissolved in liquids are a measure of their tendency to escape. If a sample of blood with a $P_{CO_2}$ of 45 mmHg (6 kPa) is exposed to air at the same partial pressure, there will be no 'net' movement of $CO_2$ between

33

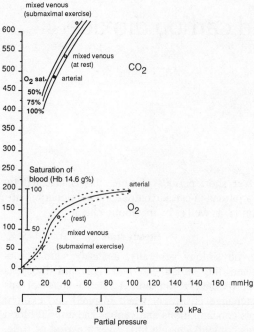

Fig. 3.1. Oxygen and carbon dioxide adsorption–dissociation curves in whole blood. Ordinate, content of $O_2$ and $CO_2$ in ml per litre of whole blood (the traditional units of vol% x 10). Abscissa, partial pressure of $O_2$ and $CO_2$ in blood. The relationship between $O_2$ content and $Po_2$ below full saturation is affected by temperature, pH, $Pco_2$ and other factors. The effect of $Pco_2$ (acting by changing pH) is known as the Bohr shift and is illustrated in the lower curve (Bohr, Hasselbalch & Krogh, 1904). Blood with a haemoglobin level of 14.6 $g\cdot dl^{-1}$ has an $O_2$ capacity of 200 $ml\cdot l^{-1}$. The dissociation curve for $CO_2$ is affected by the ratio of oxygenated to total haemoglobin ($O_2$ saturation). This is known as the C-D-H effect (Christiansen, Douglas & Haldane, 1914).

air and blood. $CO_2$ is much less soluble in water than in blood, so that a sample of water with $Pco_2$ of 90 mmHg (12 kPa) contains less $CO_2$ per ml than blood at 45 mmHg (6 kPa). If these are brought into contact but separated by a membrane which allows the diffusion of $CO_2$ gas, the $CO_2$ will pass into the blood from the water where the partial pressure is higher, although the concentration is lower.

Gases dissolve in liquids according to Henry's law:

$$\text{Gas content} = \text{partial pressure} \times \text{solubility} \qquad (3.1)$$

Solubility is constant at any given temperature.

Oxygen combines chemically with haemoglobin by a complex series of reactions: when these are complete each molecule of haemoglobin carries four molecules of $O_2$. The capacity of the blood to combine with $O_2$ is determined by its haemoglobin concentration (approximately 1.36 ml of $O_2$ per gram of haemoglobin). When fully saturated, blood containing 15 g/dl, 9 $mmol\cdot l^{-1}$, carries 200 ml $O_2$ per litre of blood in combination with haemoglobin, and a small fraction of this dissolved in the plasma (0.03 ml $O_2$ for each mmHg partial pressure, 0.23 ml per kPa).

Haemoglobin is fully saturated at a partial pressure of about 200 mmHg (25 kPa). At 100 mmHg (13 kPa), which is the usual alveolar $Po_2$, the ratio of oxyhaemoglobin to reduced haemoglobin is 96.4/3.6. This ratio is usually expressed as the percentage saturation of haemoglobin (oxyhaemoglobin/total haemoglobin), and changes very little with partial pressure until this falls to 60 mmHg (8 kPa), below which the uptake or delivery of large volumes of oxygen are reflected by small changes of $Po_2$.

The reaction between oxygen and haemoglobin is affected by temperature, by pH and by the intracellular concentrations of organic phosphates, especially 2:3-diphosphoglycerate, which compete with $O_2$ for binding sites on the haemoglobin molecule (Severinghaus 1958; Kelman & Nunn, 1966). These variations are usually described as shifts to the left or right of the $O_2$ dissociation curve. A shift to the left means that there is an increased affinity of blood for $O_2$: this enhances oxygen uptake in the lungs, but delivery of any given volume of $O_2$ to the tissues must be at a lower $Po_2$. The general shape of the curve is preserved during these changes which are usefully described by $P_{50}$, the partial pressure at which the blood is 50% saturated with oxygen. This is determined experimentally by the analysis of tonometered samples of blood. Tonometry is the traditional technique of equilibrating blood with flowing gases of known concentrations (partial pressures) in gently oscillating chambers at the required temperature.

Table 3.1. *Composition of dry atmospheric air*[a]

| Gas | Mole % |
|---|---|
| Oxygen | 20.95 |
| Carbon dioxide | 0.0310 |
| Nitrogen | 78.09 |
| Argon[b] | 0.93 |

[a] Adapted from Gilbert (1964).
[b] Including krypton, neon, helium and other inert gases.

Dissociation curves for $CO_2$ and the carriage of $CO_2$ or bicarbonate and carbamino-haemoglobin are well described in physiological texts. Pulmonary $CO_2$ exchange is influenced by two characteristics of these curves, which are illustrated in Fig. 3.1.

1. The dissociation curve for $CO_2$ is relatively linear above and below the normal range found in the arterial blood. Therefore, if alveolar $CO_2$ pressure falls by hyperventilation, the blood will continue to give up $CO_2$ in large amounts. A corresponding rise of alveolar $Po_2$ causes little increase in oxygen uptake, since the blood is almost saturated with oxygen at normal alveolar partial pressures.
2. The $CO_2$ dissociation slope of blood is steep, about the normal range of arterial $Pco_2$. Relatively large volumes of $CO_2$ may combine with blood with small resultant changes of partial pressure. In repose, when metabolic rate is about 200 ml of oxygen or carbon dioxide per minute, the difference between arterial and venous $Pco_2$ is about 4 mmHg (0.5 kPa). The corresponding difference for $O_2$ is 40–50 mmHg (5.5–7 kPa).

## Measurement of carbon dioxide output and oxygen uptake

Air, without its variable content of water vapour, consists of about 21% oxygen and 79% nitrogen. The exact constitution of room air is given in Table 3.1.

Since there is almost no $CO_2$ in the inspired air, the determination of $CO_2$ output over a period of time is simple:

$$CO_2 \text{ output} = \text{ventilation/time} \times \text{fractional expired } CO_2 \text{ concentration} \quad (3.2)$$

$$\dot{V}_E CO_2 = \dot{V}_E \times F_E CO_2 \quad (3.2a)$$

Oxygen consumption is the difference between the number of molecules of oxygen breathed in and the number breathed out in a given time. $\dot{V}o_2$ and $\dot{V}co_2$ are expressed conventionally in moles or in volumes reduced to STPD.

$$O_2 \text{ consumption} = (\text{inspired volume} \times O_2 \text{ concentration}) - (\text{expired volume} \times \text{expired } O_2 \text{ concentration}) \quad (3.3)$$

$$= (\dot{V}_I \times F_I O_2) - (\dot{V}_E \times F_E O_2) \quad (3.3a)$$

A simpler equation applies when R is equal to 1, that is, when oxygen consumption is equal to $CO_2$ output. Then, inspired and expired concentrations of all gases excluding water vapour are also equal. In this simplified condition, the equation then becomes

$$\dot{V}o_2 = \dot{V} \times (F_I O_2 - F_E O_2) \quad (3.4)$$

$$\text{Oxygen uptake} = \text{ventilation} \times (\text{fraction of oxygen removed from respired air}) \quad (3.4a)$$

### Accurate measurement of oxygen uptake from expired ventilation

When ventilation and gas exchange are proceeding in a steady state, the amount of nitrogen in the lungs and the tissues remains constant. This fact may be used to calculate oxygen uptake by estimating inspired ventilation from expired ventilation:

$$\underset{\substack{\text{Amount of } N_2 \\ \text{breathed in}}}{\dot{V}_I \times F_I N_2} = \underset{\substack{\text{Amount of } N_2 \\ \text{breathed out}}}{\dot{V}_E \times F_E N_2} \quad (3.5)$$

and

$$F_E N_2 = 1 - (F_E O_2 + F_E CO_2) \quad (3.6)$$

This information can be used to derive the formula:

$$\dot{V}o_2 = \frac{\dot{V}_E \times (F_I O_2 \cdot F N_2 - F_E O_2)}{F_I N_2} \quad (3.7)$$

The right hand term of Eq. 3.6 can be substituted for $F_I N_2$ if this is not measured.

For accurate measurements in the non-steady

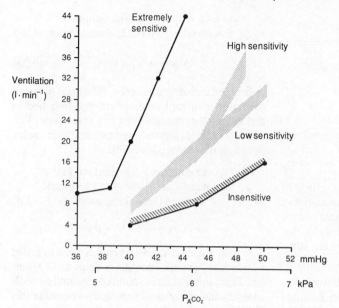

Fig. 3.2. Ventilatory response to the inspiration of gas of increasing $CO_2$ concentration measured in the steady state.

state, both inspired and expired ventilation have to be measured.

## Pulmonary gas exchange

In the following consideration of alveolar gas exchange, the difference between inspired and expired ventilation is ignored to simplify the presentation.

### Interpretation of the results of blood gas analysis

Arterial blood is sampled to discover whether pulmonary gas exchange is achieving a normal $Pco_2$ and $Po_2$. Respiratory failure is defined in these terms, arbitrary limits being set (as renal failure is said to be present when blood urea exceeds 7 mmol·l⁻¹).

#### Elevation of arterial $Pco_2$: ventilatory failure

Ventilatory control mechanisms set arterial $Pco_2$ within close limits (36–44 mmHg, 5–6 kPa). In the artificial situation where a gas mixture enriched with $CO_2$ is inhaled, there is a brisk increase in the rate and depth of breathing in over 90% of normal subjects (Fig. 3.2). This response

may be damped by training and is reduced in most, but not all, respiratory diseases notably chronic bronchitis, kyphoscoliosis and disorders of the inspiratory muscles (Chapter 14). Patients with these chronic conditions may experience asymptomatic increases of $Pco_2$ in life. When they suffer an acute deterioration of pulmonary function, $Pco_2$ can rise to very high levels. This is conveniently termed ventilatory failure.

Patients who normally have well-preserved lung function and intact ventilatory response to $CO_2$ are found to have an elevated $Pco_2$ only when the maximum breathing capacity falls below the level required to excrete the $CO_2$ produced by metabolism at normal alveolar concentrations. This is a life-threatening situation requiring treatment with assisted ventilation unless the condition can be improved and oxygen administered within a short time, usually less than 1 hour. In contrast, elevation of arterial $Pco_2$ in patients who do not appear to be acutely ill indicates diminution of the normal ventilatory response to $CO_2$ retention, a form of acclimatisation which may make life tolerable for patients with reduced ventilatory capacity. Examination of published data suggests that this occurs when resting ventilation would have to be greater than 12 l/min to maintain normal $Pco_2$ (Robin & O'Neill, 1983; Johnson *et al.*, 1983; Bégin & Grassino, 1991)

## Low arterial $P_{O_2}$

Abnormally low levels of arterial $P_{O_2}$ may be found in several situations: low inspired $P_{O_2}$ (e.g. high altitudes), and conditions which cause reduction of alveolar ventilation or impairment of pulmonary gas exchange.

Acute falls of arterial $P_{O_2}$ may occur during elevation to high altitudes or during illnesses which disturb gas exchange. Ventilation normally increases rapidly as arterial $P_{O_2}$ falls below 60 mmHg (8 kPa). This physiological response, which is mediated by impulses from the carotid body, may also be damped by acclimatisation. As chronic lung disease progresses, there is adjustment to a gradual deterioration of both $P_{CO_2}$ and $P_{O_2}$ to abnormal levels which would cause intellectual deterioration if the changes were acute. The finding of an arterial $P_{O_2}$ of 50 mmHg (7 kPa) and an arterial $P_{CO_2}$ of 50 mmHg (7 kPa) is common in ambulant patients with chronic respiratory failure.

Arterial $P_{O_2}$ and arterial $P_{CO_2}$ may, therefore, be interpreted separately with some knowledge of the patient's history and clinical state at the time the sample was taken.

Patients with respiratory disorders who are breathing room air, may be found to have:

1. Oxygen saturation which is within normal limits or low.
2. Arterial $P_{CO_2}$ which is low, normal or high.

This is because increasing the rate or depth of breathing can result in a low $P_{CO_2}$ from alveolar hyperventilation. Examination of the oxygen dissociation curve shows that hyperventilation has a very slight effect on $O_2$ saturation, because the blood is 95% saturated at normal alveolar $P_{O_2}$. Increasing alveolar ventilation twofold results only in a 2% rise of saturation, while $P_{CO_2}$ is halved (Fig. 3.1).

## Relationship of $P_{O_2}$ to $P_{CO_2}$

The section which follows shows, by considering the relationship between $P_{O_2}$ and $P_{CO_2}$, how ventilation and metabolic rate define the normal range of arterial $P_{O_2}$. The process is logically similar to the definition of abnormal blood urea concentration, when a slightly 'high' level may indicate renal failure or may merely reflect a high catabolic rate of protein.

At this stage it is worth going back to look at the significance of the ventilation/perfusion ratio and of variability of the ratio between different groups of alveoli, which was mentioned at the end of Chapter 1. Most readers will have met these ideas before, perhaps in a variety of different presentations. Some arithmetic is needed; the purpose of the approach used here is to explain the classical concepts and at the same time to demonstrate how to use all the information available.

## Gas exchange analysed as though ventilation and perfusion were uniform

First consider what would happen if the gas and blood leaving a single alveolus could be collected. The oscillations of breathing will be ignored and it will be assumed that there is a steady state of respiration in which the $O_2$ and $CO_2$ exchanged in the tissues matches that in the lungs. At any instant $P_{O_2}$ and $P_{CO_2}$ in the effluent blood are the same as in the 'alveolus'.

Alveolar and arterial $P_{CO_2}$ and $P_{O_2}$ are determined by alveolar ventilation (and by barometric pressure $P_{BAR}$)

$$P_{CO_2} (P_{BAR} - P_{H_2O}) = CO_2 \text{ output/ventilation} \tag{3.8}$$

and

$$\frac{\text{Inspired } P_{O_2} - \text{alveolar } P_{O_2}}{(P_{BAR} - P_{H_2O})} = \tag{3.9}$$

$$\frac{O_2 \text{ consumption}}{\text{Ventilation}}$$

Blood travels to the tissues of the body containing $CO_2$ and $O_2$. The amount depends on the arterial $P_{O_2}$ and $P_{CO_2}$ and the dissociation curve.

In the tissues, $O_2$ is consumed and diffuses out of the blood because arterial $P_{O_2}$ is higher than tissue $P_{O_2}$. The passage of $O_2$ continues until the partial pressures equalise or the blood leaves the capillary (the distance between capillary and mitochondrion is such that they probably do not equalise). The removal of this $O_2$ depends on tissue consumption; if it is rapid, the gradient of $P_{O_2}$

from blood to tissue is greater and gas exchange proceeds to a lower capillary $Po_2$. The $O_2$ content of the blood falls, yielding venous blood.

When $O_2$ consumption increases, tissue $Po_2$ falls and so, therefore, does venous $Po_2$. This is partly counteracted by an increase in cardiac output. If 1 litre of $O_2$ is removed from 10 litres of arterial blood, the venous $O_2$ content and $Po_2$ are higher than if the same amount is removed from 5 litres. When metabolic rate is increased by exercise, arousal or fever, the normal heart increases its output, but not enough to keep venous $Po_2$ and $Pco_2$ constant.

The blood returning to the lungs (mixed venous blood) has a lower $Po_2$ and higher $Pco_2$ than the arterial blood. While pulmonary ventilation continues, fresh air is drawn into the lungs and $O_2$ uptake and $CO_2$ output occur because of the partial pressure differences. The cycle is complete.

If the steady state is disturbed temporarily:

1. Cessation of effective pulmonary ventilation (breath-holding, rebreathing, asphyxia) results in a progressive fall in alveolar $Po_2$ and rise in $Pco_2$. These changes occur exponentially towards the mixed venous $Po_2$ and $Pco_2$. Recirculation of abnormal blood causes tissue, venous and alveolar $Po_2$ to fall rapidly. In less than 4 minutes, alveolar $Po_2$ falls below the level required to sustain life. The rise of $Pco_2$ during arrested breathing is much more gradual because, although $CO_2$ production continues, it is buffered in most tissues (Farhi, 1964).

2. If there is a reduction of ventilation without any change of tissue metabolic rate, alveolar $Po_2$ falls and $Pco_2$ rises, until a new steady state is achieved. Arterial $Po_2$ and $O_2$ content fall, and therefore venous $Po_2$ and tissue $Po_2$ would be expected to fall, but this is counteracted by a rise of cardiac output (Tenney & Lamb, 1965).

3. Hyperventilation without any change of tissue metabolic rate causes alveolar $Pco_2$ to fall. Arterial $Pco_2$ and $CO_2$ content also fall, followed by mixed venous $Pco_2$ and $CO_2$ content. Although alveolar and arterial $Po_2$ rise, arterial $O_2$ content rises very little, because the $O_2$ dissociation curve is flat above normal $Po_2$. The extra $O_2$ breathed in is simply breathed out again. Therefore mixed venous $O_2$ content and $Po_2$

change very little. There is a temporary increase of $CO_2$ output with very little increase of oxygen uptake, which results in a temporary increase of R to levels above the RQ and often above 1.0. The volume of air breathed out is greater than that breathed in. The physiological response of cardiac output to hyperventilation is variable, but it falls if respiratory alkalosis is profound.

## Calculation of pulmonary and systemic blood flow

$O_2$ uptake and $CO_2$ output in the lungs are calculated from the changes of their concentration in the gas ventilating the lungs; tissue gas exchange may be calculated in the same way from measurements of blood flow and changes of gas concentrations in the incoming and outgoing blood.

Thus:

$$CO_2 \text{ output (ml} \cdot \text{min}^{-1}) = \text{ventilation (l} \cdot \text{min}^{-1}) \times (\text{expired - inspired } CO_2 \text{ concentration (ml} \cdot \text{l}^{-1}))$$
(3.10)

Similarly:

$$CO_2 \text{ output (ml} \cdot \text{min}^{-1}) = \text{blood flow (l} \cdot \text{min}^{-1}) (\text{venous - arterial } CO_2 \text{ content (ml} \cdot \text{l}^{-1}))$$
(3.11)

and

$$O_2 \text{ consumption (ml} \cdot \text{min}^{-1}) = \text{blood flow} (\text{l} \cdot \text{min}^{-1}) \times (\text{arteriovenous } O_2 \text{ content (ml} \cdot \text{l}^{-1}))$$
(3.12)

Under steady state conditions, these formulae may be used to measure cardiac output, from measurements of the arterial and mixed venous (pulmonary arterial) $O_2$ contents.

$$\text{Blood flow (cardiac output)} = O_2 \text{ uptake} \times (\text{arteriovenous } O_2 \text{ content difference})$$
(3.13)

This is the well-known 'Fick equation' (Fick, 1870) which was first applied for this purpose some years later in animals by Zuntz & Hagemann (1898). They realised that it worked well in practice employing oxygen as the test gas, but not $CO_2$. $CO_2$ output from the lungs is affected immediately by very minor changes of ventilation while $O_2$ uptake is not, so attempts to measure tissue $CO_2$ output from blood gas exchange data usually fail.

Cardiac output at rest is about 5 l·min$^{-1}$; assuming oxygen uptake to be about 250 ml·min$^{-1}$, arteriovenous content difference is 50 ml·l$^{-1}$, that is a fall in saturation of 25%.

The $O_2$ dissociation curve (Fig. 3.1) shows that the mixed venous partial pressure corresponding to the mixed venous content of 140 ml·l$^{-1}$ is about 40 mmHg (5.5 kPa) (which is about 50 mmHg (7 kPa) less than the arterial value).

### Summary of oxygen and carbon dioxide exchange in the uniformly ventilated and perfused lung

1. In the steady state, metabolic rate is constant.
2. The arterial $O_2$ and $CO_2$ pressures and contents are determined by the ratio of ventilation/metabolic rate.
3. The arteriovenous $O_2$ and $CO_2$ content (and pressure) differences are determined by the ratio of perfusion/metabolic rate.

## Abnormalities of the exchange of oxygen

Arterial oxygen saturation normally lies between 94% and 97%. This corresponds to a wide range of normal arterial $Po_2$ (70–100 mmHg (9.5–15 kPa)). When $Pao_2$ is less than 60 mmHg (8 kPa), a pathological condition is present. Either:

1. total pulmonary ventilation is inadequate, or,
2. alveolar gas exchange is inefficient.

Theoretically, inefficiency of gas exchange leading to arterial hypoxaemia or an abnormally wide alveolar–arterial $Po_2$ difference is of two types:

1. Imperfect equilibration between alveolar gases and pulmonary capillary blood such that the blood leaves the lungs at a lower $Po_2$ than that in the individual alveoli ('diffusion defect').
2. Uneven distribution of ventilation ($\dot{V}$) and perfusion ($\dot{Q}$) causing part of the pulmonary blood to receive a relatively low share of the alveolar ventilation ('$\dot{V}/\dot{Q}$ imbalance').

While all these mechanisms can occur, clinically important hypoxaemia is caused almost entirely by total hypoventilation, by regional hypoventilation, or by a combination of both. It will be analysed as though these are the only abnormalities present. Methods of quantifying diffusion defects are discussed in Chapter 14.

## Gas exchange in lungs with non-uniform distribution of alveolar ventilation and perfusion

The real lung contains millions of alveoli, all ventilated and perfused at their own rate. To study the overall effects of breathing and gas transport, only the following can be analysed:

1. Inspired air.
2. Mixed venous blood.
3. Expired air, which is a mixture of all alveolar gases, plus tracheo-bronchial dead space gas.
4. Arterial blood, which is a mixture of all end-capillary bloods, plus any blood bypassing the lungs (for example, through an atrial septal defect).

The next step is to propose a model, with numerous alveoli, all of which are ventilated with 'inspired' air, and receive a portion of the mixed venous blood. Each alveolus, however, has a different ventilation/perfusion ratio ($\dot{V}/\dot{Q}$).

1. No ventilation ($\dot{V}/\dot{Q} = 0$). The end-capillary $Pco_2$ and $Po_2$ are the same as in the mixed venous blood.
2. No perfusion ($\dot{V}/\dot{Q}$ = infinity). Gas leaves this alveolus with its composition unchanged.
3. Finite $\dot{V}/\dot{Q}$.

In each alveolus, alveolar exchange is the same as blood gas exchange. By using an $O_2/CO_2$ diagram (Fig. 3.3) (Fenn, Rahn & Otis, 1946; Riley and Cournand, 1951), it can be shown that alveolar gas concentrations can be predicted from a knowledge of inspired gas concentration, mixed venous blood concentration and the respiratory exchange ratio, R.

R(blood) = R(gas) in each alveolus. At any value of R(gas), the partial pressures of the alveolar gases ($P_A$) must allow the alveolar air equation to be solved;

$$R = \frac{P_A co_2 - P_I co_2}{P_I o_2 - P_A o_2} \quad (3.14)$$

This is a simple linear relationship; the gas R lines are easily drawn (Fig. 3.3a).

(The use of the full equation, which corrects for the difference between the volume of oxygen

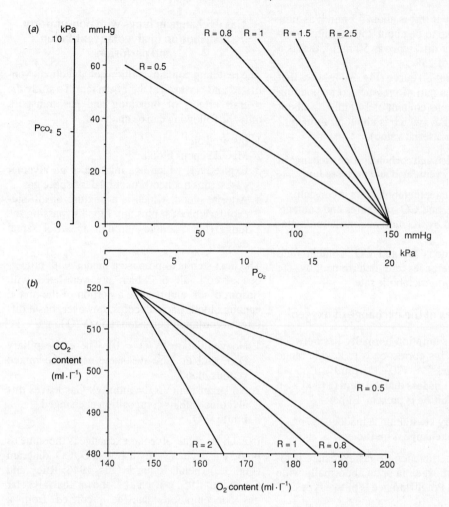

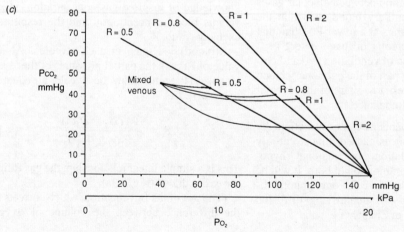

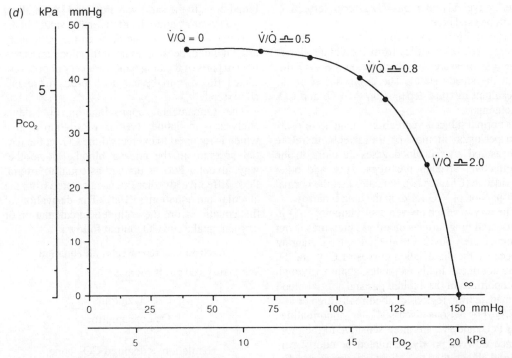

Fig. 3.3. (a) 'Gas R lines'. The relationship between alveolar $Po_2$ and $Pco_2$ at different values of R inspired $Po_2$ and $Pco_2$ are taken to be 150 mmHg (20 kPa) and 0 respectively. This is not quite rigorous, because it ignores the final portion of the previous expirate which is inspired again.

(b) Blood R lines show the relationship between $Po_2$ and $Pco_2$ in the oxygenated mixed venous blood. The oxygen content is assumed to be 144 ml·l$^{-1}$ and $CO_2$ content to be 520 ml·l$^{-1}$.

(c) Blood R lines converted to $Po_2$ and $Pco_2$ (by the use of standard dissociation curves) have been superimposed on gas R lines. X indicates the unique solutions for alveolar $Pco_2$ and $Po_2$ at different values of R in a single alveolus. NB: Different starting values of mixed venous and inspired gas concentrations result in different families of R lines.

(d) The points on (c) may be joined to form a line on which all values of alveolar $Po_2$ must be at different values of ventilation–perfusion ratio (the $\dot{V}/\dot{Q}$ line). This shows that in resting subjects alveolar $Pco_2$ varies by very little over a wide range of normal and low ventilation/perfusion rates. High ventilation/perfusion ratios (between 1.0 and 2.0) have the same effect on $CO_2$ as on oxygen.

absorbed and the volume of $CO_2$ excreted (p.35) makes a small difference.)

Blood R lines are curvilinear and to draw them it is necessary to know the relationship between $Pco_2$ and $Po_2$ and their respective contents in the blood. The points at which the same gas and blood R lines interact on the $O_2/CO_2$ diagram are the only possible values for alveolar gas pressures under those conditions (Fig. 3.3b, c and d). The line joining these points is known as the $\dot{V}/\dot{Q}$ line.

The 'effective' alveolar $Pco_2$ and $Po_2$ may be determined from the $O_2/CO_2$ diagram knowing the composition of the inspired air, the mixed venous gas pressures (or arterial pressures and cardiac output) and the dissociation curves of the patient's blood. Because these are not usually all available, the diagram has had more educational than practical value. Detailed consideration of these concepts is time-consuming, though interesting (Riley & Permutt, 1965; Farhi, 1966), but some general conclusions are important and will be discussed in depth.

1. If ventilation and perfusion were uniform throughout the lung, arterial and alveolar $Pco_2$ would lie on the line of measured 'R'. This has been called 'ideal' alveolar gas, or, better,

'effective' alveolar gas. The term 'effective' will be used here.

2. Arterial blood and expired alveolar gas are composed of mixtures from individual alveoli the gas pressures of which lie on the $\dot{V}/\dot{Q}$ line (in the steady state). The composition of the resultant mixture depends on their $O_2$ and $CO_2$ contents.

3. In normal subjects ventilation is matched closely to perfusion in most of the alveoli, therefore measured arterial blood gases lie close to the 'effective' alveolar pressures. This, and other evidence (Chapter 14), indicates that the normal dispersion of $\dot{V}/\dot{Q}$ ratios in the lung is narrow.

4. The way in which uneven distribution of $\dot{V}/\dot{Q}$ in diseased lungs affects blood gas pressures is not immediately obvious from the $Po_2/Pco_2$ diagram because the dissociation curves of $CO_2$ and $O_2$ are not linear. In disease states, abnormally high proportions of the expired gas and arterial blood emanate from regions of abnormally high or low $\dot{V}/\dot{Q}$. For reasons discussed later, abnormalities of $Pco_2$ and $Po_2$ are more sensitive to the presence of very poorly ventilated or poorly perfused alveoli than to a slight increase in the dispersion of $\dot{V}/\dot{Q}$ ratios (Chapter 14).

## Interpretations of $Pco_2/Po_2$ relationships in the arterial blood in clinical practice

The approach most used is that of Riley & Cournand (1951).

### Riley's three-compartment model

The analysis of the evenness of distribution of pulmonary ventilation and perfusion known as Riley's three-compartment model was introduced in Fig. 1.4. Any set of measurements of arterial blood gas, expired gas and cardiac output, can be interpreted as though all the oxygen uptake and $CO_2$ output occurred in one group of alveoli with a uniform ventilation and blood flow, which are called here the effective alveoli. These alveoli have the same respiratory exchange ratio, R, as that measured in the expired gas. Expired air consists of effective alveolar gas diluted with dead space gas from areas which do not receive a share of the pulmonary

blood flow. In the same way $Pco_2$ and $Po_2$ in blood from a systemic artery lie between the values in the effective alveolar gas and those in the pulmonary arterial blood, because some of the blood is distributed to parts of the lung which are very poorly ventilated. Blood from these regions results in 'venous admixture'.

The fundamental approximation of Riley's analysis is to define alveolar ventilation as that which is required to excrete all the $CO_2$ at the partial pressure in the arterial blood. Put another way, alveolar $Pco_2$ is defined as equal to arterial $Pco_2$. Effective alveolar $Po_2$ is calculated from the alveolar air equation (3.19a). The derivation of this equation from the arithmetical calculation of oxygen uptake and $CO_2$ output follows.

### Derivation of the alveolar air equation

When inspired gas is room air,

$$R = \frac{CO_2 \text{ output}}{O_2 \text{ consumption}} =$$

$$\frac{\text{ventilation} \times \text{expired } CO_2 \text{ conc.}}{\text{ventilation} \times \text{inspired - expired } O_2 \text{ conc.}}$$

$$(3.15)$$

Cancelling:

$$R = \frac{F_E CO_2}{F_I O_2 - F_E O_2} \qquad (3.16)$$

A similar equation defines the gas concentrations within the effective alveoli:

$$R = \frac{\text{alveolar } CO_2 \text{ conc.}}{\text{inspired } O_2 \text{ conc.} - \text{alveolar } O_2 \text{ conc.}}$$

$$R = \frac{F_A CO_2}{F_I O_2 - F_A O_2} \qquad (3.17)$$

Note that when R = 1, the increase of alveolar $CO_2$ equals the fall of $O_2$, whether measured as molecules, percentage concentrations or partial pressures.

Substituting pressures in the equation gives

$$R = \frac{P_A CO_2}{P_I O_2 - P_A O_2} \qquad (3.18)$$

Rearranging gives an expression for alveolar $P_{O_2}$ ($P_{A}O_2$)

$$P_A O_2 = P_I O_2 - \frac{P_A CO_2}{R} \qquad (3.19)$$

In other words:

$$\frac{\text{Alveolar } P_{O_2} = \text{Inspired } P_{O_2} - \text{Alveolar } P_{CO_2}}{R}$$

$$(3.19a)$$

**Measurement of dead space and alveolar–arterial $P_{O_2}$ difference**

There are five steps:

1. Arterial blood and expired gas are collected simultaneously over several breaths: tidal volume is measured. $P_{O_2}$ and $P_{CO_2}$ are measured in gas and blood.
2. R is calculated from inspired and expired $P_{CO_2}$ and $P_{O_2}$.
3. The assumption is now made that all the gas exchange takes place in the 'effective alveoli' in which R is the same as in the expired gas.
4. The fraction of the total ventilation which is wasted (dead space/tidal volume) is calculated from the expired and the arterial $P_{CO_2}$ (Rossier & Bühlmann, 1955). Effective alveolar $P_{CO_2}$ is defined as being the same as arterial $P_{CO_2}$. Therefore, 'effective alveolar ventilation' is the proportion of the total ventilation which excretes all the $CO_2$ produced by metabolism at the partial pressure in arterial blood.

Then:

$$\frac{\text{Dead space}}{\text{Tidal volume}} = \frac{\text{Wasted ventilation}}{\text{Total ventilation}} =$$

$$\frac{\text{Arterial - expired } P_{CO_2}}{\text{Arterial - inspired } P_{CO_2}} = \frac{P_a CO_2 - P_E CO_2}{P_a CO_2 - P_I CO_2}$$

$$(3.20)$$

When room air is inspired, $P_I CO_2 = $ zero and

$$V_D/V_T = \frac{P_a CO_2 - P_E CO_2}{P_a CO_2} \qquad (3.21)$$

This is most easily understood by examining two examples. If there is no dead space, expired $P_{CO_2}$ equals arterial $P_{CO_2}$, so the numerator is zero. If as much as 50% of the ventilation is wasted, then effective alveolar gas at $P_{CO_2} = 40$ mmHg (5.2 kPa) is diluted with equal volumes of dead space gas ($P_{CO_2} = 0$) to yield expired gas of 20 mmHg (2.6 kPa). Then:

$$V_D/V_T = 40 - 20/40 \text{ or } 5.2 - 2.6/5.2 = 50\%$$

Smaller values of $V_D/V_T$ yield less difference between expired and arterial $P_{CO_2}$.

This measurement of dead space includes the volume of the respiratory valve, the trachea and bronchi and unperfused alveoli. Normal values are available for dead space measured by this formula at various rates and depths of breathing, as well as for tracheo-bronchial volumes. In general, dead space is less than 30% of tidal volume at rest and less than 20% in exercise (Bradley et al., 1976). A correction must be made for the volume of the collecting valve.

5. Calculation of the alveolar–arterial $P_{O_2}$ difference.

Effective alveolar $P_{O_2}$ is calculated from the alveolar air equation (3.19). This is invariably higher than the measured arterial $P_{O_2}$, because systemic arterial blood is a mixture of blood from the ventilated and perfused compartment, with blood from alveoli which receive blood but have only poor ventilation. These contribute unsaturated haemoglobin to the arterial blood, reduce the $P_{O_2}$ and thereby create a positive 'alveolar–arterial $P_{O_2}$ difference'. The alveolar-arterial $P_{O_2}$ difference is often reported as a pulmonary function test. It is important to remember that the difference is between the 'effective' alveolar $P_{O_2}$ which is conceptual and the arterial $P_{O_2}$ which is measured.

The analysis may be taken further by calculation of the 'venous admixture', the fraction of the cardiac output which is perfused but not ventilated. This requires the measurement of cardiac output or mixed venous oxygen content (Fig. 3.4).

Alveolar–arterial $P_{O_2}$ difference is less than 15 mmHg (2.0 kPa) in normal young and middle-aged subjects of average build, breathing air while seated in a chair. In normal subjects it falls with exercise (Harris et al., 1976). Obesity, old age, recumbency and sleep are some normal

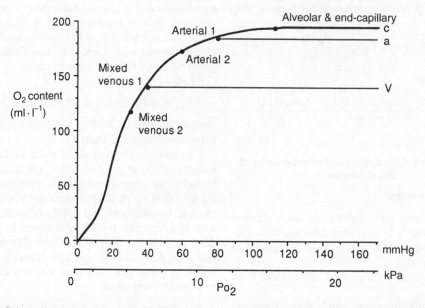

Fig. 3.4. Calculation of venous admixture from the $O_2$ dissociation curve. For patient 1 the alveolar–arterial $Po_2$ difference is 15 mmHg (2.0 kPa). The end-capillary oxygen content is 195 ml·l⁻¹. The mixed venous content is 140 ml·l⁻¹ and the arterial content is 187 ml·l⁻¹. The venous admixture is 195–187/195–140 = 0.17 (17%). Patient 2 has the same ventilation, cardiac output and thus arteriovenous difference for $O_2$. Arterial $Po_2$ is only 60 mmHg (8 kPa). Venous admixture is 195–175/195–125 = 0.40 (40%). This approach shows the importance of cardiac output in determining arterial $Po_2$ and alveolar–arterial $Po_2$ difference. If cardiac output were to fall by about half to give a mixed venous $CO_2$ of 100 ml·l⁻¹, a 17% shunt would dilute the end-capillary blood ($O_2$ content 195 ml·l⁻¹) to yield an arterial $O_2$ content of about 180 ml·l⁻¹. Arterial $Po_2$ would therefore be 63 mmHg (8.4 kPa) (not illustrated).

rated (although there is sometimes a tendency for the alveoli to shrink to the point of collapse when all the nitrogen has been removed). When totally unventilated blood reaches the systemic circulation, arterial desaturation is found during the breathing of pure oxygen. Such shunts typically occur through the communications between the right and left sides of the heart when pulmonary pressures are high. The failure of 100% oxygen to raise arterial saturation to 100% in patients with pulmonary disease but without cardiac lesions usually indicates intrapulmonary 'true shunt', with the caution that 10% of the population have a patent foramen ovale.

situations which increase the difference. Delay in performing the analysis of blood gas pressures produces an error. About 20 mmHg (approximately 2.5 kPa) may be a more realistic estimate of the upper limit of normal in clinical practice.

### Anatomical shunt: right-to-left cardiac shunt

Areas of lung which have a very low ventilation–perfusion ratio cause hypoxaemia during the breathing of air. When pure oxygen is inspired, blood leaving all ventilated alveoli is fully satu-

## Theoretical disadvantages of the calculation of dead space and shunt by Riley's three-compartment analysis

The use of arterial $Pco_2$ to estimate mean alveolar $Pco_2$ (Riley's first approximation) leads to errors when there is a large shunt, when arterial $Pco_2$ is greater than effective alveolar $Pco_2$. Because of the steep $CO_2$ dissociation curve, quite large changes of $CO_2$ content cause small changes of $Pco_2$. Therefore, small alveolar–arterial $Pco_2$ differences do not have an important effect on the alveolar air equation (Eq. 3.17). When venous admixture is greater than 30%, significant errors arise. The value of shunt can be recalculated, first working out the effective $PCO_2$ which, in the presence of the measured shunt, would yield the arterial $PCO_2$. Alveolar $PO_2$ is then recalculated using this 'second approximation' to the alveolar $PCO_2$. Further approximations usually make very little difference.

Such refinements of this technique are no longer usually applied because of the numerous difficulties with the use of over-simplified models in clinical practice. Another obvious objection to Riley's analysis is that the three-compartment model of the lung will not saturate arterial blood if given $O_2$ to breathe. This is because in practice anatomical or 'true' shunt (zero $\dot{V}/\dot{Q}$) behaves differently from areas of very low $\dot{V}/\dot{Q}$. Important limitations to remember when reading work employing this analysis are:

1. Alveolar–arterial $PO_2$ difference is not proportional to venous admixture. The same shunt yields a smaller difference at low values of $PO_2$ (because the $O_2$ dissociation curve is steeper).
2. Changes of inspired $PO_2$ have to be allowed for when calculating shunt.

### Effect of $\dot{V}/\dot{Q}$ imbalance on carbon dioxide exchange

Re-examining the $\dot{V}/\dot{Q}$ curve (Fig. 3.3) it can be seen that arterial $PCO_2$ varies only slightly over a wide range of $\dot{V}/\dot{Q}$ ratios. This justifies Riley's first approximation. It is not however true, as is often stated, that $\dot{V}/\dot{Q}$ imbalance has no effect on $CO_2$ exchange. An alveolar–arterial $PCO_2$ difference of 1 mmHg (0.15 kPa) makes little difference to the calculation of $O_2$ shunt, but it represents about 20% of the difference between mixed venous and effective alveolar $PCO_2$. Arterial $PCO_2$ can be kept normal in the face of deteriorating $\dot{V}/\dot{Q}$ disturbance by increasing total ventilation and thus the contribution from high $\dot{V}/\dot{Q}$ blood. $O_2$ uptake cannot be increased in this way, because areas of high $\dot{V}/\dot{Q}$ are on the flat part of the dissociation curve.

### Blood gas analysis in clinical practice

Normal arterial $PO_2$ varies widely. If the respiratory exchange ratio, R, is measured at the same time as the arterial blood, the alveolar–arterial $PO_2$ difference may be calculated, thus narrowing the normal range of arterial $PO_2$ to 10 mmHg (1.5 kPa). Table 3.2 shows the variation under a variety of physiological conditions in healthy lungs. If R is not measured, it is possible to allow for $PCO_2$ by adding arterial $PCO_2$ and $PO_2$. Under ideal conditions the sum should be the partial pressure of inspired oxygen when R=1. Allowing for the physiological variation of R and the alveolar–arterial $PO_2$ difference in health, arterial $PO_2$ and $PCO_2$ should add up to within 25 mmHg (2.5 kPa) of inspired $PO_2$.

Arterial blood must be sampled carefully if it is to be subjected to such detailed analysis. Alveolar–arterial $PO_2$ difference must be calculated from samples of blood and gas drawn painlessly at the same time over several breaths. If the breath is held after a period of hyperventilation, arterial $PO_2$ falls rapidly and R falls, so the interpretation can only be made on arterial blood alone if the patient has breathed steadily throughout the period of sampling (Morgan *et al.*, 1979).

*Example*. A previously healthy patient attends hospital complaining of acute dyspnoea, but no signs of bronchial asthma, pneumonia or heart failure are present and simple ventilatory tests are normal. The diagnosis may be either an acute hyperventilation attack or an acute pulmonary embolus.

A typical result, breathing air, is:

$P_aCO_2$,          27 mmHg (3.5 kPa)
$P_aCO_2$,          75 mmHg (10.0 kPa)
$P_aCO_2+P_aO_2$,   102 mmHg (13.5 kPa)
                (abnormally low).

Therefore, at the $PCO_2$ found in this case, $PO_2$ is abnormally low and indicates the presence of a disturbance of pulmonary gas exchange. This provides indirect evidence of a pulmonary abnormality compatible with acute pulmonary embolism, which causes hyperventilation with an increase of the alveolar–arterial $PO_2$ difference. The lowest 'normal' $PO_2$ at this $PCO_2$ is 100 mmHg (13.3 kPa).

When arterial $PCO_2$ is elevated, the same calculation may be used to determine whether the degree of hypoxaemia present is due to lung damage. A patient, unconscious because of an over-

Table 3.2. *Normal values of arterial $P_{O_2}$ under varying conditions*

| Condition | $P_{I}O_2$ | | $P_aCO_2$ | | R | $P_AO_2$ | | Lower normal limit of arterial $P_{O_2}$ | | Ambient air $P_{O_2}$ $-P_aO_2+P_{CO_2}$ | | $P_aO_2+P_aCO_2$ | |
|---|---|---|---|---|---|---|---|---|---|---|---|---|---|
| | mmHg | kPa | mmHg | kPa | | mmHg | kPa | mmHg | kPa | mmHg | kPa | mmHg | kPa |
| Fasting, $P_{CO_2}$ at upper limit of normal | 150 | 20 | 44 | 5.9 | 0.7 | 87 | 11.6 | 72 | 9.6 | 34 | 4.8 | 116 | 15.2 |
| Resting, average normal $P_{CO_2}$ | 150 | 20 | 40 | 5.5 | 0.8 | 100 | 13.2 | 85 | 11.2 | 25 | 3.2 | 125 | 11.8 |
| Carbohydrate feeding, average normal $P_{CO_2}$ | 150 | 20 | 40 | 5.5 | 1.0 | 110 | 14.5 | 95 | 12.5 | 15 | 2.0 | 135 | 18.0 |
| Resting, low normal $P_{CO_2}$ | 150 | 20 | 35 | 4.6 | 0.8 | 106 | 14.2 | 90 | 12.2 | 25 | 3.2 | 125 | 16.8 |
| Acute hyperventilation to low normal $P_{CO_2}$ | 150 | 20 | 35 | 4.6 | 1.2 | 122 | 16.2 | 107 | 14.2 | 8 | 1.2 | 142 | 18.8 |
| Severe acute hyperventilation e.g. anxiety | 150 | 20 | 30 | 4.0 | 1.3 | 127 | 17.0 | 112 | 15.0 | 8 | 1.2 | 142 | 18.8 |

Calculated values of alveolar $P_{O_2}$ under differing physiological conditions in healthy subjects breathing room air at sea level. The upper limit of normal for alveolar–arterial $P_{O_2}$ difference is assumed to be 15 mmHg (2 kPa). From this, the lower limit of normal for arterial $P_{O_2}$ is calculated to be 12 mmHg (9.6 kPa) when $P_{CO_2}$ is on the high side and R is low; values below this suggest an abnormality of gas exchange. The lower limit of normal for arterial $P_{O_2}$ is much higher (over 100 mmHg, 13.5 kPa) when $P_{CO_2}$ is low and R is high.

dose of opiate drugs, is mildly cyanosed. Arterial blood gas analysis shows:

| | |
|---|---|
| $P_aCO_2$, | 60 mmHg (8.0 kPa) |
| $P_aO_2$, | 64 mmHg (8.5 kPa) |
| $P_aCO_2+P_aO_2$, | 124 mmHg (16.5 kPa) (normal). |

Although ventilatory control is impaired in this case, the degree of hypoxaemia is explicable by underventilation and no gas exchange defect is present. After several hours, hypostatic pneumonia may develop, with a consequent fall in $Po_2$. As a result, $Pco_2$ may fall slightly because of increasing hypoxic drive, with the following results:

| | |
|---|---|
| $P_aCO_2$, | 53 mmHg (7 kPa) |
| $P_aO_2$, | 53 mmHg (7 kPa) |
| $P_aCO_2+P_aO_2$, | 106 mmHg (14 kPa) (abnormally low). |

When arterial $Po_2$ falls below 60 mmHg (8 kPa), venous admixture has a smaller effect on $Po_2$ because the slope of the oxygen dissociation curve becomes steeper and any measurable alveolar–arterial $Po_2$ difference is caused by defective gas exchange. Subtle analyses are not required for clinical purposes when arterial $Po_2$ is low enough to require treatment in its own right. Then, the physician needs to know the degree of hypoxaemia and whether arterial $Pco_2$ is high (indicating ventilatory failure) or 'normal'.

Ventilatory failure may be caused by the loss of the normal neural drive to breathing, or by loss of a very high proportion of functioning alveoli. In the presence of low arterial $Po_2$, the finding of $Pco_2$ at the upper end of the normal range should probably be regarded as the beginning of ventilatory failure, because the normal response to hypoxaemia is hyperventilation. Patients with very severe reductions of ventilatory capacity may not be able to achieve normal levels of arterial $Pco_2$, especially when there are gas disturbances such as those shown in the example. Moreover, increasing the inspiratory effort may increase the metabolic rate, thus increasing the $CO_2$ load and ventilatory requirement without any improvement in arterial $Pco_2$. A fall of cardiac output compounds the ventilatory problem.

### Blood gases in ventilatory failure and during oxygen therapy

Ventilation can achieve a normal arterial $Pco_2$ when ventilatory capacity is reduced to a very small fraction of normal provided that ventilation and blood flow are evenly distributed. In the presence of an impairment of the efficiency of gas exchange, characterised by 50% physiological shunt and 50% dead space, $Pco_2$ may remain normal if the ventilatory capacity is about one third of normal. Put another way, at least one sixth of the normal lung volume must be capable of ventilating to the normal maximum and must receive at least half of the cardiac output, if $Pco_2$ is to remain normal.

A patient with chronic respiratory disease breathing air cannot theoretically have an arterial $Pco_2$ much higher than 80 mmHg (10.5 kPa) (Campbell, 1965). This follows logically from the alveolar air equation. The lowest arterial $Po_2$ compatible with life is about 20 mmHg (2.5 kPa) and the majority of patients who are as hypoxic as this at sea level have large alveolar–arterial $Po_2$ differences of the order of 45 mmHg (5.5 kPa). Therefore, working upwards from arterial $Po_2$

| | | |
|---|---|---|
| Arterial $Po_2$ | 20 mmHg | 2.5 kPa |
| Alveolar–arterial difference | 45 | 5.5 |
| Alveolar $Po_2$ | 65 | 8.0 |
| Inspired $Po_2$ | 150 | 20.0 |
| Inspired-alveolar $Po_2$ difference (=alveolar $Pco_2$/R) | 85 | 12.0 |
| Assuming R = 0.8 | | |
| Alveolar $Pco_2$ | 68 | 9.6 |

Therefore, it is theoretically impossible for a patient breathing room air at sea level to have a mean alveolar $Pco_2$ of greater than 68 mmHg (9.6 kPa). Arterial $Pco_2$ is somewhat higher than effective alveolar $Pco_2$ in the presence of a large shunt. Thus it is possible to have an arterial $Pco_2$ of around 80 mmHg (10.5 kPa) breathing room air, but is generally true that if it is higher than this, the patient must have been breathing oxygen-rich gas.

Admixture of blood with high $Pco_2$ from poorly ventilated areas can be counterbalanced by blood of low $Po_2$ and $CO_2$ content from effective alveoli.

### Gas exchange in severely damaged lungs

As an extreme case, consider the $CO_2$ exchange of a patient with 50% venous admixture whose metabolic rate is high because of the high work of breathing, but whose cardiac output and veno-arterial $P_{CO_2}$ differences are normal. Remembering that arterial blood is considered to consist of blood at effective alveolar $P_{CO_2}$ mixed with a shunted fraction at mixed venous $P_{CO_2}$ and assuming the $CO_2$ dissociation slope to be linear:

$$(P_{\bar{v}}CO_2 \times \text{shunt fraction}) + [P_A CO_2 \times (1 - \text{shunt fraction})] = P_a CO_2 \quad (3.22)$$

If the shunt fraction is small, $P_a CO_2$ is close to the effective value.

*Example*

| Assume | venous admixture | 50% |
|---|---|---|
| Assume | mixed venous $P_{CO_2}$ | 50 mmHg (6.5 kPa) |
| Assume | arterial $P_{CO_2}$ | 40 mmHg (5.5 kPa) |
| Assume | $CO_2$ output | 0.600 l·min⁻¹ |
| Assume | linear $CO_2$ dissociation slope | |
| Calculate | effective alveolar $P_{CO_2}$ | 30 mmHg (4.5 kPa) |
| Therefore | effective alveolar $CO_2$ concentration | 4% = 0.04 |
| and | effective alveolar ventilation | 0.600/0.04 = 15 l·min⁻¹ |
| Assuming | wasted ventilation, i.e. dead space/tidal volume | 50% = 0.5 litre |
| Calculate | total ventilation | 15/0.05 = 30 l·min⁻¹ |

In other words, when shunt and dead space are high (50%) $P_{CO_2}$ can remain normal during spontaneous breathing, if the patient is capable of breathing at 30 l.min⁻¹.

*Example*

If the patient in the example is sedated and given artificial ventilation, metabolic rate falls, so the ventilatory requirement falls:

| Assume | $CO_2$ output | = only 0.200 l·min⁻¹ |
|---|---|---|
| Recalculate | effective alveolar ventilation | = 0.200/0.04 |
| | | = 5 l·min⁻¹ |
| | total ventilation | = 10 l·min⁻¹ |

*Example*

If cardiac output falls, but the same proportion is distributed to ventilated alveoli, effective alveolar ventilation must increase to maintain systemic arterial $P_{CO_2}$, because the veno-arterial difference widens.

| Assume | arterial $P_{CO_2}$ = 40 mmHg (5.5 kPa) |
|---|---|
| Assume | cardiac output falls to 50% of previous level, metabolic rate constant 0.600 l·min⁻¹ |
| Calculate | veno-arterial $P_{CO_2}$ difference increases × 2 |
| Therefore | mixed venous $P_{CO_2}$ = 60 mmHg (8.0 kPa) |
| Recalculate | effective alveolar $P_{CO_2}$ = 20 mmHg, (3.0 kPa) |
| | effective alveolar $CO_2$ concentration 3% = 0.03 |
| | effective alveolar ventilation 0.600/0.03 = 20 l·min⁻¹ |
| Again | wasted ventilation, i.e. dead space/tidal volume = 50% = 0.5 |
| Calculate | total ventilation 20/0.5 = 40 l·min⁻¹ |

In this last example, if artificial ventilation is given so that $CO_2$ output falls to 0.200 l·min⁻¹, the ventilatory requirement falls to 13 l·min⁻¹. This illustrates that a fall of cardiac output to half its previous value can increase the ventilation needed to keep arterial $P_{CO_2}$ normal by 30%

# References

Bégin, P. & Grassino A. (1991). Inspiratory muscle dysfunction and chronic hypercapnia in chronic obstructive pulmonary disease. *American Review of Respiratory Disease*, **143**, 905–912.

Bernard, C. (1865). Introduction à l'étude de la médecine expérimentale. Paris: Baillière.

Bohr, C., Hasselbalch, K.A. & Krogh, A. (1904). Über einer in biologischer Beziehung wichtigen Einfluss, den die Kohlensäurenspannung des Blutes auf dessen Sauerstoffbindung übt. *Scandinavian Archives of Physiology*, **16**, 402–412.

Bradley, C.A., Harris E.A., Seelye, E.R. & Whitlock, R.M.L. (1976). Gas exchange during exercise in healthy people. I: The physiological dead-space volume. *Clinical Science and Molecular Medicine*, **51**, 575–582.

Campbell, E.J.M. (1965). Respiratory failure. *British Medical Journal*, **i**, 1451–1460.

Christiansen, J., Douglas, C.C. & Haldane, J.S. (1914). The adsorption and dissociation of carbon dioxide by human blood. *Journal of Physiology (London)*, **48**, 244–277.

Farhi, L.E. (1964). Gas stores of the body. In *Handbook of Physiology*, Section 3, vol.1, ed. W. O. Fenn & H. Rahn, pp 873–886. Baltimore: APS.

Farhi, L.E. (1966). Ventilation–perfusion relationship and its role in alveolar gas exchange. In *Advances in*

*Respiratory Physiology*, ed. C.G.Caro. London: Edward Arnold.

Fenn, W.O., Rahn, H. & Otis, A.B. (1946). A theoretical study of the composition of alveolar air at altitude. *American Journal of Physiology*, **146**, 637–653.

Fick, A. (1870). Über die Messung den Blutquantums in den Herzventrickeln. *Sitzber. Physik. Med. Ges. Würzburg*, **36**.

Gilbert, D.L. (1964). Cosmic and geophysical aspects of the respiratory gases. In *Handbook of Physiology*, Section 3, vol.1, ed. W. O. Fenn & H. Rahn, p. 154. Baltimore: APS.

Harris, E.A., Seelye, E.R. & Whitlock, R.M.L. (1976). Gas exchange during exercise in healthy people. II: Venous admixture. *Clinical Science and Molecular Medicine*, **51**, 335–344.

Johnson, M.A., Woodcock, A.A., Rehan, M. & Geddes, D.M. (1983). Are 'pink puffers' more breathless than 'blue bloaters'? *British Medical Journal*, **286**, 179–182.

Kelman, G.R. & Nunn, J.F. (1966). Nomograms for correction of blood $P_{O_2}$, $P_{CO_2}$, pH and base excess for time and temperature. *Journal of Applied Physiology*, **21**, 1484–1490.

Morgan, E.J., Baidwan, B., Petty, T.L. & Zwillich, C.W. (1979). The effects of unanaesthetised arterial puncture on $P_{CO_2}$ and pH. *American Review of Respiratory Disease*, **120**, 795–798.

Riley, R.L. & Cournand, A. (1951). Analysis of factors affecting partial pressure of oxygen and carbon dioxide in gas and blood of lungs: theory. *Journal of Applied Physiology*, **4**, 77–101.

Riley, R.L. & Permutt, S. (1965). The four quadrant diagram for analysing the distribution of gas and blood in the lung. In *Handbook of Physiology*, Section 3, vol.2 , ed. W. O. Fenn & H. Rahn, pp 1413–1424. Baltimore: APS.

Robin, E.D. & O'Neill, R.P. (1983). The fighter versus the non-fighter: control of ventilation in chronic lung disease (1983). *Archives of Environmental Health*, **72**, 125–127.

Rossier, P.H. & Bühlmann, A. (1955). The respiratory dead space. *Physiological Reviews*, **35**, 860–876 (Historical review).

Severinghaus, J.W. (1958). Oxyhaemoglobin dissociation curve corrections for temperature and pH variations in human blood. *Journal of Applied Physiology*, **12**, 485–486.

Tenney, J.M. & Lamb, T.W. (1965). Physiological consequences of hyperventilation and hypoventilation. In *Handbook of Physiology*, Section 3, vol.2 , ed. W. O. Fenn & H. Rahn, pp 979–1010. Baltimore: APS.

Zuntz, N. & Hagemann, O. (1898). Untersuchungen über den Stoffwechsel des Pferdes bei Luke und Arbeit. *Landwirtschaftliches Jahrbuch 2, Wiss Landwirtschaft*, **27**, Suppl. 3, 1–450. Quoted in J.S. Haldane & J.G. Priestley (1935). *Respiration*, 2nd edn, p. 493. London: Oxford University Press.

# 4 Gas transfer

Oxygen is present in the inspired air at a higher partial pressure than in the blood returning to the lungs. It reaches the tissues of the body by:

1. Ventilation.
2. Diffusion.
3. Combination with haemoglobin.
4. Transport by the circulating blood.

## Ventilation

The volume of air in the lungs at the end of expiration is about 2.5 litres. The volumes of trachea and bronchi constitute about 0.25 litre. A tidal breath of 0.5 litre is therefore drawn only a short way into the alveolar (gas exchanging) volume. Gas reaches distal alveoli by diffusion: proximally situated alveoli are served better (Fig. 4.1).

### Diffusion within the alveolar gas

Mixing of gases within the alveoli depends on diffusion. The 'daughter' branches of dividing airways have a greater total cross-sectional diameter than the parent; the ratio is about 1.3:1. This means that the velocity of airflow becomes progressively less as air is drawn into the terminal branches. There are up to seventeen bronchial divisions and up to six further divisions of the respiratory bronchioles and alveolar ducts in the adult lung (Weibel, 1963); in the last few divisions diffusion is more rapid than inspiratory airflow, for a distance of between 1 and 5 mm (Fukuchi et al., 1976; La Force & Lewis, 1970; Cumming, Horsfield & Preston, 1971). It is possible to oxygenate the pulmonary blood when breathing air with a tidal volume which is less than that of the trachea, and if higher concentrations of oxygen are instilled into the trachea, no ventilation is required at all (apnoeic oxygenation). $CO_2$ is not eliminated adequately during apnoeic oxygenation because the partial pressure gradients are smaller.

Gases diffuse according to their density and partial pressure gradient and according to the other gases present (North & Piiper, 1978; Chang, 1987). Density is proportional to molecular weight at a fixed barometric pressure and temperature (Graham's Law). It is possible to show differences in the rate of intrapulmonary diffusion of gas of very high density (sulphur hexafluoride, molecular weight 146) and very low density (helium, molecular weight 4) (Kawashiro et al., 1976). The differences are very small indeed in the range 4 to 44 which includes the physiological gases and many anaesthetic gases. Oxygen diffuses into nitrogen at 0.25 cm·s⁻¹, and more rapidly into helium. As well as diffusion outward from a straight front, gas mixing occurs by agitation of the parabolic front of a newly entered stream of gas. During this type of dispersion, known as Taylor laminar dispersion, $O_2$ passes more rapidly into gases of high density and molecular weight (Piiper & Scheid, 1987). In experimental animals during tidal ventilation, Taylor dispersion and agitation of the lung by cardiac impulses may be important. During breath-holding, simple diffusive mixing appears to dominate $O_2$ exchange, aided by cardiac oscillations (Engel et al., 1973). The Taylor effect is probably not very important in the human lung.

50

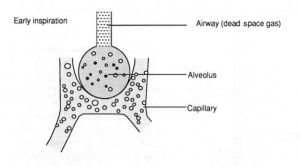

Early inspiration

Airway (dead space gas)

Alveolus

Capillary

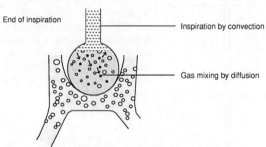

End of inspiration

Inspiration by convection

Gas mixing by diffusion

End of expiration

Mixed alveolar gas

Fig. 4.1. During quiet breathing (tidal volume = 0.5 litre, FRC = 3.5 litres) the tidal air is drawn by convection into the bronchi for a relatively short distance. Oxygen reaches the alveoli by diffusion through the respiratory bronchioles. $CO_2$ is excreted by the reverse process. Proximally placed alveoli receive more than their share of $O_2$, distal alveoli less. Ventilation–perfusion mismatching is prevented by local regulation of pulmonary blood flow, as has been demonstrated experimentally (Grant *et al.*, 1976).

### Diffusion across the alveolar membrane

The alveolar gas is separated from blood by the alveolar and capillary walls and their basement membranes, which are less than 1 micrometre thick over much of their surface in health, but may be 10 times thicker when there is oedema or an inflammatory exudate into the alveolar interstitium. The surface area available for gas exchange is the major determinant of the diffusing capacity of the whole lung.

The speed at which any single gas diffuses through a liquid or a tissue is proportional to its solubility ($\alpha$) and inversely proportional to its molecular weight. These properties determine its diffusion constant (d):

$$d = \frac{\text{Solubility}}{\text{Molecular weight}} \quad (4.1)$$

The flow ($\dot{V}$) of gas through a sheet of fluid or tissue is determined by this constant, by the driving force (the partial pressure gradient across the sheet), by the amount of tissue to be traversed (thickness), and by the space to move (area) (Fig.4.1).

$$\text{Gas flow} = \frac{d \times \text{Area} \times \text{Pressure gradient}}{\text{Thickness}}$$

$$(4.2)$$

This is Fick's law of diffusion.

### Combination with haemoglobin

Oxygen and carbon monoxide (CO) are transported in chemical combination with haemoglobin. The reactions are not instantaneous and constitute approximately half of the delay in equilibration between the alveolar and pulmonary capillary gas pressures (Klocke, 1980). Oxygen uptake by the red cells is complete in 0.1 to 0.15 seconds. $CO_2$ is released by a more complicated series of reactions, summarised in Fig. 4.2. These are:

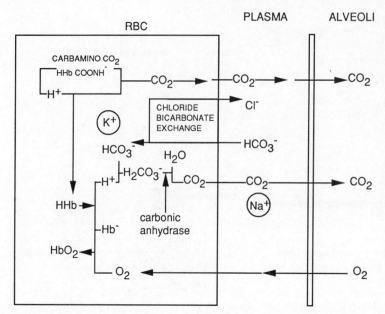

Fig. 4.2. The excretion of $CO_2$ from red cells in the lung and the influence of $O_2$ uptake. The arrows show the predominant direction of the reactions during $O_2$ uptake and $CO_2$ excretion. $O_2$ uptake releases hydrogen ions from haemoglobin, thus acidifying the blood. This (1) aids the conversion of bicarbonate ion to carbonic acid, and (2) liberates $CO_2$ from carbamino-haemoglobin. The $CO_2$ carrying capacity of the blood ($CO_2$ dissociation slope) is increased by the rapid entry of bicarbonate ion into the red cells from plasma, in exchange for chloride ion, which results in the excretion of the greatest possible amount of $CO_2$ for the smallest change of $Pco_2$.

1a. Fall of $Pco_2$ by diffusion from red cells and plasma.
1b. Conversion of red cell $HCO_3^-$ to $H_2CO_3$ followed by dehydration to $CO_2$.
1c. Transfer of $HCO_3^-$ from plasma to red cells.
2a. Release of $CO_2$ from carbamino-haemoglobin when haemoglobin is oxygenated.

The speed of the reactions between haemoglobin and $O_2$ or CO in vitro can be determined quite accurately by measuring the colour changes spectrophotometrically (Sirs & Roughton, 1963). The techniques for determining the reaction rates of $CO_2$ are much less simple (Klocke, 1987). The reactions of $CO_2$ in blood and plasma and their interactions with oxygen uptake should theoretically form an oscillating system which probably does not reach full equilibrium for several seconds, because there is no carbonic anhydrase in plasma. However, the bulk of the evidence suggests that 90% equilibration is achieved in about 0.4 second. Estimates of the volume of blood in the pulmonary capillaries (Vc) of healthy adults using CO (Chapter 5) vary from 50 to 90 ml at rest, and from 90 to 160 ml in heavy exercise. The average time spent by blood in the pulmonary capillary is simply calculated as Vc/Q̇ and is about 1 second at rest and about 0.4 seconds in heavy exercise. Any change of red cell and plasma pH and $Pco_2$ after the blood leaves the capillaries must be very small.

'Inert' gases and anaesthetic gases are carried in simple solution in the blood and red cells and their uptake is therefore not affected by any chemical reactions in the blood.

## Transport by circulating blood

Oxygen uptake and $CO_2$ output are limited by the ability of the circulating blood to transport gas rather than by the ventilatory capacity (Chapter 1).

### Limitation of gas transfer by blood flow and by diffusion

Foreign gases such as nitrous oxide, $N_2O$, which do not react chemically in blood, reach partial pressure equilibrium within the transit of the blood through the pulmonary capillary. As soon as the gas has the same partial pressure in the blood as in the alveolar gas, no further uptake can occur until the blood moves on and some more blood, free of the foreign gas, arrives. CO, on the other hand, does not reach equilibrium with the pulmonary capillary blood before it leaves the lungs; in fact, the capacity of the haemoglobin to combine with CO is so great that the partial pressure of free CO within the red cells barely rises above zero when trace quantities are drawn into the alveoli (Fig. 4.3). In consequence, the uptake of CO continues for several seconds at the same proportional rate regardless of whether the blood is flowing or not. The uptake of CO is therefore limited not by blood flow but by the rate at which it can diffuse into the red cells and combine with them to form carboxyhaemoglobin.

Diffusion equilibrium for any gas is therefore *favoured* by a high diffusion constant. Conversely it is *delayed* if the capacity for chemical combination between the gas and the blood is large: the blood then acts as a sink which absorbs large quantities of the gas (Wagner & West, 1972).

These points are illustrated in Fig. 4.4 by means of a 'hydraulic model'. The first figure illustrates the case for $N_2O$ if this added to the 'alveolar' cistern on the left. The diffusion coefficient is relatively large for a water soluble gas of low molecular weight; in this model, this is represented by a large aperture between the alveolar cistern and the blood cistern. The capacity of the blood cistern is small, because it can hold only what will enter into physical solution in the pulmonary capillary blood; at the same partial pressure this is one hundredth of the pulmonary $N_2O$ content at functional residual capacity if Vc, the pulmonary capillary blood volume, is 90 ml. In the double water-cistern model, there is free passage between the two reservoirs and the second reservoir is small so it fills rapidly. As there is no chemical reaction to consider, the diffusion of $N_2O$ into the blood from the alveolar gas depends on the diffusing capacity of the pulmonary capillary membrane. From measurements of this capacity (Chapter 5) it is possible to calculate the theoretical time course of partial pressure change within the pulmonary capillary; such calculations predict 99% equilibration in 0.01 seconds (Forster, 1964).

The very large capacity of the pulmonary blood to combine with CO is represented on the hydraulic model as a large second reservoir four times the size of the alveolar cistern. The resistance to gas transfer caused by the chemical reac-

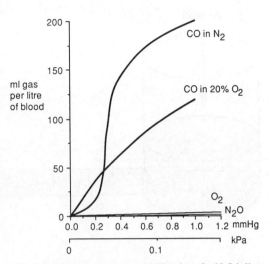

Fig. 4.3. Dissociation slopes. (1) The slope for $N_2O$ is linear and flat because the gas dissolves in water but does not combine chemically with the protein constituents of the blood. (2) The slope for CO. Carbon monoxide competes with oxygen for haemoglobin (Hb), the affinity of Hb for CO at normal values of $PO_2$ being about 250 times that for oxygen.

tion is represented by a narrowing of the diffusion pathway, that is, a reduction of the total diffusing capacity. Addition of CO to the alveolar cistern results in slow equalisation of the pressures in the blood cistern. The model can be refined by introducing a plasma compartment of low capacity. At the partial pressure employed during the test of CO diffusion, the saturation of carboxyhaemoglobin does not rise above 5%; at this saturation the partial pressure of CO is effectively zero. Diffusion equilibrium is not reached because the passage will not admit the quantity required in the time available.

## Breath-holding and rebreathing tests of pulmonary gas exchange

Foreign gases of varying densities and solubilities are used to show how gas is transported from the mouth to the tissues through diseased lungs. Single and multiple breath tests are available. These techniques have been refined since the

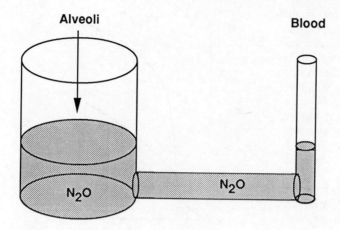

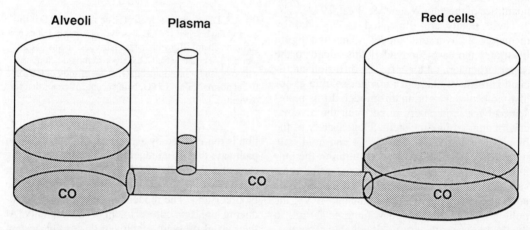

Fig. 4.4. Hydraulic models to explain the rapid diffusion of CO from alveoli into red cells. See text for details.

advent of respiratory mass spectrometers capable of rapid simultaneous analysis of several gases on very small samples.

In the simplest form of breath-holding test, the subject inspires a known volume of foreign gas and breathes out after various known times. The expired gas concentration reflects:

1. Dilution by the accessible residual lung volume.
2. Solution in lung tissue.
3. Uptake and removal by pulmonary blood.

The expirate may be measured continuously using a rapid analyser (Fig. 4.5). The test may be modified to a simple rebreathing procedure, where the subject empties a bag containing the tracer gas and sufficient oxygen. Rebreathing permits sampling of the mixed alveolar gas which is then reinspired; for most gases the results can apparently be analysed as a closed system of constant volume without much inaccuracy.

Three different types of foreign gases may be added to the inspirate and analysed in the expired air after a period of breath-holding or during rebreathing.

1. Insoluble foreign gases remain in the alveoli and make possible the study of diffusion of gas into the alveolar volume. The remainder of this

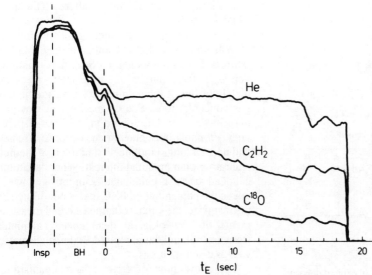

Fig. 4.5. Tracings obtained from a respiratory mass spectrometer sampling continuously during exhalation. The sample inlet was placed in a lobar bronchus via a fibreoptic bronchoscope. The test gas, a mixture of helium (He), acetylene ($C_2H_2$) and a stable isotope of CO in air ($C^{18}O$), was inhaled (Insp) and subsequently exhaled after a short period of breath-holding (BH). (Reprinted from Scheid, 1983, with permission.)

chapter will be concerned with the information that can be derived from these tests.

2. Carbon monoxide permits the study of diffusion of gas across the alveolar membrane (Chapter 5).
3. Soluble inert gases permit the measurement of pulmonary blood flow and pulmonary tissue volume. Their solubility in blood is sufficient to be able to detect their removal from alveolar gas by the blood over a short period of time (Chapter 14).

### Insoluble inert gases

Helium, neon and argon are sufficiently insoluble in water and may be used to measure the alveolar volume and the diffusion of gases into the alveoli. In normal lungs, the whole alveolar volume is filled by a single inspirate of insoluble gas within 3–4 seconds. Slow equilibrium, which may take several minutes, is characteristic of chronic airflow obstruction. The measurement of the alveolar volume during breath-holding should agree to within 0.7 litre with the measurement obtained using an equilibrium technique (Chapter 2).

#### Multiple breath tests of alveolar gas exchange

If the whole alveolar volume is readily accessible to inspired gas, there is rapid equilibrium when any change is made in the concentration of respired gases. This may be tested by 'nitrogen wash-out'. Pure oxygen is inspired in open circuit and the falling concentration of $N_2$ is measured in the expirate. Inaccessible portions of the lung exchange slowly. $N_2$ wash-out curves are discussed on p. 222. Quite minor abnormalities of gas distribution may be demonstrated by this technique.

There are several methods of reporting the results, the original being that of Cournand et al. (1941) who showed that normally, $N_2$ concentration fell to below 2.5% after 7 minutes of breathing oxygen. All take into account the average ventilation of each unit of lung volume. The lung clearance index is the volume of oxygen which will lower the end-tidal concentration of $N_2$ to 2% (normally 5–9 litres) (Becklake, 1952). The lung $N_2$ decay curve is a plot of the decline of expired $N_2$ concentration as a function of the expired volume, the latter being expressed as a cumulative fraction of lung volume (turnover = 1 volume equivalent to FRC) (Prowse & Cumming, 1973).

A more complex approach used the mathematical technique known as moment analysis. This is a method of examining the tail of the wash-out curve for minor abnormalities. This may be a useful procedure for detecting minor abnormalities in children (Fleming et al., 1980).

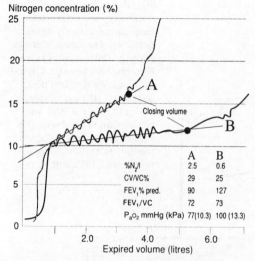

Fig. 4.6. Rapid continuous analysis of expired nitrogen
concentration at the lips after a slow inspiration of 100%
$O_2$ (or a mixture of oxygen and argon). (A) a patient with
ventilation–perfusion mismatching (emphysema), (B) a
normal subject. The first segments of the curve represent
the wash-out of expired air from the dead space (trachea
and those proximal bronchi which participate little in pulmonary gas exchange). The alveolar plateau in the normal
subject is relatively flat, showing oscillations with each
heart beat. The plateau reflects the relatively uniform concentration of $N_2$ in alveoli which empty early and those
which empty later in expiration. The change of $N_2$ concentration between 0.75 and 1.25 litres of expiration is normally less than 1% (nitrogen index). In the patient shown,
the index is 2.5%, an abnormal figure. Quite often the
expired $N_2$ trace is curvilinear and no definite end points
can be identified. Towards the end of expiration the
plateau tilts upwards to form the fourth phase of the curve;
cardiogenic oscillations usually disappear and the concentration of nitrogen rises rapidly. The explanation is that
this gas is emanating from alveoli which were beyond
closed airways when the nitrogen-free gas was inhaled, so
that the expired concentration is closer to that in the air that
was present before the experiment. (After Hughes, 1990,
with permission.)

Similar indices may be derived from the rate of
equilibration of helium during closed-circuit
spirometry with the disadvantage that every circuit has a mixing rate of its own. Normal values
have therefore to be described for each apparatus
and may vary if the setting of the fan mixing the

gas within the apparatus is altered (Bates &
Christie, 1950).

Slow equilibration of inert gases within the
alveoli may be attributed either to 'regional' or
'stratified' inhomogeneity. Stratified inhomogeneity is the failure of the inspirate to reach the
distal portion of the acinus, causing a gradient of
gas concentrations. Such a mechanism was proposed by Krogh & Lindhard in 1912 but disputed
later. Probably both phenomena occur in diseased
and normal lungs, and the distinction is of theoretical rather than practical interest. When 'anatomical dead space' is calculated from nitrogen wash-
out as the percentage of FRC that is not diluted by
the inspirate, the values obtained exceed measurements of physiological dead space calculated
from arterial and from expired $P_{CO_2}$, in normal as
well as diseased lungs.

This shows how effective is the mechanism for
redirecting pulmonary blood flow to well-ventilated regions, probably by the hypoxic vasoconstrictor reflexes. Uneven ventilation, therefore,
does not necessarily mean uneven distribution of
perfusion or of pulmonary diffusing capacity with
respect to ventilation.

## Single breath nitrogen test

Expired $N_2$ is analysed after inspiration of a single
breath of pure oxygen, or argon and oxygen, and
plotted against lung volume. In the standard test,
expiration is slow but the breath is not held after
inspiration (Fig. 4.6) (Fowler, 1949; Comroe &
Fowler, 1951). Information is obtained from two
phases of the test:

1. The volume expired which consists of pure oxygen. This is the 'anatomical dead space'.
   Theoretically, this corresponds to the volume of
   the airways between the gas-exchanging surface
   and the mouth (Aitken & Clark-Kennedy 1928),
   and can be shown to vary with changes of
   bronchial calibre induced by bronchoconstrictors. Excretion of $CO_2$ during a single breath is a
   more elegant way of measuring anatomical dead
   space; the results differ consistently because of
   the different diffusivities (Sikand et al., 1976)
   but agree to within a few millilitres.

2. The alveolar plateau. Theoretically, if there is perfect mixing of inspired and residual gas and if all the alveoli empty at once, the alveolar plateau should be flat; that is, the concentration of alveolar $N_2$ should be constant and should depend on the dilution of residual air. In fact, it slopes upward as illustrated in Fig. 4.6: this slope is used as an index of imperfect gas exchange.

There are several reasons for the presence of this slope. Firstly, the respiratory exchange ratio tends to fall as expiration proceeds because $P_{CO_2}$ approaches the mixed venous value and the respiratory exchange ratio falls. Secondly, there is in all lungs some degree of ventilation–perfusion imbalance, such that the more poorly ventilated zones, which have lower R and therefore higher $P_{N_2}$, empty last.

The single breath $N_2$ index is calculated from the change in $N_2$ concentration between 0.75 and 1.25 litres of expired gas. It should not exceed 2% (Fowler, 1949). The slope is grossly increased in the presence of severe airways obstruction, and may be abnormal when simple ventilatory tests are within normal limits. This procedure was one of the first sensitive indicators of abnormality to be recommended for use in screening programmes to detect early airflow obstruction. It can detect early changes caused by cigarette smoking (Tattersall et al., 1978; Roberts et al., 1990). In addition to the contribution of alveolar stratification and regional inhomogeneity of gas composition, the upslope of the nitrogen plateau may be ascribed in part to the effect of continuing gas exchange (the R effect) (Cormier & Belanger, 1983). $CO_2$ output falls as alveolar $P_{CO_2}$ approaches the level in the mixed venous blood, while oxygen consumption is more or less constant throughout the breath, as long as alveolar $P_{O_2}$ remains above 60 mmHg (8.5 kPa). As a result, R falls and $P_{N_2}$ rises. This effect is exaggerated when the effective alveolar volume is small, for example, in chronic airflow obstruction when many of the alveoli communicate poorly with the major airways. In this case $P_{N_2}$ rises rapidly.

The slope of the alveolar plateau is flatter after long periods of breath-holding. This can be explained on the basis of all the mechanisms given. Differences in the shape of the alveolar plateau employing gases of different densities have been used to demonstrate the presence of stratification of gaseous diffusion (Sikand et al., 1976).

The single breath nitrogen test was much used between 1950 and 1965 to study changes in anatomical dead spaces and has recently been reinstated in epidemiology. It should be regarded as an indicator of abnormality rather than of presence of any particular physiological disturbance.

## 'Closing volume'

During expiration to residual volume, airways close sequentially. In subjects with normal or nearly normal lung function, airway closure occurs mainly at the bases, because pleural pressures are more negative at the apices and the lungs contain less fluid.

Airway closure explains the last phase of the single breath test (Fig. 4.6) (Dolfuss et al., 1967; Engel, Grassino & Anthonisen, 1975). After the plateau (Phase III), normal subjects show a sharp rise of $N_2$ concentration towards the end of expiration. Similar results are obtained when 50 ml boluses of insoluble foreign gases are given at the start of a slow deep inspiration and then exhaled slowly. After the usual three phases, there is an upturn of concentration of the foreign gas which may be quite sharp. The lung volume at which this occurs is called 'closing volume'. Boluses of radioactive xenon given at the start of inspiration and counted over the chest are distributed preferentially to the upper zones because some basal units are behind closed airways at that time. During slow expiration, after the alveolar dead space has been washed out, the lung empties uniformly at first. As the point of airway closure is reached, the upper alveoli to which the inspired bolus had access, contribute more of the expirate. The concentration of foreign gas therefore rises. Boluses of argon, helium and radioactive xenon may be used to measure closing volume. They are injected at the beginning of inspiration and distributed preferentially to the apex. Phase IV is magnified and cardiogenic oscillations more obvious than with the nitrogen method.

Closing volume (CV) increases with age and smoking habit (Teculesu *et al.*, 1990). It is less than 10% of VC at the age of 20. 'Closing capacity' (CC, which is CV + RV) is greater than FRC in men over 50 years of age. This means that airway closure occurs even during normal breathing. The consequent regional hypoxaemia is probably sufficient to account for the slight increase of resting arterial $Po_2$ with age (Harris, Seelye & Whitlock, 1976).

Airway closure may be detected during the measurement of airways resistance during body plethysmography. Below FRC, there is a sharp angulation of the loop obtained by plotting airflow against box pressure caused by a sudden increase of apparent airways resistance during expiration. This is caused by the reduction of the number of parallel channels available for airflow and by compression of the non-connecting lung.

Closing volume and occasionally closing capacity have been used since 1970 as tests of the patency of small airways. There are good theoretical reasons for believing that the technique might detect early lesions of chronic bronchitis. Studies of radioactive gas distribution suggest that the airflow obstruction seen in this condition occurs mainly at the bases (Hughes *et al.*, 1972). The majority of studies have shown significant differences between smokers and non-smokers, though only if middle-aged subjects are included.

Measurements of closing volume have contributed to our understanding of the pathophysiology of lung disease (Anthonisen, 1986), but do not add useful information to the standard battery of tests in the investigation of individual patients. They are adequately reproducible under ideal conditions, but the results vary with expiratory flow rate. Closing volume cannot invariably be measured in subjects with abnormal lungs.

# References

Aitken, R.S. & Clark-Kennedy, A.E. (1928). On the fluctuation of the composition of the alveolar air during the respiratory cycle in muscular exercise. *Journal of Physiology (London)*, **65**, 389–411.

Anthonisen, N.R. (1986). Tests of mechanical function. In *Handbook of Physiology*, section 3, vol. III, ed. P.T. Macklem & J. Mead, pp. 774–776. Bethesda: APS.

Bates, D.V. & Christie, R.V. (1950). Intrapulmonary mixing of helium in health and disease. *Clinical Science*, **9**, 17–27.

Becklake, M.R. (1952). A new index of the intrapulmonary mixture of inspired air. *Thorax*, **7**, 111–116.

Bidani, A., Crandall, E.D. & Forster, R.E. (1978). Analysis of postcapillary pH changes in blood in vivo after gas exchange. *Journal of Applied Physiology*, **44**, 778–781.

Chang, H.K. (1987). Diffusion of gases. In *Handbook of Physiology*, section 3, vol. IV, ed. L.E. Farhi & S.M. Tenney, pp. 46–47. Bethesda: APS.

Comroe Jr, J.H. & Fowler, W.S. (1951). Lung function studies VI: Detection of uneven alveolar ventilation during a single breath of oxygen. *American Journal of Medicine*, **10**, 408–413.

Cormier, Y. & Belanger, J. (1983). Quantification of the effect of gas exchange on the slope of phase III. *Bulletin Européen Physiopathologie Respiratoire*, **19**, 13–16.

Cournand, A, Baldwin, E. de F., Darling, R.C. & Richards, D.W. (1941). Studies on intrapulmonary mixture of gases. IV: The significance of pulmonary emptying rate and a simplified open circuit measurement of residual air. *Journal of Clinical Investigation*, **20**, 681–689.

Cumming, G., Horsfield, K. & Preston, S. (1971). Diffusion equilibrium in the lung examined by nodal analysis. *Respiration Physiology*, **12**, 329–345.

Dolfuss, R.E., Milic-Emili, J. & Bates, D.V. (1967). Regional ventilation of the lung studied with boluses of Xenon-133. *Respiration Physiology*, **2**, 234–46.

Engel, L.A., Grassino, A. & Anthonisen, N.A. (1975). Demonstration of airway closure in man. *Journal of Applied Physiology*, **38**, 1117–1125.

Engel, L.A., Menkes, H., Wood, D.H., Utz, G., Joubert, J. & Macklem, P.T. (1973). Gas mixing during breath-holding studies by intrapulmonary gas sampling. *Journal of Applied Physiology*, **35**, 18–24.

Fleming, G.M., Chester, E.H., Saniie, J. & Saidel, G.M. (1980). Ventilation inhomogeneity using multibreath nitrogen wash-out: comparison of normal ratios with other indexes. *American Review of Respiratory Disease*, **121**, 789–794.

Forster, R.E. (1964). Diffusion of gases. In *Handbook of Physiology*, section 3, vol. I, ed. W.O. Fenn & H. Rahn, pp. 839–872. Washington D.C.: APS.

Fowler, W.S. (1949). Lung function studies. III: Uneven pulmonary ventilation in animal subjects and subjects with pulmonary disease. *Journal of Applied Physiology*, **2**, 283–299.

Fukuchi, Y., Roussos, C.S., Macklem, P.T. & Engel, L.A. (1976). Convection, diffusion and cardiogenic mixing of inspired gas in the lung: an experimental approach. *Respiration Physiology*, **26**, 77–90.

Grant, B.J.B., Davies, E.E., Jones, H.A., & Hughes, J.M.B. (1976). Local regulation of pulmonary blood flow and ventilation perfusion ratios in the coatimundi. *Journal of Applied Physiology*, **40**, 216–228.

Harris, E.A., Seelye, E.R. & Whitlock, R.M.L. (1976). Gas exchange during exercise in healthy people. II: Venous admixture. *Clinical Science and Molecular Medicine*, **51**, 335–344.

Horsfield, K. & Cumming, G. (1968). Functional consequences of airway morphology. *Journal of Applied Physiology*, **24**, 384–390.

Hughes, J.M.B. (1990). Pulmonary gas exchange. In *Respiratory Medicine*, ed. R.A.L. Brewis, G.J. Gibson & D.M. Geddes, pp. 131–157. London: Baillière Tindall.

Hughes, J.M.B., Grant, B.J.B., Greene, R.E., Iliff, L. & Milic-Emili, J. (1972). Inspiratory flow rate and ventilation distribution in normal subjects and patients with simple chronic bronchitis. *Clinical Science*, **43**, 583–595.

Kawashiro, T., Sikand, R.S., Adams, F., Takahashi, H. & Piiper, J. (1976). Study of intrapulmonary gas mixing in man by simultaneous washout of helium and sulphur hexafluoride. *Respiratory Physiology*, **28**, 261–275.

Klocke, R.A. (1980). Kinetics of pulmonary gas exchange. In *Pulmonary Gas Exchange*, vol.1 *Ventilation, Blood Flow and Diffusion*, ed. J.B. West. New York: Academic Press.

Klocke, R.A. (1987). Carbon dioxide transport. In *Handbook of Physiology*, section 3, vol. IV, ed. L.E. Farhi & S.M. Tenney, pp. 173–195. Bethesda: APS.

Krogh, A. & Lindhard, J. (1912). Measurement of blood flow through the lungs of man. *Standard Archives of Physiology*, **27**, 100–125.

La Force, R.C. & Lewis, B.M. (1970). Diffusional transport in the human lung. *Journal of Applied Physiology*, **28**, 291–298.

North, H. & Piiper, J. (1978). Diffusion of helium, carbon monoxide and sulphur hexafluoride in gas mixtures similar to alveolar gas. *Respiration Physiology*, **32**, 155–166.

Piiper, J. & Scheid, P. (1987). Diffusion and convection in intrapulmonary gas mixing. Carbon dioxide transport. In *Handbook of Physiology*, section 3, vol. IV, ed. L.E. Farhi & S.M. Tenney, pp. 54–55. Bethesda: APS.

Prowse, K. & Cumming, G. (1973). Effects of lung volume and disease on the lung nitrogen decay curve. *Journal of Applied Physiology*, **34**, 23–33.

Roberts, C.M., Rawbone, R.G., Adams, L. & Seed, W.A. (1990). Sensitivity and specificity of small airway tests in subjects with normal conventional lung function tests. *Clinical Science*, **74**, 29P.

Scheid, P. (1983). Respiratory mass spectrometry. In *Measurement in Clinical Respiratory Physiology*, ed. G. Laszlo & M.F. Sudlow. London: Academic Press.

Sikand, R.S., Magnussen, H., Scheid, P. & Piiper, J. (1976). Convective and diffusive gas mixing in human lungs: experiments and model analysis. *Journal of Applied Physiology*, **40**, 326–371.

Sirs, J.A. & Roughton, F.J.W. (1963). Stopped flow measurement of CO and $O_2$ uptake by haemoglobin in sheep erythrocyte. *Journal of Applied Physiology*, **18**, 158–165.

Tattersall, S.F., Benson, M.K., Hunter, D., Mansell, A. & Pride, N.B. (1978). The use of tests of peripheral lung function for predicting future disability from airflow obstruction in middle-aged smokers. *American Review of Respiratory Disease*, **118**, 1035–1050.

Teculescu, D.B., Varona-Lopez, W., Bruant, A., Pham, Q.T., Locuty, J. & Deschamps, J.-P. (1990). Determinants of alveolar nitrogen slope and closing volume in healthy adolescents. *American Review of Respiratory Disease*, **142**, 607–615.

Wagner, P.D. & West, J.B. (1972). Effects of diffusion impairment in $O_2$ and $CO_2$ time courses in pulmonary capillaries. *Journal of Applied Physiology*, **33**, 62–71.

Weibel, E.R. (1963). *Morphometry of the Human Lung*. Berlin: Springer-Verlag.

# 5 Carbon monoxide uptake

Carbon monoxide (CO) combines with haemoglobin. CO uptake can therefore be used to measure the capacity of the whole lung to transfer gas between haemoglobin and inspired air. The removal of trace amounts of CO added to inspired air can be used to test the integrity of the function of the whole lung.

## The single breath carbon monoxide transfer test

The single breath test of CO uptake, developed by Marie Krogh in 1915, has been standardised (Ogilvie *et al.*, 1957; McGrath & Thompson, 1959) and reference values obtained from the study of normal subjects. In addition to providing quantitative information about the gas exchanging properties of normal and diseased lungs, it is popular as a screening test of pulmonary function. This is partly because of the surprisingly narrow normal range, 2 standard deviations being represented by some 25% of the predicted mean value.

Several aspects of respiratory function must be intact to achieve normal CO uptake: the diffusion pathway through the airways (Chapter 4), the surface area of the alveolar capillary membrane (which must not be too thick), the pulmonary capillaries and the concentration of haemoglobin in the blood.

The test is useful in clinical practice, particularly when lung volumes and tests of the uniformity of distribution of inspired gas are normal. Then, impairment of CO transfer factor in the presence of a normal haemoglobin concentration indicates disease at the level of the alveoli.

### Procedure

The procedure requires detailed examination (Fig. 5.1). The subject exhales to residual lung volume and breathes in a measured volume of gas (a mixture of air, 0.3% CO and about 10% helium) to reach about 10% less than the total lung capacity. The breath is held for about 10 seconds and then exhaled. The first 0.7 litre is discarded and the next 0.6 litre collected in a bag as a representative alveolar sample, which is analysed.

#### Single breath diffusing capacity, transfer factor and transfer coefficient

The simplest view of the principle is that the two foreign gases employed, CO and helium, are both diluted by the residual air of the lungs. No measurable helium is absorbed by the blood, but the CO is taken up wherever the alveolar gas is in contact with red cells. The fraction of CO extracted over and above its dilution by the residual gas may be calculated by dividing the apparent CO dilution ratio by the helium dilution. The length of time of breath-holding determines uptake and is allowed for.

The uptake of CO in the whole lung is analysed as though it acted as a single, well-mixed gas exchanger the volume of which is defined by the dilution of the inspired helium (Fig. 1.1).

Fick's Law (Chapter 4) defines the permeability of a uniform membrane for any gas: if we rearrange it with all the 'constants' on one side we obtain a measure of the 'diffusing capacity' $DL$, of the whole unit under study.

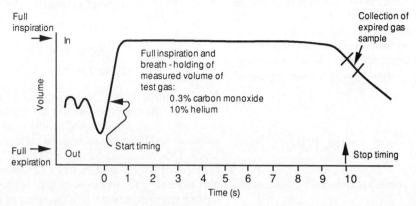

Fig. 5.1. Carbon monoxide transfer factor (single breath breath-holding method): lung volume–time trace illustrating the technique. The subject breathes in from a bag, holds the breath for about 10 seconds and then exhales. A valve opens and closes an empty bag in which the middle portion of the expirate is collected. The inspirate and expirate are analysed. The calculation of TLco is described in the text.

$$DL = \frac{\text{Gas flow across the membrane}}{\text{Pressure gradient}}$$

(5.1)

The units of the 'diffusing capacity' are $ml \cdot min^{-1}$ per mmHg pressure gradient, or, in SI units, $mmol \cdot min^{-1}$ per kPa. The uptake of CO in the whole lung is related to the average thickness of the gas exchanging surface and its surface area, as well as to the diffusion coefficient of the gas in lung tissue. The conversion of CO to carboxy-haemoglobin also takes time and adds a further barrier to the fall of Pco within the red cell. The units of gas flow/pressure drop are analogous to electrical conductance (the reciprocal of resistance); for two conductances in series:

$$\frac{1}{\text{Total diffusing capacity}} =$$

$$\frac{1}{\text{Membrane diffusing capacity}} =$$

$$\frac{1}{\text{Capillary blood volume} \times \text{rate constant of CO–Hb reaction}}$$

(5.2)

Theoretically, even the 'membrane' diffusing capacity could be subdivided in the same way to include terms for the alveolar wall, plasma and red cell wall (Roughton & Forster, 1957).

**Equation**

In a hypothetical single gas exchanger (Fig. 1.1), with no CO in the mixed venous blood, the uptake of the gas can be derived by simple calculus because uptake is exponential. At any instant, the movement of CO out of the alveolar gas is:

$$\frac{-d\,PCO}{dt} \cdot \frac{V_A}{PBAR - PH_2O}$$

(5.3)

where $V_A$ is the alveolar volume, $P_b$ the barometric pressure and $PH_2O$ the vapour pressure of water in the alveoli. In the absence of any effective back pressure of CO within the red cells, the driving pressure for diffusion across the alveolar membrane is the same as the alveolar pressure, Pco. Therefore, at any instant, the uptake of CO is determined by the diffusing capacity of the exchanger (Dco) and the alveolar Pco.

$$DCO = \left( \frac{-d\,PCO}{dt} \cdot \frac{V_A}{PBAR - PH_2O} \right) / PCO$$

(5.4)

or, rearranging, and defining $PBAR - PH_2O$ as PBARc

$$\frac{DCO \cdot PBARc}{V_A} = \frac{-d\,PCO / dt}{PCO}$$

(5.5)

The right-hand term shows that Pco is changing at a rate proportional to itself, that is, constant fraction of the total CO present is diffusing out of the alveoli at any time. This is the condition of logarithmic change with time, like a bath emptying progressively more slowly as the weight of the water falls.

By calculus

$$\frac{- \, d \, \text{Pco} / dt}{\text{Pco}} = - \, d \log_e \text{Pco} / d \, t \quad (5.6)$$

Over a measured period of time, $t_2 - t_1$, this equals

$$\frac{\log_e \text{Pco}(t_2) - \log_e \text{Pco}(t_2)}{t_2 - t_1} \quad (5.7)$$

or

$$\frac{\log_e \, (\text{Pco}(t_2) / \text{Pco} \, (t_2)}{t_2 - t_1}$$

In the more usual form of the equation, the logarithms are expressed to base 10, which requires them to be divided by 0.434.

In the single breath test (Fig. 5.1) it is assumed that the initial concentration of CO in the lungs can be calculated from the dilution of the inspired volume with CO-free residual air; the dilution ratio is obtained from that of inspired helium.

Initial CO conc. =

$$\text{Inspired CO} \cdot \frac{\text{Expired helium}}{\text{Inspired helium}} \quad (5.8)$$

Initial / final CO conc. =

$$\frac{\text{Inspired CO} \cdot \text{Expired helium}}{\text{Expired CO} \cdot \text{Inspired helium}} \quad (5.9)$$

This takes no account of the time of diffusion of the gases into the distal portions of the alveoli, but this is less important than the other approximations inherent in the approach.

The total alveolar volume is obtained from the dilution of inspired helium. It is known as the virtual alveolar volume, $V_A'$, to distinguish it from the true volume of gas in the lung.

$$V_A' = \left( \begin{array}{c} \text{Inspired volume } - \\ \text{apparatus dead space} \end{array} \right) \cdot$$

$$\frac{\text{Inspired helium}}{\text{Expired helium}} \quad (5.10)$$

If the expired helium concentration is derived from an instrument requiring $CO_2$ absorption, such as a katharometer, the expired helium must be corrected. It is sufficiently accurate to multiply by the factor 0.95, correcting for expired $CO_2$. (When an infrared analyser is used for CO, $CO_2$ absorption is also necessary for the expired gas, so the factor cancels out in equation 5.l0.) The effect of making these corrections is small and predictable.

### Transfer constant, transfer factor and transfer coefficient

CO uptake during the single breath test may be expressed in three ways:

*Marie Krogh's permeability constant, 'k'.*

$$k = \frac{\log_{10} \cdot \text{Fco}_i / \text{Fco}_e \cdot 1}{0.4343 \cdot \text{FHe}_i / \text{FHe}_e \cdot t} =$$

$$\frac{\text{Dco} \cdot \text{PBARc}}{V_A} \quad (5.11)$$

In Marie Krogh's words, the permeability constant of the lung for CO is the number of millilitres of CO, STPD, which would diffuse in from 1 ml of lung volume, STPD, if the lungs were filled with pure CO and if the capillary Pco could be kept at zero.

*The whole lung 'diffusing capacity' or 'transfer factor' for CO* (TLco).

$$\text{Dco (or TLco)} =$$

$$\frac{k \cdot V_A'}{\text{PBARc}} \, \text{ml} \cdot \text{min}^{-1} \cdot \text{mmHg}^{-1}$$

$$(5.12)$$

$$= \frac{k \cdot V_A'}{\text{PBARc} \cdot 22.4} \, \text{mmol} \cdot \text{min}^{-1} \cdot \text{kPa}^{-1}$$

where k is Krogh's constant, PBARc the barometric pressure excluding water vapour and 22.4 the factor which converts millilitres to millimoles.

The term 'transfer factor for CO' was introduced to replace 'diffusing capacity'. The purpose was to counter the widespread belief that a reduction of this value in patients with bronchopulmonary disease indicated that they had an alveolar–capillary diffusion defect. In fact, any abnormality of any of the mechanisms governing gas exchange may cause a reduction of TL. In spite of the ambiguity of the term 'transfer factor', it will be employed in this book as the accepted name of the clinical laboratory tests of CO uptake, reserving 'Dco' for theoretical discussions of diffusion and diffusing capacity. 'Diffusing capacity' is used in the USA and Australia, and increasingly, again, in European journals.

When the single breath test was first applied in clinical studies (Ogilvie *et al.*, 1957) the 'alveolar volume' was estimated from the inspired breath and the patient's previously measured residual volume. The single breath $V_A'$ gives identical results in normal lungs. It was partly for convenience that the test was modified for use as a single procedure (McGrath & Thompson, 1959; Mitchell & Renzetti, 1968). There are, however, sound theoretical reasons for using the modification, which measures the CO uptake of that portion of the lung which is ventilated during the manoeuvre. The slowly ventilated parts of the lung are not accessible to study by a simple test of this type. The use of a larger lung volume gives a larger value for 'whole lung diffusing capacity', which in effect means 'the capacity to transfer CO which the whole lung would possess if it were all accessible to the inspired gas and if the distribution of the pulmonary diffusing capacity were uniform'. When referring to published studies of TLco, especially in patients with chronic airflow obstruction, it is important to notice which test has been used.

*Transfer factor per unit lung volume*. Although this is usually described a 'Kco' this is not Marie Krogh's kCO and should be called TLco/$V_A'$. It is the CO transfer per litre of ventilated lung volume, and is supposed to indicate the gas exchanging properties of the lung while correcting for reductions of lung volume. There are certain situations in which this number is more useful than TLco.

It is important to notice the exact units in which TLco/$V_A'$ is expressed, as all the following have been used.

1. TLco/$V_A'$ ($V_A'$ in STPD units)
2. TLco/$V_A$ ($V_A$ in STPD units)
3. TLco/$V_A'$ ($V_A'$ in BTPS units): recommended
4. TLco/$V_A$ ($V_A$ in BTPS units)

Since the conversion factor from STPD to BTPS is 1.2, (1) and (3) are widely different.

## Subdivision of diffusing capacity

### Membrane diffusing capacity (Dm) and capillary blood volume (Vc)

The measurement of the subdivisions of TLco sometimes sheds light on the physiological disturbances present in diseased lungs. The method depends on two observations:

1. The rate of reaction between CO and haemoglobin (Hb) measured in vitro ($\theta$) has a linear relation to Po$_2$, the reaction being slower at high Po$_2$. The formula used at present is

$$\frac{1}{\theta} = \frac{a + b\, P_c O_2}{Hb/14.9} \qquad (5.13)$$

where a and b are constants, given the values 0.33 and 0.0057 by Roughton & Forster (1957). $P_c O_2$ is the mean pulmonary capillary Po$_2$ and is calculated as follows, from the assumption that the diffusing capacity for oxygen is $1.23 \times DLco$ (a factor calculated from the relative diffusivities of O$_2$ and CO). The formula is

$$P_c O_2 = P_A O_2 - V O_2 / 1.23\, TLco \qquad (5.14)$$

which is similar to the formula for diffusion given at the beginning of the chapter.

2. TLco falls if the subject performs the same test at higher inspired Po$_2$.

The Roughton–Forster relationship (equation 5.1) may be solved to divide the diffusing capacity into oxygen-dependent and oxygen-independent portions. It is generally assumed that the fall of TLco with increasing Po$_2$ is all due to the slowing of the rate of the chemical reaction between CO and haemoglobin, so the oxygen-independent portion is a measure of the capacity of the gas to

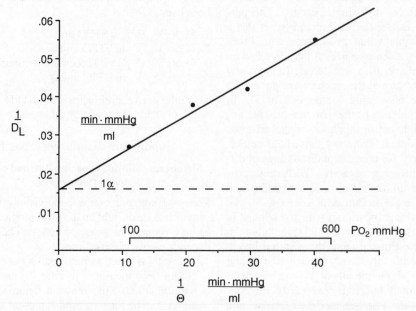

Fig. 5.2. Calculation of the oxygen-dependent ($\theta$.Vc) and oxygen-independent (Dm) components of the whole lung diffusing capacity. Dm, the diffusing capacity of the alveolar membrane; $\theta$, the reaction rate between haemoglobin and CO; Vc, the volume of red blood corpuscles available at any instant for CO exchange (the 'pulmonary capillary blood volume'). 1/Dm is the intercept of the straight line drawn through values of 1/TLco measured at various values of inspired $Po_2$. $\theta$ is calculated from equation 5.13. Vc is calculated from the slope of the line because

$$1/D_L = 1/Dm + 1/\theta.Vc$$

and

$$1/D_L = 1/Dm + 1/\theta.\tan \alpha$$
$$1/Vc = \cotan \alpha$$

In these equations, the term $D_L$ is used to represent the theoretical diffusing capacity of a single alveolus.

reach contact with the red cells. In a uniform system with perfect gas mixing, this is the membrane diffusing capacity (Dm).

In practice, TLco is measured during breath-holding at different levels of $Po_2$. The principle of the calculation is shown in Fig. 5.2. Most laboratories use two, some three levels of $Po_2$. The measurement is rather unreproducible, less so if more points are obtained.

The accumulation, after a single breath-hold, of 0.3% CO is very small (less than 1%) but signifi-

cant back pressure is found in heavy smokers, whose arterial COHb saturation may reach 10%. Back pressure, expressed as gas concentration in the rebreathing bag, is subtracted from the estimated 'alveolar' concentrations, both initial and final. This step is usually neglected in the simple measurement of TL and may cause underestimation in heavy smokers (Knudson, Katterborn & Burrows, 1987; Mohsenifar & Tashkin, 1979; Gulsvik *et al.*, 1992). The formula is:

$$\% \text{ reduction TLco} =$$
$$0.97 \text{ COHb\%} + 0.33\% \qquad (5.15)$$

Calculation of the 'back pressure' of CO is therefore necessary for the refined measurement of Dm and Vc. There is no standard way of measuring it. An approximate technique is to rebreathe from a bag containing air or oxygen for 30 seconds and measure Pco and $Po_2$ in the bag. Cotes (1979) suggests ignoring the back pressure at low levels of $Po_2$ and measuring it by rebreathing suitable mixtures of $O_2$, with $CO_2$ absorption, for 4 minutes.

Dm, calculated in this way, yields much lower results than morphometric methods in experimental animals (Weibel, 1984; Crapo *et al.*, 1988). Which is true cannot be determined, but considerable uncertainty is introduced by the assumptions used to calculate $\theta$ in equation 5.13.

### Standardisation of inspired gas concentration, breath-holding time and topographical factors during the measurement of TLCO

Most reference values have been obtained employing mixtures of helium (10%), CO (0.3%) and air which result in an inspired oxygen concentration of about 18%. Although mixtures containing 21% cause less desaturation in patients with defective $O_2$ transfer, they are much more expensive and are rarely used (Crapo & Gardner, 1987). Since CO uptake is enhanced by hypoxaemia, there is a theoretical possibility that CO transfer is overestimated in hypoxaemic patients. It is possible to correct TLCO for expired $Po_2$ but it is not certain that this has any clinical value.

The determination of the time of breath-holding has conventionally been taken from one third of the initial inspired volume to the time when one half of the expired sample has been collected. These times have been chosen after careful experiments showed that they gave a similar result after various breath-holding times in normal subjects: in other words, the closest approximation to an exponential fall of alveolar PCO (Jones & Meade, 1961). An alternative method was chosen by the American Thoracic Society (Ferris, 1978) whereby timing started halfway through the first inspirate. This gives results which are 7% higher (Leech et al., 1985). Arbitrary standards have been set for rate of inspiration, which should be complete in 2.5 seconds in subjects without airflow obstruction and not longer than 4.0 seconds when there is airflow obstruction (Crapo & Gardner, 1987).

In the standard technique, TL is measured between 90% and 100% of full inspiration (Crapo & Gardner, 1987). In clinical practice, an inspired volume of 85% of vital capacity is acceptable. TL is sufficiently independent of lung volume when it is measured at a lung volume between 90% and 100% of TLC, varying by 4% in the majority of subjects. $TLCO/V_A$ varies rather more with lung volume near TLC, by about 8%. Changes in the volume of the lung during breath-holding are therefore an important source of error when comparing one reading with another (Frans et al., 1979; Stam, Kreuzer & Versprille, 1991). Below

90% of TLC, TLCO is reduced and $TLCO/V_A$ increased (Lipscomb, Patel & Hughes, 1978). A 30% error is introduced if $V_A$ is only 70–80% of TLC, and a 13% error between 80% and 90%. In the upright position at rest, the diffusion coefficient $TLCO/V_A$ at the lung base is about twice that in the apex which are determined by the uptake of radioactive CO measured over the thorax (West et al., 1962). The gradient is not affected by oxygen, so Dm and Vc probably vary in the same proportion. These findings explain the technical observations that have had to be overcome by standardisation of the procedure:

1. The removal of alveolar CO during breath-holding is not exponential at rest in the upright position (Newth, Cotton & Nadel, 1977), although it is in exercise and in the supine position.
2. The calculation of TL is affected by the exact volume of sampling of expired gas: analysis of the first portion of the expired gas which comes from the upper zones gives a lower value of TL than the later portion of the expirate, except for the very end of expiration.

## Significance of the breath-holding TLCO

If a healthy subject inhales a trace of CO, holds the breath for 10 seconds and breathes out, the amount of CO extracted will depend on the size and vascularity of the lungs. The 96% limits of normality are approximately ± 25% of the population normal value, predicted from regression equations which take into account height, age, ethnic origin and sex, when CO extraction is calculated as TLCO in the manner just described.

### Low TLCO

Some of the ways in which disease can reduce TLCO are true reductions of 'diffusing capacity' while others are disturbances of the distribution of ventilation and perfusion.

1. Loss of lung tissue, by surgical removal or obliteration by disease. This reduces the surface area for gas exchange, although the pulmonary capillary bed may distend and compensate partly for the loss. TLCO, Dm and Vc are reduced; $TLCO/V_A$ may be normal or high.

2. Increase of the intra-alveolar diffusion pathway: TLco is reduced, TLco/$V_A$ normal.
3. Increased thickness of the alveolar membrane; TLco, TLco/$V_A$ and Dm are reduced.
4. Decreased volume of blood in the pulmonary capillaries (Vc): this reduces TLco and TLco/$V_A$.
5. Reduced haemoglobin concentration: TLco, TLco/$V_A$ and Vc are reduced. The best correction factor for this is from Cotes (1979).

$$TLco \text{ (corrected)} = TLco \text{ } (14.6 \text{ } a + [Hb]/1 + a \text{ } [Hb] \quad (5.16)$$

where a = Dm/Vc and is taken to be 0.7.

(see also Dinkara *et al.*, 1970; Knudson *et al.*, 1987).

6. Regional inhomogeneity of ventilation and perfusion: these cause inefficiency of gas transfer. In general, an area of lung having good ventilation but a reduced vascularity or surface area may also have a high ratio of ventilation to perfusion; although blood flow and vascularity do not have a constant relationship. Such regions will dilute both inspired helium and CO, and cause a reduction of TLco and TLco/$V_A$. The correlation between 'dead space' and reduction of TLco can be predicted theoretically but not in practice because there may be compensatory increases of TLco/$V_A$ in other areas of the lung. Areas of poor ventilation which have a share of the pulmonary blood volume are not freely accessible either to inspired CO or to helium. These areas will tend to reduce TLco and $V_A'$ but not TLco/$V_A'$. This point, although obvious now, is stressed because many papers, especially those written between 1951 and 1965, have attempted to distinguish between 'diffusion defects' and 'distribution defects' (of ventilation and perfusion) on the basis of tests of so-called diffusing capacity.

## Elevation of TLco

CO uptake during the standard test is increased when there is an unusually large volume of haemoglobin within the lungs. This may be intravascular or extravascular; the presence of recent extravasation of blood in the lungs in Goodpasture's syndrome may be demonstrated by a raised (or rising) TLco/$V_A$ (Ewan *et al.*, 1976; Greening & Hughes, 1981). TLco/$V_A$ is increased when there is pulmonary plethora, notable in patients with left-to-right shunts (Bedell & Adams, 1962).

## Variation of TLco in normal subjects

Under optimal conditions, TLco varies in a single individual by about 5%. If the test is not performed in a standard manner, the variation is much greater (apart from analytical errors) and reproducibility could be improved by standardising the inspiratory part of the test (Graham, Mink & Cotton, 1981).

Variations of TL at constant lung volume are probably caused either by increased filling of the pulmonary vessels, or by recruitment of previously empty channels. Exercise increases single breath TLco by 25% (Kendrick *et al.*, 1986) when measured in the upright position. Lying down increases TL in young subjects (Ogilvie *et al.*, 1957; Stam, Kreuzer & Versprille, 1991), by increasing the filling of upper lobe blood vessels to an extent which mimics the rise produced by exercise. In elderly subjects, the change is slight.

## Exercise

Exercise increases TLco by recruitment of empty capillaries or by increased capillary engorgement. Single breath TLco can be measured without difficulty and breath-holding time is shortened to 6 seconds (Neville, Kendrick & Gibson, 1984). With maximal exercise, TLco is greater than at rest by a factor of 1.25. The relationship of TLco to oxygen uptake probably shows a plateau at higher loads. This suggests that the blood vessels are maximally recruited at high loads; unfortunately detailed interpretation is hampered by the number of assumptions inherent in the calculations (Kendrick *et al.*, 1986). During breath-holding in exercise, alveolar $Po_2$ changes rapidly. This problem can be overcome by $Po_2$ analysing of the expirate and correcting the value obtained by a factor determined experimentally (Kanner & Crapo, 1986). The effects of pH on CO uptake is not known. It is therefore difficult to draw conclusions about the changes and physiological state of the gas exchanging surface from measurements of

TLco made when the biochemical state of the blood is changing.

It is unusual to find instances where exercise TLco is abnormal when resting TLco is normal, or indeed where exercise TLco is the only abnormality (Kendrick & Laszlo, 1991; Kendrick, 1991). The measurement of single breath TLco in exercise has therefore not contributed many useful clinical insights to the investigation of disease.

### Interpretation

Patients with non-uniform pathological processes which tend to reduce TLco may also have pulmonary plethora in other parts of the lung resulting in TLco which is not necessarily low. In isolation, the statement that a patient has a TLco which is less than 75% of 'predicted normal', means only that there is a 95% chance that there is a bronchopulmonary disorder if there is no haematological disturbance. If $TLco/V_A$ is very high, there probably is pulmonary plethora.

TLco contributes to the diagnostic process in clinical practice if it is interpreted quantitatively, in conjunction with all the available information, rather like the use of the erythrocyte sedimentation rate in haematology. It is part of the standard routine of investigation and receives considerable attention in the clinical chapters.

## Alternative methods of measuring TLco

1. *Rebreathing*. This is the same, in principle, as the breath-holding technique, but the expirate is rebreathed for a period of a few seconds (Lewis *et al.*, 1959; Marshall, 1977). The result is not affected by respiratory rate. The results are comparable to those obtained by breath-holding in patients with a wide variety of diseases and the procedure is easier for the breathless. Patients who are very ill and who cannot hold their breath are usually able to rebreathe from a small bag of known volume at FRC (Clark, Jones & Hughes, 1978). This procedure has been used to determine changes of $TLco/V_A$ in the investigation of pulmonary haemorrhage (Ewan *et al.*, 1976).
2. *Rebreathing with continuous analysis of CO*. Mass spectrometers cannot analyse CO in the presence of $N_2$ as they both have the same mass. It requires stable isotopes of CO which are very expensive, so physiological, rather than clinical, information has been obtained by this method. By mixing the expirate frequently, regional variations of $TLco/V_A$ are averaged and Pco falls exponentially with time in normal, upright subjects (Sackner *et al.*, 1975). The numerical results are somewhat larger than the single breath procedure performed in the standard manner but the difference is less than 10%.

3. Analysis of a single expirate (Newth, Cotton & Nadel, 1977). This has not so far been exploited.

4. Steady state methods (TLco,ss). These have been used widely in clinical laboratories. The patient breathes a mixture of CO in air or $O_2$ from a large bag in a box, the excursions of which are recorded on a spirometer. The expirate is collected in a second bag in the same box. CO uptake is calculated as

$$V_I \cdot F_I co - V_E \cdot F_E co \qquad (5.16)$$

Alveolar Pco is obtained in one of two ways

1. Calculation of 'alveolar Pco' from measured $CO_2$ dead space and mixed expired Pco (Filley, Mackintosh & Wright, 1954). Dead space is obtained from arterial $Pco_2$ and expired $Pco_2$ by Bohr's formula. Alveolar Pco calculated from it is analagous to 'effective' alveolar $Po_2$ (Chapter 3). The formula is:

$$P_A co = P_{BAR} \cdot \frac{F_E co - V_D / V_T \cdot F_I co}{1 - V_D / V_T} \qquad (5.18)$$

2. A variant is to obtain alveolar $Pco_2$ indirectly. Values obtained from end-tidal samples (Bates, Boucot & Dormer, 1955) are satisfactory in normal subjects. Back pressure must be estimated. A rebreathing estimate of mixed venous $Pco_2$ may be used.

These techniques are very sensitive to non-uniformity of ventilation and perfusion, and vary considerably with the rate and depth of breathing, particularly at rest. Clinical studies employing them should be viewed with caution.

The method of allowance for 'dead space' in the calculation of PACO is critical: in fact, the Kroghs (1909) abandoned the steady state technique for this reason.

Normal limits are narrower in exercise: the rise of TLCO,ss is an important indicator of normality.

There are not many studies comparing the breath-holding (TLCO,sb) and steady state (TLCO,ss) methods in patients with lung diseases. The topic is reviewed by Kanaev & Laskin (1980) who showed that similar numerical results were obtained for TLCO by both methods in patients with damage to the pulmonary circulation. Normal subjects and those expected to have intact pulmonary vasculature had higher values for CO uptake during breath-holding at TLC. The probable explanation is that in these patients, increasing the depth of breathing does not distribute inspired gas more uniformly to the pulmonary blood vessels as occurs normally. The information gained from the exercise TLCO,ss was similar to that obtained from the resting single breath procedure (Bedell & Ostiguy, 1967).

Useful information can be obtained by measuring the fractional CO uptake

$$\frac{F_ICO - F_ECO}{F_ICO} \qquad (5.19)$$

which is a useful indicator of normality if greater than 50%, but is critically dependent on ventilation. It can be improved by relating it to $O_2$ extraction (Ameratunga & Harris, 1988). This method, like all steady state techniques, is not now as widely used as it was, but those experienced with it find it valuable in the assessment of patients with airflow obstruction and small lungs (Chapters 6 and 7).

## Conclusion

The Kroghs used the measurement of whole lung diffusing capacity to investigate the physiology of breathing: from their results, they concluded that 'diffusion' did not limit oxygen uptake in normal man. Interesting physiological information about alveolar–capillary transfer continues to emerge from studies of TLCO, 'Dm' and 'Vc' in physiological stress and in disease. Defective gaseous diffusion, uneven distribution of ventilation and of diffusing capacity can all cause reduction of TLCO below the expected value.

In clinical practice, TLCO and TLCO/$V_A$ are useful indicators of the vascularity of the well-ventilated parts of the lung. They may be reported as being high, normal or low and add to the clinical and physiological profiles which characterise lung disorders.

## References

Ameratunga, R. & Harris, E.A. (1988). The alveolar carbon monoxide fraction, a simple, alternative measure of carbon monoxide transfer factor. *European Respiratory Journal*, **1**, 115–118.

Bates, D.V., Boucot, N.G. & Dormer, A.E. (1955). The pulmonary diffusing capacity in normal subjects. *Journal of Physiology (London)*, **129**, 237–252.

Bedell, G.N. & Adams, R.W. (1962). Pulmonary diffusing capacity at rest and in exercise: a study of normal persons and persons with atrial septal defect, pregnancy and pulmonary disease. *Journal of Clinical Investigation*, **41**, 1908–1914.

Bedell, G.N. & Ostiguy, G. (1967). Transfer factor for carbon monoxide in patients with airways obstruction. *Clinical Science* **32**, 239–248.

Clark, E.H., Jones, H.A. & Hughes, J.M.B. (1978). Bedside rebreathing technique for measuring carbon monoxide uptake by the lung. *Lancet*, **i**, 791–793.

Cotes, J.E. (1979). *Lung Function*, 4th edn. Oxford: Blackwell Scientific Publications.

Cotes, J.E., Dabbs, J.M., Elwood, P.C., Hall, A.M., McDonald, A. & Saunders A.M. (1972). Iron deficiency anaemia: its effects on transfer factor for the lung and ventilation and cardiac frequency during submaximal exercise. *Clinical Science*, **42**, 325–335.

Crapo J.D., Crapo, R.D., Jensen, R.L., Mercer, R.R., Weibel, E.R. (1988). Evaluation of lung diffusing capacity by physiological and morphometric technique. *Journal of Applied Physiology*, **64**, 2083–2091.

Crapo, R.O., Gardner, R.M. (1987). (For the American Thoracic Society.) Single breath carbon monoxide diffusing capacity (transfer factor): recommendations for a standard technique. *American Review of Respiratory Disease*, **136**, 1299–1307.

Dinkara, P., Blumenthal, W.S., Johnston, R.F., Kauffman, L.A. & Solnick, P.B. (1970). The effect of anaemia on pulmonary diffusion capacity with derivation of a correction equation. *American Review of Respiratory Disease*, **102**, 965–969.

Ewan, P.W., Jones, H.A., Rhodes, C.G. & Hughes,

J.M.B. (1976). Detection of intrapulmonary haemorrhage with carbon monoxide uptake. *New England Journal of Medicine*, **215**, 1391–1396.

Ferris, B.G. (1978). Epidemiology standardisation project. *American Review of Respiratory Disease*, **118** (Suppl.), 62–72.

Filley, G.F., Mackintosh, D.J. & Wright, G.W. (1954). Carbon monoxide uptake and pulmonary diffusing capacity in normal subjects at rest and during exercise. *Journal of Clinical Investigation*, **33**, 530–539.

Frans, A., Francis, C.H., Stanescu, D., Nemery, J.B., Prignot, J. & Brasseur, L. (1979). Transfer factor in patients with emphysema and lung fibrosis. *Thorax*, **33**, 539–540.

Graham, B.L., Mink, J.T., Cotton, D.J. (1981). Improved accuracy and precision of single breath CO diffusing capacity measurements. *Journal of Applied Physiology*, **51**, 1306–1313.

Greening, A.P. & Hughes, J.M.B. (1981). Serial estimations of carbon monoxide diffusing capacity in intrapulmonary haemorrhage. *Clinical Science*, **60**, 507–512.

Gulsvik, A., Bakke, P., Humerfelt, S., Omenaas, E., Tosteson, T., Weiss, S.T. & Speizer, F.E. (1992). Single breath transfer factor for carbon monoxide in an asymptomatic population of never smokers. *Thorax*, **47**, 167–173.

Jones, R.S. & Meade, F. (1961). A theoretical and experimental analysis of anomalies in the estimation of pulmonary diffusing capacity by the single breath method. *Quarterly Journal of Experimental Physiology*, **46**, 131–143.

Kanaev, N.N., Laskin, G.M. (1980). Clinical significance of the ratio between breath-holding and steady state diffusing capacity in patients with chronic bronchitis and diffuse lung fibrosis. *Bulletin European Physiopathologie Respiratoire*, **16**, 309–320.

Kanner, R.E. & Crapo, R.O. (1986). Relationship between alveolar oxygen tension and the single breath carbon monoxide diffusing capacity. *American Review of Respiratory Disease*, **133**, 676–678.

Kendrick, A.H. (1991) Pulmonary transfer factor for carbon monoxide in exercise. PhD Thesis, University of Bristol.

Kendrick, A.H., Cullen, T., Green, H., Papouchado, M. & Laszlo, G. (1986). Measurement of single breath carbon monoxide transfer factor (diffusing capacity) during progressive exercise. *Bulletin European Physiopathologie Respiratoire* **22**, 365–370.

Kendrick, A.H. & Laszlo, G. (1991). Transfer coefficient (Kco) on exercise in alveolar disease. *European Respiratory Journal*, **4** (Suppl. 14), 193S.

Knudson R.J., Katterborn H.T., Knudson, P.T. &

Burrows, B. (1987). The single breath diffusing capacity: reference equations from a healthy non-smoking population and the effects of haematocrit. *American Review of Respiratory Disease*, **135**, 805–811.

Krogh, A. & Krogh, M. (1909). Rate of diffusion of CO into the lungs of man. *Standard Archives of Physiology*, 23, 236–247.

Krogh, M. (1915). The diffusion of gases through the lungs of man. *Journal of Physiology (London)*, **49**, 271–300.

Leech, J.A., Martz, L., Liben, A. & Becklake, M.R. (1985). Diffusing capacity for carbon monoxide: the effects of different durations of breath-hold time and alveolar volume and of carbon monoxide back pressure on calculated results. *American Review of Respiratory Disease*, **132**, 1127–1129.

Lewis, B.M., Lin, T-H., Noe, F.E. & Hayford-Westing, E.J. (1959). The measurement of pulmonary diffusing capacity for carbon monoxide by a rebreathing method. *Journal of Clinical Investigation*, **38**, 2073–2986.

Lipscomb, D.J., Patel, K. & Hughes J.M.B. (1978). Interpretation of increases in the transfer coefficient for carbon monoxide. *Thorax*, **33**, 728–733.

Marshall, R. (1977). A rebreathing method for measuring carbon monoxide diffusing capacity. *American Review of Respiratory Disease*, 115, 537–539.

McGrath, M.W. & Thompson, M.L. (1959). The effect of age, body size and lung volume change on alveolar capillary permeability and diffusing capacity in man. *Journal of Physiology*, **146**, 572–582.

Mitchell, U.M. & Renzetti, A.D. (1968). Application of the single breath method of total lung capacity measurement to the calculation of carbon monoxide diffusing capacity. *American Review of Respiratory Disease*, **97**, 581–584.

Mohsenifar, Z. & Tashkin, D.P. (1979). Effect of carboxyhaemoglobin on the single breath diffusing capacity: derivation of an empirical correction factor. *Respiration*, **37**, 185–191.

Morris, A.H. & Crapo, R.O. (1985). Technical note: standardisation of computation of single breath transfer factor. *Bulletin Européen Physiopathologie Respiratoire*, **21**, 183–190.

Neville, E., Kendrick, A.H. & Gibson, G.J. (1984). A standardised method of estimating Kco on exercise. *Thorax*, **39**, 823–827.

Newth, C.J.L., Cotton, D.J. & Nadel, J.A. (1977). Pulmonary diffusing capacity measured at intervals during a single exhalation in man. *Journal of Applied Physiology*, **43**, 617–625.

Ogilvie, C.M., Forster, R.E., Blakemore, W.S. & Morton, J.W. (1957). A standardised breath-holding technique for the clinical measurement of the diffusing capacity of the lung for carbon monoxide. *Journal of Clinical Investigation*, **36**, 1–17.

Roughton, F.J.W., & Forster, R.E. (1957). Relative importance of diffusion and chemical reaction rates in determining rate of exchange of gases in the human lung with special reference to the diffusing capacity of pulmonary membrane and volume of blood in pulmonary capillaries. *Journal of Applied Physiology*, **61**, 290–302.

Sackner, M.A., Greeneltch, D., Heiman, M.S., Epstein, L.S. & Atkins, N. (1975). Diffusing capacity, membrane diffusing capacity, capillary blood volume, pulmonary tissue volume and cardiac output measured by a rebreathing technique. *American Review of Respiratory Disease*, **111**, 157–165.

Stam, H., Kreuzer, F.J.A. & Versprille, A. (1991). Effect of lung volume and positional change on pulmonary diffusing capacity with its components. *Journal of Applied Physiology*, **71**, 1477–1488.

Stam, H., Versprille, A. & Bogaard G. (1983). Components of the carbon monoxide diffusing capacity in man dependent on alveolar volume. *Bulletin Européen Physiopathologie Respiratoire*, **19**, 17–22.

Weibel, E.R. (1984). The Pathway for Oxygen. Cambridge, MA: Harvard University Press.

West, J.B., Holland, R.A.B., Dollery, C.T. & Matthews, C.M.E. (1962) Interpretation of radioactive gas clearance rates in the lung. *Journal of Applied Physiology*, **17**, 14–20

# 6 Chronic airflow obstruction

Several common conditions can cause obstruction to the tidal respiratory flow of air:

1. Bronchial asthma and hyperreactivity of airways.
2. Chronic bronchitis: (a) mucus hypersecretion, (b) inflammation of small airways less than 2 mm in diameter.
3. Pulmonary emphysema.

Similar disturbances may be caused by bronchiectasis, cystic fibrosis and obliterative bronchiolitis. Airflow obstruction affects some patients with alveolar diseases involving the bronchi, especially sarcoid. It forms part of a few rare syndromes, notably lymphangioleiomyomatosis.

These disorders are clinically distinct and may generally be diagnosed as separate entities in their early stages, but can progress to a disabling condition characterised by chronic airflow obstruction and sometimes to respiratory failure. This is often called chronic obstructive lung disease or chronic airways obstruction because the underlying pathological processes often coexist and are difficult to distinguish clinically in their late stages. They have to be distinguished from narrowing of the apertures of the larynx, trachea and central airways.

Chronic or recurrent airflow obstruction accounts for most of the referrals to pulmonary function laboratories. The traditional emphasis has been to assign each patient to one or more diagnostic categories. Recently, the approach has moved towards measurement of the problems that are common to all the patients and developing treatment strategies to cope with these (Bates, 1989*b*) (Table 6.1). Nevertheless, much energy has been expended in attempting to classify the different components of chronic obstructive lung disease and the account that follows attempts to assess this work in the light of current knowledge.

## Chronic bronchitis, disease of small airways and pulmonary emphysema

### Background

Intensive research into the epidemiology, pathology and clinical physiology of chronic bronchitis and of pulmonary emphysema has led to many changes in definition, terminology and understanding of these conditions. To review critically the mass of information available on this topic, the reader needs to understand the subtle shift of emphasis that has taken place since 1960 (Thurlbeck, 1976).

The Victorians understood chronic bronchitis to be a major cause of cough and respiratory difficulty among the inhabitants of city slums. In the period 1920–1930, the major concern of chest physicians in the United Kingdom was with the eradication of pulmonary tuberculosis; in these circumstances, chronic bronchitis was regarded as benign cause of sputum production and diagnosed by exclusion when there was no evidence of phthisis. With the decline of tuberculosis more interest was shown in the problem of chronic respiratory disease, which continued to cause disability and shortening of life in a substantial section of the community. In about 1955 the British Medical Research Council initiated an intensive programme of research into chronic respiratory symptoms which provided a vital stimulus to

Table 6.1. *Approach to chronic airflow obstruction (modified from Bates, 1989b)*

*History (severity and duration)*
  Cough
  Volume of sputum
  Wheezing and chest tightness
  Dyspnoea
    Episodic, variable or constant
    Exercise grade
    Nocturnal
    Positional
  Oedema
  Exertional fatigue
  Weight loss or gain
  Intellectual/mood disturbance
  Sleep disturbance
  Daytime sleepiness
  Smoking present and past
  Alcohol
  Drugs
  Medication

*Examination*
  Breath sounds
  Wheezing or crackles
  Use of cervical accessory muscles
  Diaphragm contraction
  Venous pressure
  Oedema

*X-ray*
  Lung volume, nodularity
  Consolidation, bronchial wall thickness
  Localised transradiancy or bullae
  Pulmonary arteries: large or small, peripheral or central
  Cardiac contours

*Pulmonary function: most patients*
  Indices of flow limitation (PEF, $FEV_1$)
  (*a*)  present
  (*b*)  variability with time, exercise,
        response to bronchodilators,
        response to steroids
  Correlates of worsening disability and respiratory failure
    Vital capacity
    Hyperinflation
  Correlates of alveolar destruction ($FEV_1/VC$, $TL_{CO}$)
    Resting blood gases or estimate ($O_2$ saturation, rebreathing $P_{CO_2}$)

*Pulmonary function: some patients*
  $FEV_1$ and VC decline with time over years
  Sleep studies
  Flow volume loops and detailed tests of lung mechanics
  Assessment of disability, exercise performance

Table 6.1. *Continued*

*Other information: most patients*
ECG: right ventricular hypertrophy
Haematocrit: for polycythaemia

*Other information: some patients*
Sweat test if cystic fibrosis suspected
Pulmonary arterial pressure
Echocardiography (transoesophageal) to exclude septal defects

*CT*
Emphysema
Bronchial wall thickening
Associated pulmonary fibrosis, pleural disease

*Magnetic resonance (future development)*
Cardiac chambers

research into the assessment of pulmonary function in the laboratory and in the field.

Up to that time, expectoration of sputum from the chest was accepted as a physiological response to bronchial irritation (the normal man's cough). Chronic bronchitis was described as a condition in which the lower airways, normally sterile, became colonised by bacteria. The patient suffered from frequent chest illnesses characterised by increase in the volume and purulence of the sputum with fever and dyspnoea. Gradually, the purulence became a permanent feature and the dyspnoea failed to remit between exacerbations until cyanosis and right heart failure supervened (cor pulmonale). In most descriptions, emphysema was regarded as the inevitable consequence of this condition and was diagnosed whenever the chest appeared to be hyperinflated or barrel-shaped. The dyspnoea was assumed to be due to the emphysema. This condition was readily confirmed at post mortem to be present in the majority of lungs of patients dying of respiratory failure. While this was probably close to the truth, a number of points called for some explanation.

### The British Disease

Chronic bronchitis was thought to be very much commoner in urban England than elsewhere. However, the American medical literature contained descriptions of 'emphysema' which appeared similar to those of chronic bronchitis. Surveys in London and Chicago in 1960 showed that British bronchitis and American emphysema were similar in their clinical presentation and epidemiology (Burrows *et al.*, 1964). Chronic respiratory symptoms and airflow obstruction are now found around the world wherever they are sought, although the incidence varies.

### Pink and puffing, blue and bloated

Simpson (1968) and Dornhorst (1955) pointed out that some patients with chronic airflow obstruction presented with severe shortness of breath without hypoxaemia. Others were hardly distressed by their breathing, but developed signs of right heart failure and were often cyanosed with low resting arterial $O_2$ saturation. These distinctions were dramatised by the descriptions 'pink puffer' and 'blue bloater', soon embodied into standard medical teaching without much regard for the obvious fact that most patients showed features of both of these groups.

The pink and puffing group were equated with extensive pulmonary emphysema and the blue and bloated group with chronic 'bronchitis' without emphysema (Type A and B disease; Burrows *et al.*, 1966). Eighty per cent of the patients had features of both types of disorder (type X).

A number of careful pathophysiological studies have clarified these relationships. Although some patients with respiratory failure have no macroscopic emphysema at post-mortem, the majority of patients with respiratory failure and right heart enlargement have evidence of extensive emphysema (Thurlbeck, 1976; Biernacki *et al.*, 1989). The 'blue and bloated' group are made up of patients with progressive hypoxaemia, caused by disease of small airways which in many instances progresses in parallel with the lesions of pulmonary emphysema. There is a 'pink' group constituting about a quarter of unselected series of patients well enough to be studied in life using computerised radiographic techniques or to undergo lobectomy. They are short of breath on exertion and have extensive disease, with reduced $FEV_1$ with relatively little arterial desaturation until the disease is far advanced.

These problems would become uncommon if cigarette smoking were to cease world-wide, but only a quarter of smokers develop disabling respiratory symptoms.

The account given here describes the ways which have been developed to study the effects of chronic airflow obstruction in detail for clinical and epidemiological purposes. Because it is the easiest to summarise, the pathophysiology of emphysema will be described first and contrasted with the mixed type of chronic airflow obstruction. These distinctions are of more importance epidemiologically than for decisions about immediate treatment but they do influence prognosis.

## Definitions

### Pulmonary emphysema

Traditionally, pulmonary emphysema has been defined as a state in which alveolar spaces are enlarged, because of either dilatation or destruction of the alveolar walls. This includes hyperinflation secondary to bronchial asthma and acute bronchiolitis which may be reversible. It also includes the condition of compensatory emphysema, in which the normal lung expands to fill a space left by diseased or excised lobes, which does not affect the function of the lung. Pulmonary emphysema is now usually defined as an increased size of the air spaces distal to the terminal bronchiole with destruction of alveolar walls.

There are two main types:

1. Centriacinar (centrilobular): the lesions are most severe near the terminal bronchiole. This type of emphysema is associated with chronic bronchitis and possibly with industrial dust diseases.
2. Panacinar (panlobular): the lesions involve the whole of affected lobules, although the whole lung is not uniformly affected. This type may occur as 'primary emphysema' without chronic bronchitis.

Other patterns include paraseptal and subpleural emphysema and emphysema related to the presence of localised scars.

### Chronic bronchitis

According to the Medical Research Council of the United Kingdom (MRC), chronic bronchitis is defined as being present when there is abnormal bronchial secretion of sufficient quantity to cause expectoration of sputum from the chest (Medical Research Council, 1965). For epidemiological purposes, an arbitrary degree of involvement was set, the condition being labelled 'simple chronic bronchitis' to distinguish it from the severely disabling disorder that caused loss of work. Thus, simple chronic bronchitis is 'the regular expectoration of sputum from the chest on most days in the winter months for as much as three months of the year for at least two years'.

This condition was said to become complicated by 'chronic infection' and 'airflow obstruction' to cause the disabling illness previously recognised by doctors as chronic bronchitis. Built into this set of definitions is the hypothesis that severe chronic airflow obstruction results from a natural progression of a proportion of cases of simple chronic bronchitis. This hypothesis now needs restating because it has become clear that the rate of decline of lung function is not inevitably more rapid than normal in all individuals with bronchial hypersecretion. The definitions remain useful.

### Questionnaire of respiratory symptoms

MRC standard questionnaires provide information in a form which allows populations to be compared for the incidence of cough, sputum, haemoptysis, shortness of breath on exertion and at rest and chest pain.

With full occupational and environmental information this questionnaire (1967) and extensions of it (Ferris, 1978), form the basis of most research into the epidemiology of all types of chronic lung disease. These take about half an hour to complete.

## Pulmonary emphysema

### Clinical background

The patient who has panacinar emphysema without chronic bronchitis rarely presents any diagnostic difficulty. Symptoms begin between the ages of 30 and 55 with progressive shortness of breath on exertion. Smokers develop symptoms earlier. Sputum expectoration is scanty or absent (less than 5 ml daily). The chest appears to be large. Although a large breath may be taken, lateral expansion at the level of the nipples is usually less than 2.5 cm. The diaphragm is low and the chest expands upwards rather than outwards. Breath sounds are quiet or absent over the most affected areas and there is little noise audible at the mouth during quiet breathing. There is prolongation of forced expiration to greater than 5 seconds and there may be a fine wheeze audible in forced expiration (Lal, Ferguson & Campbell, 1964).

The chest X-ray may show hyperinflation, poor vascularisation and hypertransradiancy, with a vertical heart. Computed tomographic (CT) images are capable of demonstrating lesions larger than 4 mm and can be used to quantify the presence of these lesions in life (Goddard *et al.*, 1982; Bergin *et al.*, 1986; Müller *et al.*, 1988). Calculation of lung density based on CT is also feasible and reflects loss of alveolar walls (Gould *et al.*, 1988). Neither method is perfect, because the visual appearances of low density may reflect regional diversion of the blood flow as well as destruction of blood vessels, while calculations of lung density may be affected by hyperinflation as well as by destruction of alveolar walls (Table 6.2).

Ventilation–perfusion scans show matched defects which may be extensive but do not help to measure the extent of microscopic alveolar destruction.

### Functional disturbance

The functional disturbance of emphysema is caused by loss of alveolar walls. This has three important effects:

1. Loss of elastic recoil.
2. Lengthening of the pathway for diffusion of gases within the air passages during quiet breathing.
3. Reduction of the total area for gas exchange.

The intrinsic elasticity of the lungs is determined by the elastic tissue in the alveoli; the emphysematous zones have reduced elastic recoil and are abnormally easy to distend. The degree of destruction may not account for all the changes of lung volume (Silvers, Petty & Stubbs, 1980), but in general there is a correlation between the amount of distal air space enlargement and the elastic properties of the lung (Leaver, Tattersfield & Pride, 1973; Finucane & Colebatch, 1969; Gibson *et al.*, 1979; Paré *et al.*, 1983; Gugger *et al.*, 1991). $FEV_1$, $FEV_1/FVC$ and $FEV_1/EVC$ are good clinical indicators of the severity of emphysema. When $FEV_1/VC$ is less than 55% there is substantial air space enlargement, usually emphysema (Goddard *et al.*, 1982; Nicholson, 1980; Sakai *et al.*, 1987; Gould *et al.*, 1988). In summary, indices derived from pressure–volume curves which estimate elastic recoil are capable of demonstrating alterations of alveolar size and number (Gugger *et al.*, 1991). However, measurements of distal air space enlargement and of the amount of macroscopic emphysema that can be seen by eye at CT or pathology, both correlate well with $TLco/V_A$. The conclusion is that these two conditions generally progress together and that it is the elastic recoil which determines $FEV_1$ and RV/TLC ratio. These findings add weight to the idea that loss of elastic recoil is an important determinant of maximal expiratory flow (Chapter 2) and of airway closure.

The long diffusion pathway acts as dead space. In the normal lung during quiet breathing, a tidal inspiration draws air only into the proximal alveoli within the acinus; some gas exchange takes place by diffusion into more distal alveoli. In emphysematous areas, the inspired air has to travel further to reach gas exchanging tissue. As a

Table 6.2. *Relationship between TLco/VA and different methods of grading emphysema in life*

Study: Goddard *et al.* (1982), recalculated
Subjects: unselected clinic patients

| CT: macroscopic 'emphysema' | >50% | 25–50% | <25% | None | |
|---|---|---|---|---|---|
| | | | | Asthma | Normal |
| **TLco/V$_A$** | | | | | |
| Traditional units[a] | 2.4 | 3.6 | 4.3 | 4.8 | 4.5 |
| SI units[b] | 0.8 | 1.2 | 1.45 | 1.6 | 1.5 |
| Ratio FEV/EVC % | 37 | 48 | 53 | 68 | 82 |

Study: Gould *et al.* (1988)
Subjects: undergoing lung resection

| Pathology: macroscopic emphysema | >10% | <5% | | None |
|---|---|---|---|---|
| **TLco/V$_A$** | | | | |
| Traditional units[a] | 1.9 | 4.1 | | 4.4 |
| SI units[b] | 0.6 | 1.4 | | 1.5 |
| CT: EMI number (lowest 5% of pixels)[c] | −480 to 460 | −459 to 440 | −439 to 430 | −429 to 400 |
| **TLco/V$_A$** | | | | |
| Traditional units[a] | 1.1 | 3.8 | 3.8 | 4.4 |
| SI units[c] | 0.4 | 1.3 | 1.3 | 1.5 |

Study: Biernacki *et al.* (1989)
Subjects: Severe airflow obstruction, undergoing cardiac catheterisation

| CT: EMI number (lowest 5% of pixels) | −480 to 460 | −459 to 440 |
|---|---|---|
| **TLco/V$_A$** | | |
| Traditional units[a] | 1.5 | 2.9 |
| SI units[d] | 0.5 | 0.95 |

[a] Traditional units: ml·min⁻¹ mmHg⁻¹·l⁻¹.
[b] SI units: mmol·min⁻¹·kPa⁻¹·l⁻¹
[c] This correlated closely with the ratio of surface area of alveolar wall/alveolar volume.
[d] Calculated from % normal results assuming a normal value of 4.4 (1.5). (Recalculated: detailed results of Goddard *et al.* given by Nicholson, 1980.)

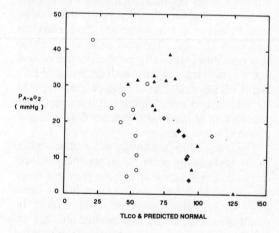

Fig. 6.1. Pathways to respiratory failure. The relationship between TLco, expressed as percentage predicted normal, and alveolar arterial Po$_2$ difference at rest. Data on 29 subjects from Nicholson (1980). Open circles, patients with more than 50% of CT lung fields affected by visible changes of emphysema; triangles, patients with chronic airflow obstruction and less than 50% disruption; diamonds, patients with bronchial asthma. There appear to be two populations, the patients with macroscopic emphysema having a much lower TLco in relation to the disturbance of oxygen exchange than patients in whom small airways disease is presumed to be the predominant disorder. In the latter, there is a strong correlation between the gas transfer deficit and the degree of resting hypoxaemia.

Table 6.3. *Mechanical stress imposed by breathing at high lung volume (from the graphical analysis by Pride, 1990)*

| Problem | Normal subject | Emphysema/ hyperinflation | Explanation |
|---|---|---|---|
| FRC increased | 50% TLC | 80% predicted TLC | Airway closure |
| TLC increased | 100% predicted | 115% predicted | Loss of elastic recoil |
| Chest wall in unfavourable position | Recoils outwards at TLC aiding inspiration | Recoils inwards at FRC, inhibiting inspiration | |
| Pressure swings needed to overcome airway resistance are increased | 2 cm $H_2O$ | 5 cm $H_2O$ | Airway narrowing |
| Total pressure swings during tidal inspiration, overcoming both resistance and elasticity $P_{tidal}$ are increased | 5 cm $H_2O$ | 20 cm $H_2O$ | Increased work to overcome chest wall recoil at high volumes |
| Highest negative pressure that can be generated at at FRC ($P_I$max) is reduced | $-100$ cm $H_2O$ | $-50$ cm $H_2O$ | Reduced efficiency due to shortening of respiratory muscles at high volume |
| Percentage of maximum inspiratory pressure reserve used during tidal breathing at rest is near fatigue level | 5% | 40% | $P_{tidal}/P_I$max |

See also Chapter 2. Exercise makes matters worse, because slow expiration makes it necessary to inspire forcefully to shorten the time taken to breathe in.

result, TLco and TLco/$V_A$ are reduced, by half in severe cases. When the disease is localised to the distal parts of the lung, TLco/$V_A$ may remain normal. Dead space is greatly increased, sometimes as high as 0.5 litre with $V_D/V_T$ ratios often exceeding 50%. The alveolar–arterial Po$_2$ difference is usually less than 20 mmHg (3 kPa). Oxygen desaturation at rest is a feature of very severe disease (Fig. 6.1).

The attenuation of the pulmonary capillary bed results in considerable reduction in the time spent by the red cell in contact with alveolar gas, when cardiac output is normal. Arterial desaturation is found during exercise in patients with emphysema when TLco is below 60% of predicted values (Owens *et al.*, 1984; Owens, Sciurba & Rogers, 1988).

Intrapulmonary gas mixing is abnormal however it is measured. Single breath tests show a steep upslope of the nitrogen plateau after a breath of oxygen or foreign gas. Wash-in and wash-out curves of inert gases reveal slow intrapulmonary gas exchange even at an early stage of the disease. This may be apparent during the measurement of lung volumes by helium dilution, when the time taken for equilibration may be much increased. In some instances quite large volumes of lung appear to be only slowly accessible to inspired gas.

These pathophysiological mechanisms cause the derangements which occur regularly in patients with advanced pulmonary emphysema: increased compliance, high resting lung volume, poor intrapulmonary gas mixing, reduced CO transfer and low expiratory flow rates with low FEV$_1$/VC ratio. However, the way in which individual patients

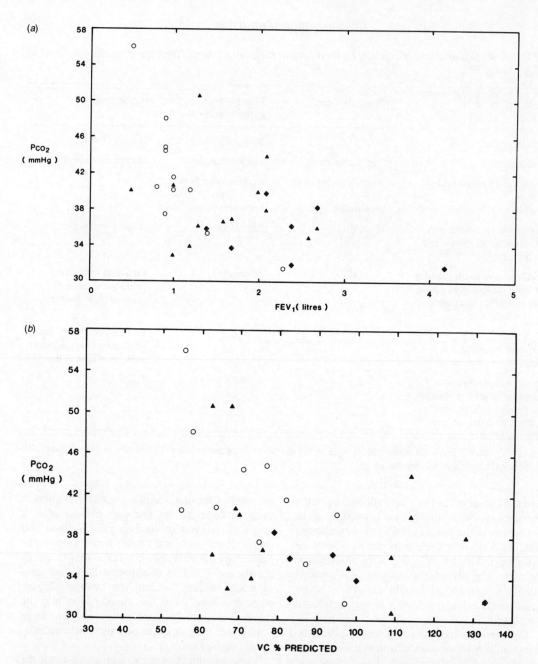

Fig. 6.2. (*a*) Relationship between FEV$_1$ and Pco$_2$ in the same series of patients, who had CT scans performed on the same day. The patients with extensive emphysema in general had the lowest values of FEV$_1$. (*b*) Relationship between arterial Pco$_2$ and vital capacity (VC) expressed as a percentage of predicted normal. Same patients and symbols as Fig. 6.1. Patients with well-preserved vital capacities tend to have normal or low values of Pco$_2$. Pco$_2$ shows a tendency to rise when vital capac-

ity falls below 75% of predicted normal, and the subjects with emphysema are distributed evenly throughout the diagram. VC appears to be the best predictor of the gas exchange disturbance in patients with chronic airflow obstruction, regardless of the amount of emphysema or hyperinflation present. Patients with severe hyperinflation have relatively low values of FEV$_1$ in relation to the severity of gas exchange disturbance, for the mechanical reasons given in the text.

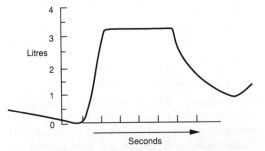

Fig. 6.3. Spirometer trace. Forced inspiration followed by forced expiration in a patient with moderate emphysema. $FEV_1 = 1.6$ litres, $FIV_1 = 3.2$ litres.

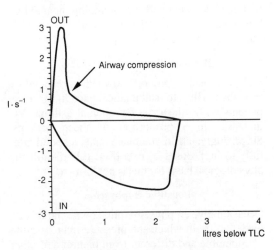

Fig. 6.4. This is similar to Fig. 6.3, but expressed as a flow–volume loop. Maximal expiratory flow rate = 3 $l \cdot s^{-1}$ (180 $l \cdot min^{-1}$), maximal expiratory flow at 50% VC = 0.56 $l \cdot s^{-1}$ (34 $l \cdot min^{-1}$), maximal inspiratory flow = 2.4 $l \cdot s^{-1}$ (144 $l \cdot min^{-1}$). $MEF_{50}/MEF = 0.2$ (normally 0.4–0.6).

breathe and the relationship of symptoms to disturbance of pulmonary function is very variable, because the disease is not uniform and there may be large volumes of more or less normal lung. Emphysema affects these in several ways:

1. By increasing the resting thoracic volume: this makes inspiration more difficult (Table 6.3).
2. By stealing air from normal lung during inspiration because emphysematous lung is easier to expand than normal lung. Because of its poor gas exchanging surface, emphysematous lung acts as dead space
3. In moderate disease there is alveolar hyperventilation (Fig. 6.2). This may partly be the result of the effect of hypoxaemia on the peripheral chemoreceptors. In some instances the reduction of $PCO_2$ is considerable, even when arterial $PO_2$ is above the level usually found to cause hyperventilation in normal subjects (about 65 mmHg, 9 kPa). The effect is to increase the ventilatory demand, which is already increased even at rest because of the increased work of breathing and the increased dead space. Resting ventilation is often increased to about 13 l/min (data from Johnson et al., 1983).
4. Because of expiratory airflow obstruction. When emphysema is uncomplicated by bronchial disease, expiratory obstruction to airflow is caused by abnormal collapsibility of the airways which are normally embedded among neighbouring alveoli and dependent on them for support (Chapter 2). This increases the time

needed for expiration and therefore reduces inspiratory time, especially in exercise.

The rate and depth of breathing depend on the patency of the small airways and the inspiratory reserve. Some patients with large VC breathe at a slow rate with a large tidal volume, while others are forced into a rapid shallow pattern.

Expiratory flow rates are reduced throughout forced expiration. Flow rates are particularly reduced at low lung volumes. Sometimes the expiratory spirogram shows rapid initial downslope followed by a rapid deceleration to a constantly obstructed slow expiration. This is attributed to collapse of the trachea or main bronchi during forced expiration (Campbell, 1967); weakening of these structures may be part of the disease (Healey, Wilson & Fairshter, 1984). Forced inspiratory flow rates are reduced but less than expiratory flow rates. The normal pattern of inspiratory flow is preserved (Figs. 6.3, 6.4).

The increased compliance of the emphysematous lung might be expected to make inspiration easier. In fact, the total effect is unfavourable, because work has to be done to overcome the recoil of the thoracic cage. Some idea of the problem may be obtained by breathing near TLC, breathing in through the nose and out through pursed lips, with a tidal volume of about 1 litre.

### Bronchodilator responsiveness

$FEV_1$ and peak expiratory flow (PEF) respond by less than 10% to salbutamol except in those patients with a history of bronchial asthma. VC increases in a proportion of these patients. Surprisingly, effort tolerance may respond usefully to high doses of nebulised salbutamol: the physiological basis for this is not known.

### Localised emphysema

Occasionally, emphysema presents as large distended cysts in which the pressure may be quite considerable and different from pleural and other local intrapulmonary pressures. Such cysts are often, but not always inaccessible to measurable quantities of inspired gas during tidal breathing. They are demonstrable by CT of the thorax (Morgan & Strickland, 1984). They may occupy considerable volumes within the thorax and increase the true FRC and thoracic gas volume. If helium or inert gases are used to measure lung volumes, the gas may fail to enter the cyst during the period of the test and the lung volumes are grossly underestimated. There is usually good correlation between measurements of lung volume in a body plethysomograph and those obtained by applying formulae to postero-anterior and lateral chest radiographs taken in full inspiration (Chapter 2). When large and tending to expand, emphysematous cysts are readily diagnosed on serial X-rays. Improvement is unpredictable (Gaensler *et al.*, 1983) and likely to follow resection or decompression if:

1. There is evidence of compression of normal lung or on X-ray or CT.
2. TLco is reduced only in proportion to the vital capacity or $TLco/V_A$ is not less than $3 \ ml \cdot min^{-1} \cdot mmHg^{-1} \cdot l^{-1}$ (1 mmol.min$^{-1}$.kPa$^{-1}$.l$^{-1}$).
3. The static compliance curve is normal.
4. CT suggests that the lesions are localised.

When these conditions are not met, the patient is probably suffering from generalised emphysema and can benefit only fractionally from removal of a segment of lung. This has the effect-

ing of reducing FRC and may be accompanied by some symptomatic relief, but this is usually short-lived and of no great benefit. The indications for surgery in the treatment of emphysema are not yet agreed.

### Alpha₁-antiprotease

Homozygous alpha₁-antiprotease deficiency, readily determined by enzymatic assay or by electrophoresis of the alpha₁-globulin fraction of the plasma proteins, accounts for a proportion of patients with emphysema (Hutchinson, 1990). The disease is almost always basal in the early stages and usually accompanied by low flat diaphragms. Defective CO transfer is an early manifestation. Some patients have bronchiectasis. Reduction of ventilation and perfusion at both bases in patients with emphysema points strongly to antiprotease deficiency, as the common types of smoking-related emphysema are found predominantly in the upper parts of each lobe (Thurlbeck, 1976).

## Chronic bronchitis (chronic mucus hypersecretion and small airways obstruction)

The clinical hallmark of chronic bronchitis is chronic mucus hypersecretion: the tendency to expectorate sputum from the bronchi on most days, at least in the winter months. When this symptom occurs, there is usually an increase in the thickness of the mucous glands in the bronchial wall. Respiratory infections frequently involve the chest and chronic infection of the normally sterile lower respiratory tract may occur. Dyspnoea on exertion occurs later, accompanied by signs of chronic airways obstruction. The chest alters in shape, in a manner somewhat similar to that seen in chronic asthma and emphysema. Chest expansion is reduced, occurs mainly in the upper half of the chest and is altered such that the chest appears to move up and down in one piece with little lateral movement of the ribs. The ribs, which normally slope downwards and forwards, are held horizontally. The lower chest may paradoxically move inwards, instead of outwards, with inspiration. Similarly the larynx and soft tissues of the neck are sucked inwards during inspiration, a sign of increased resistive mode of breathing which is not always present when emphysema is the predominant disturbance. The breath sounds are harsh and may be audible from a distance. There may be wheezing, especially during episodes of chest infection and when mucus obstructs the airways. At other times there is prolongation of the normal expiratory sounds.

### Epidemiology

These conditions are predominantly caused by smoking. At least 90% of Western patients smoke cigarettes and almost all the remainder suffer from asthma or bronchial hyperactivity or may have had respiratory disease in childhood (Samet, Tager & Speizer, 1983), leaving about 1% in whom the cause is unknown. The pathology of airflow limitation lies in the small airways.

Urban dwelling and dust exposure interact with cigarette smoking to increase the incidence of respiratory symptoms. The epidemiology of airways obstruction should change now that the levels of smoke are reduced and replaced by photochemical pollution. Domestic pollution, mainly from open cooking and heating sources, probably contributes to airflow obstruction in developing countries, where the respiratory health of women may be as bad as among men (Lalloo, 1992).

In 1955 approximately 40% of British men over 40 years of age expectorated sputum daily in the winter, the incidence in women being lower. About a quarter of these developed infective complications or respiratory failure. The incidence is now much lower and the death rate attributed to 'chronic bronchitis' or chronic obstructive pulmonary disease has halved in the United Kingdom (Royal College of Physicians, 1983).

It would be helpful to be able to predict which smokers are likely to develop the symptomatic disease; clearly not all do. Serial measurements of PEF and $FEV_1$ show a more rapid decline with age in a population of smokers than in non-smokers (Fletcher & Peto, 1977; Fletcher et al., 1976). However, this is probably due to the inclusion among the smokers of a sub-group of patients entering a phase in which they develop respiratory failure with a rapid decline of ventilatory function; the remainder are indistinguishable from normal (Fig. 6.5). Mucus hypersecretion by itself has no effect on mortality (Peto et al., 1983).

Simple measurements of PEF and $FEV_1$ made in contrasting populations have helped to identify factors which cause or contribute to the development of bronchial disease. However, major symptoms do not develop until there is considerable alteration of these tests to values below the normal range. To some extent, this may be explained by a gradual reduction of expectation of working capacity with age. Most patients with symptomatic bronchitis present after the age of 50 (Burrows et al., 1964; Jones, Burrows & Fletcher, 1967), expectation of life being reduced to an average of 65. Many young smokers who give up smoking notice immediate improvement of physical working capacity which may be related more to alterations of cardiac and muscle metabolism with reduction of blood and tissue CO levels than to changes of pulmonary function. Chronic bronchitis does not appear to cause any noticeable alteration in the breathing pattern or in respiratory sensations until airflow obstruction is moderately advanced, so the first symptom is that of breathlessness on exertion appropriate to the magnitude of the functional disturbance. The patients do not hyperventilate, but complain of dyspnoea when their maximal breathing capacity is too low to ventilate the functioning lung and the dead space (Chapter 1).

Epidemiological studies have demonstrated that populations at risk have values of PEF and $FEV_1$ which are lower than optimal but within the normal range. These tests are therefore not a very sensitive way of detecting disease in the presymptomatic stage. Physiologists have turned their attention to the development of a number of tests which purport to detect the early change attributable to smoking and associated with simple chronic bronchitis (Buist, 1984; Wright et al., 1984; Roberts et al., 1990). The most useful are:

1. Forced expiratory flow at low lung volume (Chapter 2) and the ratio $FEV_1/VC$.
2. Single breath nitrogen index (Chapter 4).

Closing volume (Chapter 4) and frequency dependence of dynamic compliance (Chapter 2) have been employed, but are less useful in practice.

These studies suggest that the earliest manifestations of bronchial obstruction affect small air-

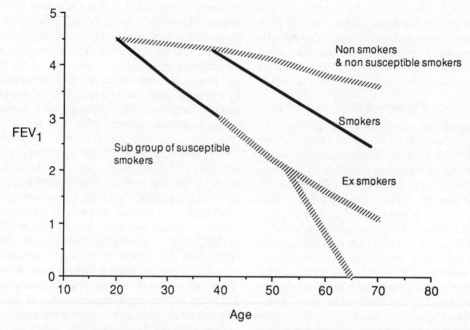

Fig. 6.5. Previous cross-sectional studies suggested that there was an accelerated decline of airway function among smokers. It is now evident that this is caused by the rapid decline of lung function among a small proportion of susceptible individuals, who develop symptomatic dyspnoea on modest exertion at around 50 years of age and develop respiratory failure at about 60. Cessation of smoking appears, in some instances, to be able to halt the decline. $FEV_1$ in healthy smokers is within normal range. (Adapted from Fletcher & Peto, 1977.)

ways. There is post-mortem evidence that young smokers show changes in alveolar macrophage structure and have respiratory bronchiolitis (Niewohner, Kleinerman & Rice, 1974; Niewohner, Knoke & Kleinerman, 1977).

The present view is that disease of small airways is the precursor of symptomatic bronchitis and that in its early stages this is a reversible process characterised by inflammation. Subsequently, there is obliteration of some air passages (Biskin et al., 1990). The alveoli distal to these do not necessarily collapse, because of collateral ventilation. Collateral drift of air may occur through pores in the alveolar walls or through channels connecting bronchioles (Menkes & Macklem, 1986).

Small airways disease is patchy (Niewohner, Kleinerman & Knoke, 1972) and predominantly basal. Radioactive gas inhaled rapidly is distributed mainly to the upper zones in patients with established chronic bronchitis. In slow inspiration it is distributed more uniformly, from which it is concluded that the bronchial obstruction is more severe at the base of the lung because obstructed airways offer more impedance to regional ventilation at high than at low inspiratory rates (Hughes et al., 1972).

It is not known whether centriacinar emphysema is responsible for some of the physiological changes.

### Functional changes associated with obstructive bronchitis

The functional disturbances of bronchial obstruction which correlate with the severity of the disease are:

1. Reduced maximal expiratory and inspiratory flow rates, especially at low lung volumes.
2. Reduced vital capacity and increased residual

volume, with, usually, preservation of a normal TLC.

3. An increase in ventilation–perfusion mismatching, proportional to the reduction of vital capacity, with widening of the alveolar–arterial $P_{O_2}$ difference and slow ventilation of a proportion of the lung volume. The latter accounts for some reduction of CO uptake with preservation of a relatively normal $T_{LCO}/V_A$ (Fig. 6.1).

4. A rise of $P_{CO_2}$ in a substantial proportion of patients whose $FEV_1$ is below 1.0 litre or VC below 70% predicted (Fig. 6.2).

5. Reduction of effort tolerance, in proportion to vital capacity and $FEV_1$ (Chapter 12).

## Ventilation–perfusion relationships in chronic airflow obstruction

Hypoxaemia in chronic airflow obstruction is caused by the presence of poorly ventilated regions of lung. These constitute the major abnormality in patients with 'Type B' disease, in contrast to 'Type A' or emphysematous subjects (Wagner et al., 1977) (see p. 73). A wide range of abnormalities is present in subjects with the intermediate type of airflow obstruction (Ringsted et al., 1989). These have mainly dead space abnormalities with increased numbers of alveoli with high ventilation–perfusion $(\dot{V}/\dot{Q})$ ratios. The effects of drugs and exercise on arterial $P_{O_2}$ and $S_{O_2}$ depend on cardiac output as well as on the distribution of blood flow and ventilation. Bronchodilators generally worsen $\dot{V}/\dot{Q}$ relationships, because although they improve the regional distribution of ventilation in responsive individuals they also dilate the pulmonary arteries, thus reducing the ability of the pulmonary circulation to regulate $\dot{V}/\dot{Q}$ relationships locally within the lung (Ringsted et al., 1989). Exercise improves $\dot{V}/\dot{Q}$ in mildly affected patients (Barbera et al., 1991). Patients with 'Type A' disease desaturate in exercise; oxygen therapy during exercise improves the ability to perform steady exercise but has little effect walking speed and none on maximal exercise performance (Swinburn, Wakefield & Jones, 1985).

### Exercise tolerance in chronic airflow obstruction

Patients with chronic airflow obstruction find exercise difficult because of dyspnoea. This is usually described as some form of difficulty with breathing in or out.

There is a crude relationship between maximum exercise ventilation and simple tests of ventilatory function (Chapter 1). Dillard, Piantadosi & Rajagopal (1985) gave

$$\text{Maximal exercise ventilation} = 28 \times FEV_1 + 18 \qquad (6.1)$$

The prediction could be improved by taking maximal inspiratory flow (MIF in litres per minute) into account; this is to be expected because at extremes of exertion the respiratory muscles are close to fatigue when breathing is hampered (Rochester et al., 1979; also Chapter 2).

$$\text{Maximal exercise ventilation} = 21 \times FEV_1 + (MIF/10) \qquad (6.2)$$

There is very little that can be done to improve maximum ventilation in patients with non-responsive chronic airflow obstruction. Retraining can achieve a little, but maximal exercise ventilation is by and large determined by mechanical factors.

Loss of ability to perform sprints, or to recover from them, is a common complaint at the onset of a slowly progressive disabling condition. Once the disability has been accepted and is established, the patient will judge its severity by the extent to which daily activity has become difficult. This is best measured by endurance at a fixed exercise load or by measuring the distance walked at a self-selected speed over a set time. These relationships are considered further in later chapters. Most papers examine only some aspects of the relationship between disability, symptoms and pulmonary function in patients with chronic airflow obstruction. Most conclude that mechanical factors at best account for only about 50% of the prediction of submaximal exercise capacity and ascribe the remainder to differences in the perception of respiratory discomfort and to psychological factors. Undoubtedly there are individuals who have inappropriate dyspnoea or who walk more slowly than would be expected from the degree of airflow obstruction for psychological reasons or because of prolonged inactivity (McGavin et al., 1978; Morgan et al., 1983; Pearce et al., 1985). Many will on detailed investigation be found to have other problems. Previous experience of bronchial asthma (unpublished data), reduction of vital capacity or an unexpected degree of hypoxaemia occasionally add to the difficulty. Supplemental oxygen may relieve dyspnoea in hypoxaemic patients (Swinburn *et al.*, 1991) and perhaps in patients with very little hypoxaemia by reducing ventilatory drive (reviewed by Bates, 1989b). Detailed assessment may reveal other conditions such as aortic stenosis, pulmonary embolism or metabolic acidosis.

### Chronic carbon dioxide retention

The current view is that patients become acclimatised to abnormal blood gases, particularly elevation of arterial $P_{CO_2}$, because the ventilation required to maintain normal levels is excessive and likely to lead to fatigue (Bégin & Grassino, 1991). The important factors are increased $V_D/V_T$, the pressure needed to initiate flow, the pressure during inspiration as a proportion of the patient's maximum and the total lung resistance (or $FEV_1$). Respiratory weakness and impairment of mechanics and gas exchange are therefore the major determinants of chronic $CO_2$ retention. The alternative view, favoured between 1955 and 1980 but first put forward much earlier, was that $CO_2$ retention was caused by impaired ventilatory responsiveness to elevation of arterial $P_{CO_2}$. This was expressed most elegantly by Robin & O'Neill (1983), who noted that some patients could voluntarily reduce arterial $P_{CO_2}$ over short periods and called them 'non-fighters'. It might be better to consider these groups as 'winners and losers'. Bégin & Grassino described the hypercapnic patients as 'wise fighters' who weigh their options and choose hypoventilation rather than respiratory muscle fatigue. Most other studies can be analysed in these terms, although the authors sometimes come to different conclusions (see also Lourenco & Miranda, 1968; Sorli *et al.*, 1978; Bellemare & Grassino, 1983; Johnson *et al.*, 1983; Light *et al.*, 1989; Rochester, 1991).

### Steroid responsiveness in chronic airflow obstruction

In a small proportion of patients presenting with chronic airflow obstruction symptoms can be improved dramatically by corticosteroids, with major increases in $FEV_1$ and VC. The best predictors of steroid responsiveness are:

1. A history of rapid deterioration within the last year.
2. Previous bronchial asthma.

Those with obvious emphysema are unlikely to respond (Weir *et al.*, 1991). Bronchial hyperreactivity and bronchodilator responsiveness (Chapter 7) are features of the non-emphysematous type of chronic airflow obstruction, and IgE levels are also higher among these patients. It remains uncertain whether these are the consequences of smoking but they probably constitute a separate risk factor for the development of chronic airflow obstruction. A previous history of asthma identifies a group of patients with a better prognosis than those with the emphysematous type of airflow obstruction (Burrows *et al.*, 1987), although there are conflicting results (Kanner, 1984).

## Secondary effects of chronic airflow obstruction

### Polycythaemia

Increased production of erythrocytes with a high red blood cell (RBC) mass is a physiological response to chronic arterial hypoxaemia. This is well known in high altitude dwellers. The correlation between resting arterial $P_{O_2}$ and $S_{O_2}$ and RBC mass is not close, mainly because $P_{O_2}$ varies widely throughout the day; there may be sleep apnoea and there is considerable individual variation in the magnitude of the response. Plots of $P_{O_2}$ and RBC mass are different for altitude dwellers and for patients with chronic airway obstruction (Shaw & Simpson, 1961; Weil *et al.*, 1968). In one study, performed in the UK (Hume, 1968), of stable bronchitics not known to be suffering from any other condition, there was fairly good correlation between arterial $P_{O_2}$ and the degree of polycythaemia, the formula being

$$\log_{10} P_{O_2} = 2.165 - 0.0029 \times \text{RBC mass \% normal} \qquad (6.3)$$

Heavy current smokers have a greater degree of polycythaemia than expected because carboxyhaemoglobin stimulates erythropoiesis (Calverley *et al.*, 1982). As a general rule, non-smoking patients in this category whose RBC mass is very much greater than would be expected from these rather modest increases usually turn out to have some other condition such as sleep apnoea syndrome, polycythaemia rubra vera, renal tumour or another cause of erythrocytosis. There may be an interaction of hypoxaemia and liver disease in the production of polycythaemia, which requires further documentation (data from Murray, 1965).

Polycythaemia rubra vera usually causes a minor degree of hypoxaemia but arterial $Po_2$ is rarely less than 70 mmHg (9.3 kPa) in these patients when ventilatory function is normal.

### Haemodynamics in chronic airflow obstruction

About half of all patients dying of chronic lung disease have increased right ventricular wall thickness and some have had episodes of right-sided heart failure. This is caused mainly by hypoxaemia. Low $Po_2$ causes pulmonary arteriolar constriction and pulmonary hypertension. Prolonged vasoconstriction results in muscularisation of the arterioles with intimal thickening. When this occurs, the pulmonary hypertension is irreversible or at best takes several weeks to recede if adequate oxygenation is established. Low arterial $Po_2$ and smoking also cause polycythaemia, which loads the circulation further (Naeye, 1967). The attenuation of the pulmonary vasculature caused by emphysema is responsible for only modest rises of pulmonary arterial pressure (Williams *et al.*, 1984).

There is some evidence that, as chronic airway obstruction develops, the progression of the cardiovascular changes depend on two factors:

1. The ventilatory response of the subject to falling $Po_2$ while the disease is at the stage where hyperventilation can lessen the effects of deteriorating pulmonary gas exchange.
2. The strength of the pulmonary vascular response to hypoxia (Weil *et al.*, 1970), which varies among individuals.

The ventilatory response to hypoxaemia and to elevated $Pco_2$ is certainly blunted in a number of these patients, but whether this is the result of acclimatisation or the cause of 'unnecessarily' profound hypoxaemia is by no means certain.

Several studies have shown a correlation between diminution of chemoreceptor drive and elevation of arterial $Pco_2$ in patients with severe airway obstruction, but a causal effect has not been shown in prospective studies.

Similar mechanisms appear to determine the acclimatisation of humans and other species to altitude, where low ambient $Po_2$ results in hypoxaemia and polycythaemia. At the same altitude, pulmonary arterial pressure may vary from 20 to 60 mmHg without any noticeable difference of effort tolerance. A few individuals develop chronic mountain sickness with right heart failure for which the only cure is to live at sea level.

### Cor pulmonale

Cor pulmonale is the name given to right ventricular hypertrophy secondary to pulmonary vascular disease, but excepting those conditions where the lung disease itself is secondary to congenital heart disease or left heart disorders (World Health Organization, 1963). The diagnosis of cor pulmonale in life is likely to become easier as techniques of radionuclide and magnetic resonance cardiac imaging improve and are validated. The use of echocardiography has been limited by the inability of the sound waves to penetrate the hyperinflated lung in front of the heart. ECG changes specific to right ventricular hypertrophy include S waves in V6 of greater than 5 mm; this change identifies only half of patients with cor pulmonale. Oedema in chronic respiratory failure is rarely caused by impaired right ventricular function, and the use of the term 'cor pulmonale' to define peripheral oedema in exacerbations of chronic lung disease is unsatisfactory (Bardsley & Howard, 1990).

Pulmonary arterial pressure varies very little over time in moderate airflow obstruction (Weitzenblum *et al.*, 1984). Those with normal pulmonary arterial pressures at rest may have mild increase in exercise, presumably because there is some destruction of the vascular bed with limitation on its ability to accommodate large increases in pulmonary blood flow. Cardiac output is normal in these subjects and increases normally. Patients without heart failure but with pulmonary hypertension (usually 20–40 mmHg) also increase their output normally when exercising to within the capability of their lungs, approximating to a normal Starling curve. Left ventricular pressures also rise, for uncertain reasons (Albert *et al.*, 1985). Those with heart failure have mean pulmonary arterial pressures above 40 mmHg and fail to increase their output normally in exercise, which causes a very sharp rise of pulmonary arterial and right atrial pressure. This carries a poor prognosis (Kawakami *et al.*, 1983; Weitzenblum *et al.*, 1984).

### Pulmonary oedema and left heart disease in association with cor pulmonale

Patients admitted with 'exacerbations' of chronic bronchitis often have widespread radiographic lung shadows which resolve rapidly with diuretic therapy and are accompanied by high values of extravascular lung water when this has been measured. There seems little doubt that in many cases the fluid retention can involve the lungs, though there is no definite evidence that this is in any sense secondary to left heart failure. There has been considerable argument as to whether cor pulmonale causes or is accompanied by left ventricular dysfunction. Experiments on excised hearts suggest that moderate reduction of $Po_2$ in the perfusate does not impair myocardial contractility. There is, however, evidence of interdependence of right and left ventricular function, as pulmonary wedge pressures are increased in patients with cor pulmonale in heart failure. There may be a 'reversed Bernheim effect' in operation, with compression of the left ventricle by the dilated right ventricle.

Studies of left ventricular function in patients with chronic airway obstruction are conflicting (Kachel, 1978). The present conclusion is that left ventricular function is normal. The great majority, all but 15% or less, of patients with impaired left ventricular performance have one or other of the diseases which might be expected to produce this result, such as coronary artery disease, alcoholism or hypertension. Many of the patients with chronic bronchitis who have the most severe congestive failure, have concomitant left ventricular disease.

Experience suggests that the combination of left ventricular disease or cardiac arrhythmia with chronic airway obstruction is more disabling than either condition would be separately. The prognosis of combined coronary artery disease and chronic airway obstruction is poor.

The effects of concomitant cardiac disease on gas exchange are uncertain. In one study patients with a higher $Pco_2$ generally had impaired left ventricular function. This could be because the pulmonary disease impairs the left ventricle or because left ventricular disease, combined with chronic bronchitis, is more likely to result in a modest elevation of arterial $Pco_2$ than chronic airflow obstruction alone (Jezek & Schrijen, 1974; Laszlo & Schrijen, 1974). Overt left ventricular hypertrophy can almost always be explained by left ventricular disease (Murphy, Adamson & Hutcheson (1974).

### The coexistence of heart failure and chronic bronchitis

Pulmonary oedema alters the mechanical properties of the lungs by increasing the elastic recoil pressure and reducing alveolar volume. Thus, TLC, FRC and RV fall as does VC. $FEV_1/VC$ ratio increases, PEF may rise or remain unaltered. The breathing pattern becomes more rapid and shallow. Even after treatment, when the radiological changes of oedema have resolved, these changes tend to persist for several weeks presumably because interstitial oedema remains.

Coincident airways obstruction and myocardial dysfunction, from whatever cause, tend to cause dyspnoea on effort which is disproportionate to the apparent severity of either when the heart and lungs are examined and tested separately (Fig. 12.3, p. 181).

The effect on blood gases is not well documented. Acute pulmonary oedema may sometimes cause respiratory failure and severe respiratory acidosis (Avery, Samet & Sackner, 1970). A secondary rise of arterial $Pco_2$ may occur after treatment of acute pulmonary oedema with morphine and oxygen, especially when a diuresis occurs and there is sufficient reduction of the pulmonary shunt to allow full arterial $O_2$ saturation. When this occurs, and indeed when $CO_2$ retention complicates pulmonary oedema at any stage, subsequent investigation usually reveals a degree of chronic obstructive bronchitis which may be quite mild.

## Other types of airway obstruction

### Obliterative bronchiolitis

Certain patients with the physiological stigmata of irreversible small airway obstruction have no emphysema, no history to suggest bronchial asthma and no history of smoking or sputum production. Histological studies of the lungs of such patients have shown obliteration of bronchioles. It is not easy to demonstrate the absence of microscopic tubes in two-dimensional sections of three-dimensional branching airways; much careful examination of normal lung material was needed to establish the expected frequency of bronchioles in lung sections obtained under various conditions. This pathological entity is well known to occur after specific viral infections in childhood and is occasionally found in adults. Chronic airflow obstruction is accompanied by varying degrees of hyperinflation according to whether the process was accompanied by alveolar inflammation or fibrosis. Low arterial $Po_2$ is usually combined with low or normal $Pco_2$, low TLco and normal $TLco/V_A$. Obliterative bronchiolitis has been described as a complication of rheumatoid arthritis and may occur in isolation (Geddes *et al.*, 1977). The physical signs were those of airway obstruction with a mid-inspiratory squeak. Tests of pulmonary function showed:

- Low PEF 85–220 $l\cdot min^{-1}$
- Low $FEV_1$ 0.4–0.7 litre
- FEV/VC ratio 40–55%, one of 60%
- RV over 3 litres, TLC normal
- TLco 3–6 $mmol\cdot min^{-1}\cdot kPa^{-1}$ (reduced)
- $TLco/V_A$ 1.4–1.9 $mmol\cdot min^{-1}\cdot kPa^{-1}\cdot l^{-1}$ (normal)
- Static compliance normal in three subjects
- $Po_2$ variable, 41–90 mmHg (5.5–12 kPa)
- $Pco_2$ normal 40–42 mmHg (5.3–5.6 kPa)

### Obstruction of the larynx, trachea and major bronchi (central airway obstruction)

Obstruction of large airways is occasionally misdiagnosed as asthma or bronchitis, because it may present with wheezing and dyspnoea. The characteristic harsh, stridulous sound heard over an obstructed trachea or larynx should be recognised quite easily. A single repeated wheeze to one or other side of the mid-line in the front of the chest alerts the physician to the possibility of a lesion obstructing a main bronchus, usually a carcinoma, but often laryngeal paralysis or a stricture, a benign tumour or foreign body. Such wheezes are often audible in inflammatory bronchitis or asthma, but the possibility of a tumour may need to be excluded by endoscopy or by contrast radiography. Tumours invading the tracheal wall may alter the inspiratory breath sounds without causing obstruction. Tracheal tumours on a pedicle may vary in their behaviour.

When obstruction is present it may be classified as:

1. Fixed obstruction of extrathoracic airways.
2. Collapsible obstruction of extrathoracic airways.
3. Fixed obstruction of the intrathoracic trachea.
4. Collapsible obstruction of the intrathoracic trachea.

Fixed obstructions affect inspiration and expiration equally. Their effect may be simulated by breathing through a narrow orifice. Expiratory and inspiratory flow are limited by the power of the respiratory muscles to force air through the narrowed orifice. When collapsible, extrathoracic obstructions do so in inspiration, by analogy with collapsible laboratory tubing to which suction is applied. Thus extrathoracic obstructions reduce inspiratory flow rates. The problem is exaggerated by exercise (Albazzaz, Grillo & Kazemi (1975).

Advanced lesions are readily recognised by examination of the spirographic trace or flow–volume loop. Their hallmark is a slow constant inspiration or expiration yielding a curve quite dissimilar from that seen in chronic bronchitis or asthma (Figs. 6.6, 6.7). The normal deceleration due to dynamic compression is seen only at the end of expiration. PEF is reduced more, proportionally, than $FEV_1$.

There is a linear relationship between PEF and $FEV_1$ in chronic airflow obstruction, although it is difficult to predict because of a wide scatter. On average

$$PEF \text{ (litres per minute)} = (150 \times FEV_1 \text{ litres BTPS)} \qquad (6.4)$$

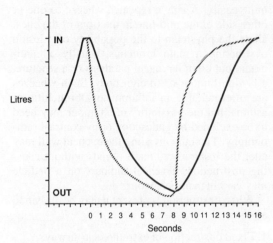

Fig. 6.6. Spirometric trace of forced expiration followed by forced inspiration in a subject with a fixed extrathoracic airway obstruction. $FEV_1 = 1.1$ litres, $EVC = 6.0$ litres, $FIV_1 = 1.0$ litres. The interrupted line shows a normal trace: $FEV_1 = 4.5$ litres, $EVC = 6.1$ litres, $FIV_1 = 4.8$ litres.

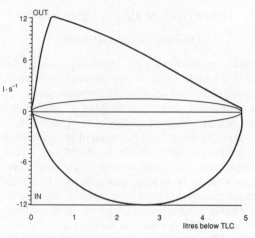

Fig. 6.7. Same as Fig. 6.6, plotted as a flow–volume loop: maximal inspiratory flow = $1.0 \, l \cdot s^{-1}$, maximal expiratory flow = $1.0 \, l \cdot s^{-1}$, maximal expiratory flow at 50% VC = $1.0 \, l \cdot s^{-1}$, $MEF_{50}/MEF = 1.0$. Normal trace: maximal expiratory flow = $12 \, l \cdot s^{-1}$, maximal inspiratory flow = $12 \, l \cdot s^{-1}$, maximal expiratory flow at 50% VC = $5 \, l \cdot s^{-1}$, $MEF_{50}/MEF = 0.4$ (normally 0.4–0.6, cf. Fig. 6.4).

(Lal, Ferguson & Campbell 1964, Vaughan *et al.*, 1989). In a series of 2000 patients (unpublished observations) of whom 1000 had chronic airflow obstruction, the relationship depended on lung volume, those with the lowest total lung capacity having a relatively higher PEF at any given $FEV_1$. The overlap between patients with fibrosing alveolitis and obstructive disorders was too great to allow the relationship to be used as an index of restrictive or obstructive disease. The lower 95% confidence limit for the prediction was close to

$$PEF = 100 \times FEV_1 \text{ litres BTPS} \qquad (6.5)$$

which means that only 5% of patients with diffuse airways obstruction had values of PEF before bronchodilator lower than this. Most of these were asthmatics and the relationship returned towards normal after bronchodilators. Routine investigation of all new patients referred to the lung function laboratory with a ratio of $PEF/FEV_1$ of less than 100 showed that 50% had central airway obstruction.

When more detailed lung function studies are performed, a number of relationships may point towards the need to investigate further:

1. High airways resistance in subjects with fairly normal $FEV_1$ (Shim *et al.*, 1972), improving if helium is breathed.
2. $FIV_1$ less than $FEV_1$ (Clark, 1970).
3. Maximal inspiratory flow rate less than maximal expiratory flow rate at 50% of vital capacity (but this also occurs in patients with stiff lungs and is only true if the obstruction is outside the thorax).
4. Maximal expiratory flow at 50% vital capacity more than 70% of peak expiratory flow.

Unless there is associated lung disease, vital capacity lung volumes and gas transfer are normal. Arterial blood gases are well preserved until the lesion produces a situation akin to strangulation. The limitation of effort tolerance may seem out of proportion to the reduction of ventilatory function, and maximum breathing capacity is reduced. Attempts at exercise, voluntary hyperventilation and forced expiration accentuate the characteristic breath sounds. It is wise to alert technicians who perform tests of ventilation as an unsupervised service to the existence of central obstruction, which is diagnosed as a result of a pulmonary function consultation about once every 4–6 months in an average laboratory serving a general hospital.

### Functional upper airway narrowing

Acute non-organic laryngeal or epiglottic obstruction is a psychiatric disorder which may occur in isolation or complicate bronchial asthma (Cormier, Camus & Desmeules, 1980; Rodenstein, Francis & Stanescu, 1983; Goldman & Muers, 1991). Fibreoptic nasendoscopy demonstrates transient opening of the glottal chink during inspiration. PEF and $FEV_1$ readings mimic central airway obstruction. $Po_2$ and arterial oxygen saturation are usually, but unfortunately not always, normal (Niven & Pickering, 1991). Until the problem is identified, patients are often sedated and ventilated. The underlying psychiatric abnormality is usually profound, and may include features of extreme anxiety, hypochondriasis, hysteria or Münchhausen's syndrome.

The narrow upper airway seen in patients with sleep apnoea syndrome may collapse intermittently during forced expiration, yielding a sawtooth appearance of oscillating airflow on the flow–volume plot (Vincken & Cosio, 1985) which is exaggerated in recumbency.

Spirometers which deliver only numerical results of $FEV_1$ and FVC are not suitable for diagnostic work, because there is a danger that central airway obstruction will be missed.

## References

Albazzaz, F., Grillo, H. & Kazemi, H. (1975). Response to exercise in upper airway obstruction. *American Review of Respiratory Disease*, **111**, 631–640.

Albert, R.K., Muramoto, A., Caldwell, J., Koepsell, T. & Butter, J. (1985). Increases in intrathoracic pressure do not explain the rise in left ventricular and diastolic pressure that occurs during exercise in patients with chronic obstructive pulmonary disease. *American Review of Respiratory Disease*, **132**, 623–627.

Avery, W.G., Samet, P. & Sackner, M.A. (1970). The acidosis of pulmonary oedema. *American Journal of Medicine*, **48**, 320–324.

Barbera, J.A., Roca, J., Ramirez, J., Wagner, P.D., Ussetti, P. & Rodriguez-Roisin, R. (1991). Gas exchange during exercise in mild chronic obstructive pulmonary disease. *American Review of Respiratory Disease*, **144**, 520–525.

Bardsley, P.A. & Howard, P. (1990). Respiratory failure. In *Respiratory Medicine*, ed. R.A.L. Brewis, G.J. Gibson & D.M. Geddes, pp. 534–536. London: Baillière Tindall.

Bates, D.V. (1989a). Exercise limitation. In *Respiratory Function in Disease*, 3rd edn, pp. 197–201. Philadelphia: Saunders.

Bates, D.V. (1989b). Severe chronic airflow limitation. In *Respiratory Function in Disease*, 3rd edn, p. 213. Philadelphia: Saunders.

Bégin, P. & Grassino, A (1991). Inspiratory muscle dysfunction and chronic hypercapnia in chronic obstructive pulmonary disease. *American Review of Respiratory Disease*, **143**, 905–912.

Bellemare, F. & Grassino, A. (1983). Force reserve of the diaphragm in patients with chronic obstructive pulmonary disease. *Journal of Applied Physiology*, **55**, 8–15.

Bergin, C, Müller, N., Nichols, D.M., Lillington, G., Hogg, J.C. Mullen, B., Grymaloski, M.R., Osborne, S. & Paré, P.D. (1986). The diagnosis of emphysema: a computed tomographic-pathologic correlation. *American Review of Respiratory Disease*, **133**, 541–546.

Biernacki, W., Gould, G.A., Whyte, K.A. & Flenley, D.C. (1989). Pulmonary haemodynamics, gas exchange and the severity of emphysema as assessed by quantitative CT scan in chronic bronchitis and emphysema. *American Review of Respiratory Disease*, **139**, 1509–1515.

Biskin, C.H., Wiggs, B.R., Paré, P.D. & Hogg, J.C. (1990). Small airway dimensions in smokers with obstruction to airflow. *American Review of Respiratory Disease*, **142**, 563–570.

Buist, A.S. (1984). Current status of small airway disease. *Chest*, **86**, 100–105.

Burrows, B., Bloom, J.W., Traver, G.A. & Cline, M.G. (1987). The course and prognosis of different forms of chronic airways obstruction in a sample from the general population. *New England Journal of Medicine*, **317**, 1309–1314.

Burrows, B., Fletcher, C.M., Heard, B.E., Jones, N.L. & Wootliff, J.S. (1966). The emphysematous and bronchial types of chronic airways obstruction: a clinico-pathological study of patients in London and Chicago. *Lancet,* **i**, 830–835.

Burrows, B., Niden, A.H., Fletcher, C.M. & Jones, N.L. (1964). Clinical types of chronic obstructive lung disease in London and Chicago: a study of one hundred patients. *American Review of Respiratory Disease*, **90**, 14–27.

Calverley, P.M.A., Leggett, R.J., McElderry, L. & Flenley, D.C. (1982). Cigarette smoking and secondary polycythaemia in hypoxic cor pulmonale. *American Review of Respiratory Disease*, **125**, 535–539.

Campbell, A.H. (1967). Definition and cause of the tracheobronchial collapse syndrome. *British Journal of Diseases of the Chest*, **61**, 1–11.

Clark, T.J.H. (1970). Upper airway obstruction. *British Medical Journal*, **iii**, 628–684.

Colebatch, H.J.H., Finucane, K.E. & Smith, M.M. (1973). Pulmonary conductance and elastic recoil relationships in asthma and emphysema. *Journal of Applied Physiology*, **34**, 143–153.

Cormier, Y.F., Camus, P. & Desmeules, M. (1980). Non-organic acute upper airway obstruction. *American Review of Respiratory Disease*, **121**, 147–155.

Dillard, T.A., Piantadosi, S. & Rajagopal, K.R. (1985). Prediction of ventilation at maximal exercise in chronic air flow obstruction. *American Review of Respiratory Disease*, **132**, 230–235.

Dornhorst, A.C. (1955). Respiratory insufficiency. *Lancet*, **i**, 1185–1187.

Empey, D.W. (1972). Assessment of upper airway obstruction. *British Medical Journal*, **iii**, 503–505.

Ferris, B.G. (1978). Epidemiology standardisation project. *American Review of Respiratory Disease*, **118** (Suppl.), 1–52.

Finucane, K.E. & Colebatch, H.J.H. (1969). Elastic behaviour of the lung in patients with airway obstruction. *Journal of Applied Physiology*, **26**, 330–338.

Fletcher, C.M., Peto, R., Tinker, C.M. & Speizer, F.E. (1976). *The Natural History of Chronic Bronchitis and Asthma: An Eight Year Study of Early Chronic Obstructive Lung Disease in Working Men in London*. Oxford: Oxford University Press.

Fletcher, C.M. & Peto, R. (1977). The natural history of chronic airflow obstruction. *British Medical Journal*, **i**, 1645–1648.

Gaensler, E.A., Angell, D.W., Knudson, R.J. & Fitzgerald, M.X. (1983). Surgical management of emphysema. *Clinics in Chest Medicine*, **4**, 443.

Geddes, D.M., Corrin, B., Brewerton, D.A., Davies, R.J. & Turner-Warwick, M. (1977). Progressive airway obliteration in adults and its association with rheumatoid disease. *Quarterly Journal of Medicine*, **46**, 427–444.

Gibson, G.J., Pride, M.B., Davis, J & Schroter, R.C. (1979). Exponential description of the static pressure-volume curve of normal and diseased lungs. *American Review of Respiratory Disease*, **120**, 799–811.

Goddard, P.R., Nicholson, E.M., Laszlo, G. & Watt, I. (1982). Computed tomography in pulmonary emphysema. *Clinical Radiology*, **33**, 379–387.

Goldman, J. & Muers, M. (1991). Vocal cord dysfunction and wheezing. *Thorax*, **46**, 401–404.

Gould, G.A., MacNee, W., McLean, A., Warren, P.M., Redpath, A., Best, J.J.K., Lamb, D. & Flenley, D.C. (1988). CT measurements of lung density in life can quantitate distal airspace enlargement – an essential defining feature of human emphysema. *American Review of Respiratory Disease*, **137**, 380–392.

Gugger, M., Gould, G., Sudlow, M.F., Wraith, P.K. & MacNee, W. (1991). Extent of pulmonary emphysema in man and its relation to the loss of elastic recoil. *Clinical Science*, **80**, 353–358.

Healey, F., Wilson, A.F. & Fairshter, R.D. (1984). Physiologic correlates of airway collapse in chronic airflow obstruction. *Chest*, **85**, 476–487.

Hughes, J.M.B., Grant, B.J.B., Greene, R.E., Iliff, L. & Milic-Emili, J. (1972). Inspiratory flow rate and ventilation distribution in normal subjects and patients with simple chronic bronchitis. *Clinical Science*, **43**, 583–595.

Hume, R. (1968). Blood volume changes in chronic bronchitis and emphysema. *British Journal of Haematology*, **15**, 131–139.

Hutchinson, D.C.S. (1990). Proteases and antiproteases. In *Respiratory Medicine*, ed. R.A.L. Brewis, G.J. Gibson & D.M. Geddes, pp. 485–496. London: Baillière Tindall.

Jezek, V. & Schrijen, F. (1973). Left ventricular function in chronic obstructive pulmonary disease with and without cardiac failure. *Clinical Science and Molecular Medicine*, **45**, 267–279.

Johnson, M.A., Woodcock, A.A., Rehan, M. & Geddes, D.M. (1983). Are 'pink puffers' more breathless than 'blue bloaters'? *British Medical Journal*, **286**, 179–182.

Jones, N.L., Burrows, B. & Fletcher, C.M. (1967). Serial studies of 100 patients with chronic airways obstruction in London and Chicago. *Thorax*, **22**, 327–335.

Kachel, R.G. (1978). Left ventricular function in chronic obstructive pulmonary disease. *Chest*, **74**, 286–290.

Kanner, R.G. (1984). Relationship between airways responsiveness and chronic airflow limitation. *Chest*, **86**, 54–57.

Kawakami, Y., Kishi, F., Yamamoto, H. & Miyamoto, K. (1983). Relation of oxygen delivery, mixed venous oxygenation and pulmonary hemodynamics to prognosis in chronic obstruction pulmonary disease. *New England Journal of Medicine*, **308**, 1045–1049.

Lal, S., Ferguson, A.D. & Campbell, E.J.M. (1964). Forced expiratory time: a simple test for airways obstruction. *British Medical Journal*, **i**, 814–817.

Lalloo, U.G. (1992). Respiratory health survey in an Indian South African community. Thesis submitted for M.D., University of Natal, Durban, South Africa.

Laszlo G. & Schrijen, F. (1974). Left ventricular function in chronic obstructive pulmonary disease with and without cardiac failure. *Clinical Science and Molecular Medicine*, **46**, 281–282 (letters).

Laws, J.W. & Heard, B.E. (1992). Emphysema and the chest film; a retrospective radiological pathological study. *British Journal of Radiology*, **419**, 750–761.

Leaver, D.G., Tattersfield, A.E. & Pride, N.B. (1973). Contributions of loss of lung recoil and enhanced airways collapsibility to the airflow obstruction of chronic bronchitis and emphysema. *Journal of Clinical Investigation*, **52**, 2117–2128.

Light, R.W., Mahutte, C.K. & Brown, S. (1989). Etiology of carbon dioxide retention at rest and during exercise in chronic airflow obstruction. *Chest*, **94**, 61–67.

Lourenço, R.V. & Miranda, J.M. (1968). Drive and performance of the ventilatory apparatus in chronic obstructive lung disease. *New England Journal of Medicine*, **279**, 53–59.

McGavin, C.R., Artvinli, M., Naoe, H. & McHardy, G.J.R. (1978). Dyspnoea disability and distance walked: a comparison of estimates of exercise performance in respiratory disease. *British Medical Journal*, **ii**, 241–243.

Medical Research Council (1965). Definition and classification of chronic bronchitis for clinical and epidemiological purposes. *Lancet*, **i**, 775–779.

Menkes, H.A. & Macklem, P.T. (1986). Collateral flow. In *Handbook of Physiology*, section 3, vol. 1, ed. P.T. Macklem & J. Head, pp. 337–353. Bethesda: APS.

Miller, R.D. & Hyatt, R.E. (1973). Evaluation of obstructing lesions of the trachea and larynx and flow volume curves. *American Review of Respiratory Disease*, **108**, 475–481.

Morgan, A.D., Peck, D.F., Buchanan, D.R. & McHardy, G.J.R. (1983). Effects of attitudes and beliefs on exercise tolerance in chronic bronchitis. *British Medical Journal*, **286**, 171–173.

Morgan, M.D.L. & Strickland, B. (1984). Computed tomography in the assessment of bullous lung disease. *British Journal of Diseases of the Chest*, **78**, 10–25.

Müller, N.L., Staples, C.A., Miller, R.R. & Abboud, R.T. (1988). Density mask: an objective method to quantitate emphysema using computed tomography. *Chest*, **94**, 782–787.

Murphy, M.L., Adamson, J. & Hutcheson, F. (1974). Left ventricular hypertrophy in patients with chronic bronchitis and emphysema. *Annals of Internal Medicine*, **81**, 307–313.

Murray, J.F. (1965). Arterial studies in primary and secondary polycythaemic disorders. *American Review of Respiratory Disease*, **92**, 435–449.

Naeye, R.L. (1967). Polycythaemia and hypoxia. *American Journal of Pathology*, **50**, 1027–1033.

Nicholson, E.M. (1980). The diagnosis of pulmonary emphysema in life. Thesis for M.D., University of Bristol.

Niewohner, D.E., Kleinerman, J. & Knoke, J.D. (1972). Regional chronic bronchitis. *American Review of Respiratory Disease*, **105**, 586–593.

Niewohner, D.E., Kleinerman, J. & Rice, D.B. (1974). Pathologic changes in the peripheral airways of young cigarette smokers. *New England Journal of Medicine*, **291**, 755–758.

Niewohner, D.E., Knoke, J.D. & Kleinerman, J. (1977). Peripheral airways as a determinant of ventilatory function in the human lung. *Journal of Clinical Investigation*, **60**, 139–151.

Niven, R. McL. & Pickering, C.A.C. (1991). Vocal cord dysfunction and wheezing. *Thorax*, **46**, 688.

Owens, G.R., Rogers, R.M., Pennock, B. & Levin, D. (1984). The diffusing capacity as a predictor of arterial oxygen saturation during exercise in patients with chronic obstructive pulmonary disease. *New England Journal of Medicine*, **310**, 1218–1221.

Owens, G.R., Sciurba, F.C. & Rogers, R.M. (1988). $D_{L}CO$ in COPD. *Chest*, **94**, 897.

Paré, P.D., Brookes, L.A., Bates, J., Lawson, K.M., Nelems, J.M.B., Wright, J.L. & Hogg, J.C. (1983). Exponential analysis of the lung pressure volume curve as a predictor of pulmonary emphysema. *American Review of Respiratory Disease*, **126**, 54–61.

Pearce, S.J., Posner, V., Robinson, A.J., Barton, J.R. & Cotes, J.E. (1985). 'Invalidity' due to chronic bronchitis and emphysema: how real is it? *Thorax*, **40**, 828–71.

Peto, R., Speizer, F.E., Cochrane, A.L., Moore, F., Fletcher, C.M., Tinker, C.M., Higgins, I.T.T., Gray, R.G., Richards, S.M., Gilliland, J. & Norman-Smith, B. (1983). The relevance of airflow obstruction but not mucus hypersecretion to mortality from chronic lung disease. *American Review of Respiratory Disease*, **188**, 491–500.

Phelan, P.D. (1987). Does adult chronic obstructive lung disease really begin in childhood? *British Journal of Diseases of the Chest*, **78**, 1–9.

Pride, N.B. (1990). Chronic obstructive pulmonary disease: pathophysiology. In *Respiratory Medicine*, ed.

R.A.L. Brewis, G.J. Gibson & D.M. Geddes, p. 516. London: Baillière Tindall.

Ringsted, C.V., Eliasen, K.V., Andersen, J.B., Heslet, L. & Qvist, J. (1989). Ventilation–perfusion distributions and central haemodynamics in chronic obstructive pulmonary disease. Effects of terbutaline administration. *Chest*, **96**, 976–983.

Roberts, C.M., Rawbone, R.G., Adams, L. & Seed, W.A. (1990). Sensitivity and specificity of small airway tests in subjects with normal conventional lung function tests. *Clinical Science*, **78**, 29P.

Robin, E.D. & O'Neill, R.P. (1983). The fighter versus the non-fighter. Control of ventilation in chronic lung disease. *Archives of Environmental Health*, **72**, 125–127.

Rochester, D.F. (1991). Respiratory muscle weakness. Pattern of breathing and $CO_2$ retention in chronic obstructive pulmonary disease. *American Review of Respiratory Medicine*, **143**, 901–903.

Rochester, D.F., Arora, N.S., Braun, N.M.T. & Goldberg, S.K. (1979). The respiratory muscles in chronic obstructive pulmonary disease (COPD). *Bulletin Européen Physiopathologie Respiratoire*, **15**, 821–837.

Rodenstein, D.O., Francis, C. & Stanescu, D.C. (1983). Emotional laryngeal wheezing: a new syndrome. *American Review of Respiratory Disease*, **127**, 354–356.

Royal College of Physicians (1983). *Health or Smoking*. London: Pitman.

Sakai, F., Gamsu, G., Im, J-G. & Ray, C.S. (1987). Pulmonary function abnormalities in patients with CT-determined emphysema. *Journal of Computer Assisted Tomography*, **11**, 963–968.

Samet, J.M., Tager, I.R.A., Speizer, F.E. (1983). The relationship between respiratory illness in childhood and chronic airflow obstruction in adulthood. *American Review of Respiratory Disease*, **127**, 508–523.

Shaw, D.B. & Simpson, T. (1961). Polycythaemia in emphysema. *Quarterly Journal of Medicine*, New Series, **30**, 135.

Shim, C., Corro, P., Park, S.S. & Williams, M.H. (1972). Pulmonary function studies in patients with upper airways obstruction. *American Review of Respiratory Disease*, **106**, 233–238.

Silvers, G.W., Petty, T.L. & Stubbs, S.E. (1980). Elastic recoil changes in early emphysema. *Thorax*, **35**, 490–495.

Simpson, T. (1968). Chronic bronchitis and emphysema with special reference to prognosis. *British Journal of Diseases of the Chest*, **62**, 57–69.

Sorli, J., Grassino, A., Lorang, G. & Milic-Emili, J. (1978). Control of breathing in patients with chronic obstructive lung disease. *Clinical Science and Molecular Medicine*, **54**, 295–304.

Swinburn, C.R., Mould, H., Stone, T.N., Corris, P.A. & Gibson, G.J. (1991). Symptomatic benefit of supplemental oxygen in hypoxaemic patients with chronic obstructive pulmonary disease. *American Review of Respiratory Disease*, **143**, 913–915.

Swinburn, C.R., Wakefield, J.M. & Jones, P.W. (1985). Performance, ventilation and oxygen consumption in three different types of exercise test in patients with chronic obstructive lung disease. *Thorax*, **40**, 581–586.

Thurlbeck, W.M. (1976). *Chronic Airflow Obstruction in Lung Disease*. Philadelphia: Saunders.

Thurlbeck, W.M. (1979). Post mortem lung volumes. *Thorax*, **34**, 735–739.

Vaughan, T.R., Weber, R.W., Tipton, W.R. & Nelson, H.S. (1989). Comparison of PEF and $FEV_1$ in patients with varying degrees of airway obstruction. *Chest*, **95**, 558–562.

Vincken, W. & Cosio, M.G. (1985). Flow oscillations on the flow volume loop. A non-specific indicator of upper airway dysfunction. *Bulletin Européen Physiopathologie Respiratoire*, **21**, 559–567.

Wagner, P.D., Dantzker, D.R., Duek, R., Clausen, J.L. & West, J.B. (1977). Ventilation–perfusion inequality in chronic obstructive pulmonary disease. *Journal of Clinical Investigation*, **59**, 203–211.

Weil, J.V., Byrne Quinn, E., Sodal, I.E., Friesen, W.O., Underhill, B., Filley, G.F., Grover, R.F. (1970). Hypoxic ventilatory drive in normal man. *Journal of Clinical Investigation*, **49**, 1061–1071.

Weil, J.V., Jamieson, G., Brown, D.W., Grover, G.F., Balchum, O.J. & Murray, J.F. (1968). Red cell mass–arterial $O_2$ relationship in normal man. *Journal of Clinical Investigation*, **47**, 1627–1639.

Weir, D.C., Gove, R.I., Robertson, A.S. & Burge, P.S. (1991). Response to corticosteroids in chronic airflow obstruction: relationship to emphysema and airways collapse. *European Respiratory Journal*, **4**, 1185–1190.

Weitzenblum, E., Sautegeau, A., Ehrhart, M., Nammosser, M., Hirth, C. & Roegel, E. (1984). Long term course of pulmonary arterial pressure in chronic obstructive pulmonary disease. *American Review of Respiratory Disease*, **130**, 993–998.

Williams, I.P., Boyd, M.J., Humberstone, A.M., Wilson, A.G. & Millard, F.J.C. (1984). Pulmonary arterial hypertension and emphysema. *British Journal of Diseases of the Chest*, **78**, 211–216.

World Health Organization (1963). Chronic cor pulmonale. Report of an expert committee. *Circulation*, **27**, 594.

Wright, J.L., Lawson, L.M., Paré, P.D., Wiggs, B. & Hogg, J.C. (1984). The detection of small airways disease. *American Review of Respiratory Disease*, **129**, 989–994.

# 7 Bronchial asthma

## Clinical background

Bronchial asthma is a familial, inflammatory disorder of the bronchi which causes wheezing and recurrent difficulty with breathing. Variability of bronchial calibre leads to airway obstruction. This varies spontaneously or with treatment, at least in the early stages of the condition. Large and small airways may be affected.

Many individuals with bronchial asthma have genetically determined elevated serum IgE levels and some suffer intermittently from various types of rhinitis and eczema (Tollerud *et al.*, 1991).

The condition may present with chest tightness, shortness of breath, wheezing or coughing. There are different patterns of variability as some subjects deteriorate slowly while others are subject to abrupt changes in their condition (Turner-Warwick, 1977). Individuals with bronchial asthma are affected at various times in one or more of four ways:

1. Exacerbations. These are chest illnesses lasting a few days or weeks after respiratory infections or heavy exposure to allergens. Coughing may be a major feature. Response to bronchodilators may be absent, or lost.
2. Continuous variable asthma, with (*a*) diurnal variation of airway calibre with nocturnal deterioration; (*b*) exercise-induced asthma; (*c*) asthma triggered by hyperventilation.
3. Acute attacks provoked by individual trigger factors which may include infection, domestic and environmental allergens, sensitisers, pollutants, industrial sensitisers and pharmacological triggers such as aspirin. Climatic changes affect the liberation and the physical characteristics of airborne allergens, pollutants and infectious particles. Emotional changes are mediated through hyperventilation, exercise and probably by vagal efferent fibres in the airways. Acute attacks may be short-lived and respond to treatment or they may progress to become severe, sometimes leading to unconsciousness. They usually, but not invariably, occur in patients who are in a phase of moderate chronic airflow obstruction.
4. Some patients progress over the years to a condition of irreversible airflow obstruction, with loss of variability. They present with shortness of breath on exertion.

A number of pathological processes are responsible for the symptoms and the airflow obstruction. In some measure they affect all the airways in all types of attack and may be detected in remission.

*Rapidly reversible*: bronchial smooth muscle contraction; mucosal oedema.
*Slowly reversible*: increased respiratory secretions, sometimes forming plugs, in small airways; shedding of the mucosal cells and inflammation, often with eosinophil, neutrophil and activated T cell invasion of the bronchiolar walls.
*Irreversible*: (presumed) obliteration of small airways.

The role of immunological mechanisms in the pathogenesis of airway narrowing is not discussed further (Moreno, Hogg & Paré, 1986; Barnes & Holgate, 1990).

93

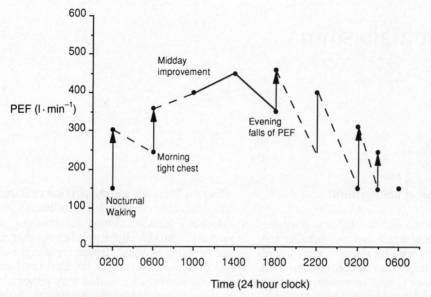

Fig. 7.1. Variation of peak expiratory flow rate (PEF) in an individual with poorly controlled asthma who has access to a bronchodilator inhaler. Unless exercise is taken, the condition improves at midday, but morning and evening symptoms are common and nocturnal waking is the rule if the episodes of bronchoconstriction are sufficiently severe to cause arousal. Diurnal variation occurs in the absence of treatment. This example indicates very poor control, because symptom relief is sought (by the use of a bronchodilator) 6 times in one 24-hour period. Sleep is disrupted, and the lowest values of PEF are associated with significant blood gas disturbances and leave little margin for further deterioration.

## Physiological disturbances in bronchial asthma

### Airflow obstruction

The tests which measure or indicate increased airways resistance are:

1. Direct measurement of airway resistance (Raw) or specific conductance (SGaw).
2. Peak expiratory flow rate (PEF).
3. Maximum expiratory flow rate at lung volumes below TLC.
4. $FEV_1$, when it is an abnormally low fraction of the total lung capacity.

Remembering that all these tests may be abnormal for other reasons, any one of them may be used to measure variations in the severity of bronchial asthma when this is the only condition present causing airflow obstruction. Measurements of inspiratory flow are also affected and variable. Large numbers of simple measurements, generally $FEV_1$ and PEF, have been used to explore the pattern of variability in individual asthmatics. More detailed tests help to identify other causes of airflow obstruction, and detect minor abnormalities which persist in remission (Cade & Pain, 1973).

### Variability

Many of the responses of asthmatic airways are exaggerations of the normal variability of bronchial calibre.

#### Diurnal variation of peak flow

Fig. 7.1 shows the most characteristic pattern of diurnal variation of PEF. The readings may dip sharply in the night or early in the morning. They tend to be highest between 10 o'clock in the morning and 12 noon, with a slight fall towards the end of the working day and frequent further fall during relaxation in the evening. All these oscillations, even morning dips, may be interrupted by bronchodilator drugs taken prophylactically or in response to symptoms. When asthma deteriorates, bronchodilator responsiveness tends to be lost. The nocturnal symptoms are related to sleep; their timing and severity may change rapidly in shift workers and travellers. Sleeping upright does not alter the pattern (Connolly, 1979; Hetzel & Clark, 1979, 1980; Hetzel, 1981).

### Portable peak flow meters and home readings

The use of peak flow readings in the home has made assessment of the variability of bronchial asthma very much easier. The use of diary cards in conjunction with home peak flow readings became standard practice both for testing new drugs and for assessing the response of individual patients to steroids and cromoglycate. Diary cards of many kinds are in use. Some suffer from lack of proper evaluation of the questions asked: these usually relate to nocturnal waking, coughing, effort limitation and number of doses of prescribed agents taken. More elaborate questionnaires regarding quality of life are available for clinical trials (Juniper et al., 1992).

It is not always useful to give a patient a diary card when first trying a new treatment. There are two pitfalls which must be avoided in interpretation of subjective and objective measurements made by the patient at home. Firstly, trends of peak flow readings may themselves influence the diary entries (Higgs et al., 1986). Secondly, patients who have not performed the tests under supervision may at times forget the importance of full inspiration when performing peak flow measurements at home with the result that the readings may be unreliable during the first few days. Home observations are more reliable when performed by experienced patients.

### Antigen challenge

Measurements of $FEV_1$, PEF or airways resistance may be performed after the inhalation of sensitisers or extracts of them (Newman Taylor & Davies, 1982).

Measurements made after antigen challenges in a relatively small number of volunteers have contributed largely to our knowledge of the mechanisms of all forms of bronchial asthma: particu-

larly by highlighting the prolonged multiphasic inflammatory response that follows exposure of a susceptible individual to a single agent. Apart from research applications, clinicians are likely to refer patients to laboratories specialising in antigen challenges when they need to establish which of a number of possible sensitisers is responsible for a series of episodes of bronchoconstriction. In practice this is necessary most frequently in the detection of work-related asthma.

Hypersensitivity reactions in the bronchi occur in three phases (Fig. 7.2). Each of these is self-limiting if it is mild:

1. Immediate, occurring 10–60 minutes after challenge.
2. Late, starting about 4 hours after the challenge and lasting 24–48 hours
3. A prolonged period during which the bronchi are abnormally sensitive to all constricting stimuli (an account of this follows). Diurnal variation may also increase in severity.

Until fairly recently it was thought that different basic immunological mechanisms were responsible for these phases. It is now accepted that a single initiating event can liberate a cascade of inflammatory mediators invoking several parts of the immune system which vary in their speed of onset and their duration (Barnes & Holgate, 1990).

It follows that antigen challenge cannot be undertaken lightly. The reactions which follow may be prolonged, may require treatment at any time for several days after the procedure and are occasionally severe. They cannot safely be performed during clinical asthma: baseline $FEV_1$ has to be better than 90% of predicted at the start of the challenge and the pattern of diurnal variation during the preceding days known to avoid confounding errors.

### Work-related asthma

Reactions to industrial sensitisers may be studied in the workplace. Frequent readings of peak flow provide the most graphic illustration of the events, if the individual can be relied on to produce accurate readings (Fig. 7.3) (Brooks, 1982; Perrin et al., 1992). The measurements should be requested by the clinician as soon as the condition

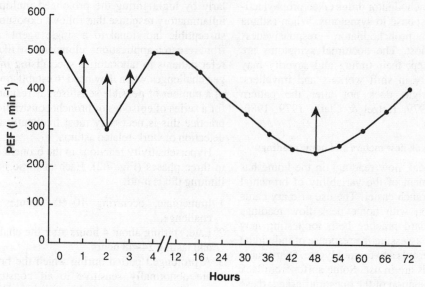

Fig. 7.2. PEF readings from an asthmatic exposed for a short time to an allergen. The immediate reaction can be reversed or prevented by the use of bronchodilator drugs (arrows). Many, but not all individuals show a late response, of longer duration. This has more profound effects on airway inflammation and is poorly reversible. Allergen challenges are followed by a prolonged period of increased sensitivity and reactivity of the airways, with worsening of nocturnal and exercise-induced asthma.

is suspected, if possible before treatment. Industrial medical officers are generally thwarted in their attempts to establish a diagnosis accurately, by treatment and by subtle changes in working practice which may mask but not solve the problem (Henneberger *et al.*, 1992; Rosenman 1992). Frequent spot checks of $FEV_1$ are usual in potentially hazardous environments. The occa-

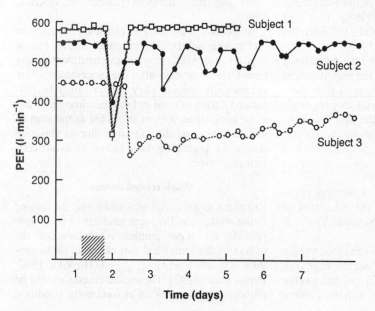

Fig. 7.3. Home reading of PEF by three sensitised subjects exposed on one occasion to toluene di-isocyanate (hatched column) at work. Subject 1 showed an immediate hypersensitivity reaction but recovered quickly. Subject 2 also reacted immediately but experienced a dual reaction and the symptoms of asthma persisted for several days. Subject 3 experienced only late symptoms, 8 to 12 hours after exposure. The diagnosis of work-related asthma presenting in this way is often delayed. When there is doubt about the reliability of the readings, repeated supervised tests of ventilatory function are necessary.

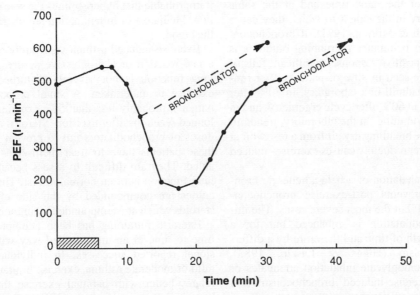

Fig. 7.4. Asthma provoked by 6 minutes of intensive exercise, sufficient to raise the pulse rate to 160 beats per minute. PEF rises after 6 minutes of exercise. After 5 minutes' rest it begins to fall. This occurs more rapidly in children. In the most severely affected, bronchoconstriction occurs during exercise. The episode wears off spontaneously in 45–60 minutes and may be terminated by a dose of beta-adrenergic bronchodilator, after which further exercise can usually be taken without any recurrence (see text).

sional measurement of $FEV_1$ before the first shift, after a break, at the end of the shift and before reporting for work the next day will identify many incipient problems.

Challenge tests are indicated (Newman Taylor, 1986):

1. Where the pattern of respiratory disease is new or unusual.

2. In previously unrecognised situations.

3. When multiple agents are involved.
They may be performed occasionally:

4. When reactions at the workplace are so severe that small doses are needed to establish the cause of the bronchoconstriction.

5. When the cause of the asthma remains in doubt and there are strong reasons for investigating possible precipitating factors.

## Bronchoconstriction induced by exercise or hyperventilation at constant $P_{CO_2}$

Fig. 7.4 shows the results of a typical exercise test. Peak flow rises after 5 or 6 minutes of running at a sufficient speed to elevate the pulse rate to the permitted maximum (170 beats per minute in young adults, see Chapter 13) (Eggleston & Guerrant, 1978). Peak flow then falls, usually within 5 minutes. Observations are continued for 20 minutes before the test is considered negative. If bronchoconstriction is not severe and the attack is not terminated with a bronchodilator, it usually begins to improve 20 minutes after the end of exercise. In the next hour or two, further exercise causes little or no bronchoconstriction and the response remains diminished for up to 4 hours (Silverman & Anderson, 1972; Anderson et al., 1975; Edmunds, Tooley & Godfrey, 1978).

There is less information about the effects of more prolonged running. Bronchoconstriction occurs during exercise, but some asthmatics can run through their bronchoconstriction and warming up can help (Ruff et al., 1989).

Exercise-induced asthma is influenced by the state of the airways and often improves when the patient is in remission. It is enhanced by cold air which may itself induce asthma (Strauss et al., 1978). Different forms of exercise, even when performed for the same time and at the same intensity, vary in the extent to which they cause asthma (Fitch & Morton, 1971). If bronchoconstriction after 6 minutes of running outdoors is defined as a positive response, significant falls of peak flow are seen in 90% of patients after running on a treadmill in a laboratory, in 70% after horse riding, in 60% after cycle ergometry, and in 40% after swimming. In the laboratory, treadmill running while breathing dry air from a reservoir at a fixed load reproducibly causes exercise-induced asthma.

A single inhalation of a beta-adrenergic bronchodilator prevents post-exercise bronchoconstriction in all but the most severe cases. The initial bronchodilatation is enhanced but for a different length of time and therefore by a different mechanism (Higgs & Laszlo, 1983). Disodium cromoglycate inhalation attenuates or abolishes exercise-induced bronchoconstriction in the majority of patients, in some cases after a single dose. Forty milligrams is sufficient to prevent symptoms from developing in about 50% of adults with exercise-induced asthma. The proportion may be higher in children even when the standard dose of 20 mg is given. Corticosteroids in single doses do not prevent exercise-induced asthma, but regular treatment may induce a sufficient degree of remission to abolish or reduce the response (Hartley, Charles & Seaton, 1977; Henriksen & Dahl, 1983). Other bronchodilator drugs (alpha-adrenergic blockers, vagal inhibitors, calcium channel antagonists, antihistamines, frusemide) may reduce but do not consistently prevent bronchoconstriction in exercise (table 1 in Anderson, 1988). Oral bronchodilators, taken regularly or as a single dose, appear to have no effect (Smith *et al.*, 1990; Anderson *et al.*, 1976).

The mechanisms of exercise-induced asthma (and the mode of action of the pharmacological agents which inhibit it) are still being debated. Hypotheses include cooling followed by hyperaemia of the bronchial circulation (McFadden, 1990) and drying of the airways accompanied by changes of osmolality (Anderson, 1988; Anderson & Smith, 1989). There is some evidence for all of these, although the development of asthma during severe cold air challenges makes it improbable that hyperaemia is the sole explanation. Mediators of inflammation are liberated into the blood.

Exercise-induced asthma very rarely results in a late reaction or a progressive severe attack if lung function is not severely disturbed before exercise is undertaken. A small proportion of patients, probably less than 5%, experience prolonged reactions after exertion. Steroids and high doses of bronchodilators fail to prevent this and these patients have to treat themselves as disabled. They are difficult to assess because their lung function is often normal at rest. Their difficulties are compounded by the side effects of steroids which are compounded by immobility.

Exercise retraining has been attempted from time to time in an uncontrolled way with occasional reported successes. In individuals with mild or moderate asthma, exercise limitation correlates better with habitual exercise than with bronchial hyperreactivity or $FEV_1$ (Garfinkel *et al.*, 1992).

The magnitude of exercise-induced changes of airway calibre have been expressed in several ways. The most reliable exercise lability index is

$$\frac{\text{Highest PEF - lowest PEF}}{\text{Initial PEF}} \times 100 \ (\%)$$

$$(7.1)$$

The exercise–bronchodilator lability index may also be calculated. The test is then conducted as usual, but after the trough of PEF has been reached or the test terminated by the clinical need for a bronchodilator, salbutamol is administered and a further 1 minute period of exercise taken at 5 minutes. After a further 5 minutes, lung function is measured again. Normal individuals vary by less than 10%, the change being mainly exercise-induced bronchodilatation.

Subjects who have had hay fever with wheezing may have responses which are intermediate (Deal *et al.*, 1980). Liability of 20% or more is diagnostic of bronchial asthma.

### Repeated forced expiration

Repeated prolonged forced expiratory efforts may provoke asthma, which is why repeat PEF measurements are safer than those of FVC and to a

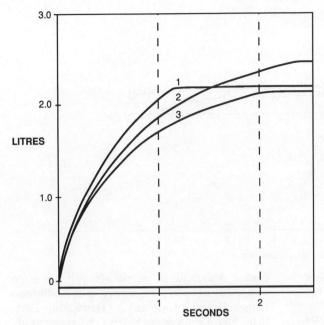

Fig. 7.5. Bronchoconstriction caused by repeated expiratory efforts. Tests showing this phenomenon have to be terminated. It rarely occurs after bronchodilators.

lesser extent $FEV_1$. This effect is blocked by bronchodilators (Fig. 7.5).

### Asthma and respiratory heat exchange

The bronchoconstriction caused by exercise is exaggerated by cold air (Heaton, Henderson & Costello, 1984). Voluntary hyperventilation with cold air at normal $P_{CO_2}$ also induces bronchoconstriction (Deal *et al.*, 1979a, b). This observation led to a number of experiments which suggested that the heat loss required to cause a similar degree of bronchoconstriction was the same in both tests. Voluntary hyperventilation does not cause an initial bronchodilatation, presumably because this is a result of adrenaline circulating as a response to exercise. Bronchoconstriction caused by cold air is prevented by premedication with salbutamol and cromoglycate in the same subjects, but rather variably by other agents. The pattern of refractoriness is also rather different. Observations of this type suggest that the mechanism of bronchoconstriction is not identical in the two procedures.

The cold air test is nevertheless a useful procedure in the investigation of bronchial lability especially for elderly subjects who cannot easily exercise. A full dose–response to respiration heat exchange is cumbersome and expensive to set up, requiring complex gas mixing equipment. The procedure has been simplified and it is known that transient bronchoconstriction can reliably be achieved using a dry gas containing 4.8% $CO_2$, provided that about 80% of MVV can be sustained (Philips *et al.*, 1985).

### Response to physiological and pharmacological bronchoconstrictor and bronchodilator agents: 'non-specific airway reactivity'

Histamine and methacholine are bronchoconstrictors in all individuals. In normal subjects the response is limited and reaches a plateau. In patients with bronchial asthma, the effect is greatly exaggerated (Woolcock, Salome & Yan, 1984). Dose–response curves to one or other of these agents, employing standard methods, have been studied extensively to obtain a measurement of 'bronchial reactivity'. The subject inhales aerosols of either agent in increasing concentrations. Inhalations from a dosimeter device are theoretically ideal for dose–response studies (Chai *et al.*, 1975), but adequate results have been obtained simply by inhaling increasing concentrations of the agent by deep inspiration or tidal breathing from a mouthpiece from a standard nebuliser (Ryan *et al.*, 1981; Yan, Salome &

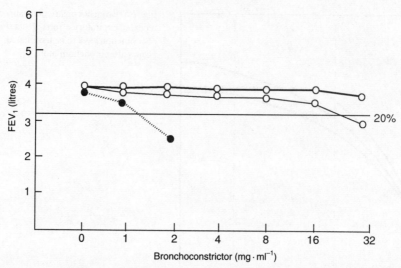

Fig. 7.6. Bronchoconstrictor effect of the inhalation of increasing (doubling) concentrations of histamine or methacholine. Open symbols, normal subjects. In one, the test was terminated without an endpoint. In the second, $FEV_1$ fell by more than 20% after the inhalation of 32 mg/ml. $PC_{20}$, the provocation concentration causing a 20% fall of the measured variable, is calculated by interpolation as a measure of bronchial sensitivity. Bronchial reactivity is, strictly, the slope of the descending portion of the dose–response curve. (The term reactivity is used generically to describe the response of airways to bronchoconstrictor challenges in general.) Filled symbols, asthma. Reactivity is enhanced. $PC_{20}$ is reduced.

Woolcock, 1983; Sterk *et al.*, 1993; Britton, Mortagy & Tattersfield, 1986).

Bronchoconstriction is usually measured by $FEV_1$. Bronchial sensitivity is usually defined by the provocation dose which causes a 20% fall of $FEV_1$ ($PD_{20}$) or the concentration which provokes a 20% fall of $FEV_1$ ($PC_{20}$) (Fig. 7.6). These measurements have become standard, in preference to reactivity which is the slope of the descending portion of the dose–response curve (Orehek *et al.*, 1976; Malo *et al.*, 1985). Reactivity may be more discriminatory in epidemiological studies (Abramson, Saunders & Hensley, 1990). A 20% bronchoconstrictor response to the inhalation of histamine or methacholine in low concentration ($\leqslant$ 8mg/ml) identifies almost all current asthmatics. About 5% of individuals with few or no symptoms have hyperreactivity in the asthmatic range (Hargreave, Ryan & Thompson, 1981; Schachter, Doyle & Beck, 1984; Sekizawa *et al.*, 1986; Pattemore *et al.*, 1990; Trigg *et al.*, 1990; Zhong, 1990). Although there is a crude relationship between the severity of asthma and $PD_{20}$, it can vary without any major change in the background asthma (Josephs *et al.*, 1987). Changes in non-specific reactivity may partly be responsible for worsening of asthma after episodes which provoke bronchoconstriction. This has led some researchers to equate hyperreactivity with background airway inflammation. There is probably more than one mechanism involved. Airways resistance is more sensitive if measured by forced oscillation or body plethysmography using increasing doses of bronchoconstrictor sufficient to achieve a 35–40% fall, but there is some overlap between normal subjects and asthmatics. When changes of reactivity in individuals are to be measured as part of a physiological study (for example, the effects of infection on the airways), this is not a problem and the more sensitive tests may save time, drugs and discomfort.

There is little to choose between histamine and methacholine. Histamine is more stable and therefore more convenient but methacholine causes less itching and discomfort. Both agents provoke alterations of $Po_2$, lung volumes and the other manifestations of asthma described later.

### Osmotic challenge

Changes in the osmolarity of the extracellular fluid in the airway induce asthma (Cheney & Butler, 1968). Two types of osmotic challenge have been studied.

1. Hypertonic saline nebulised in an ultrasonic chamber to a particle size of about 5 micrometres (Anderson & Smith, 1989). Exposure is increased in steps from 30 seconds up to 8 minutes, with a 90 second interval between exposures. In normal subjects, $FEV_1$ falls by less than 17%. A fall of 20% or greater is therefore a sensitive indicator of bronchial asthma. The response is inhibited by anti-asthmatic medication, including, in the short term, bronchodilators.

   The bronchoconstrictor effect of hypertonic saline aerosols constitutes a major hazard to scuba divers and this form of challenge may well become a standard part of the medical examination for this occupation. Hypertonic saline challenge shows promise as a laboratory test for asthma when it is not demonstrable by other means, but more standardisation is required because particle size and volume are critical and changes in the configuration of the delivery circuit can alter the results.

2. Distilled water. This provokes asthma and coughing when delivered as a mist (Allegra & Bianco, 1980). This is not recommended as a laboratory test.

Non-isotonic challenge correlates with other indicators of non-specific hyperreactivity (Anderson & Smith, 1989). It appears to act by causing the release of mediators in the airway and may therefore mimic antigen and exercise challenge but, unlike allergen challenge, there is so far no experience of any long-term increase in reactivity after the test.

### Clinical and epidemiological relevance of bronchial hyperreactivity

Increased non-specific reactivity and sensitivity of the bronchi is considered by some to be the hallmark of asthma. The concept has provided a satisfactory explanation for the similarity between the clinical manifestations of asthma and wheezing with bronchial infections that occur in non-atopic as well as in atopic people. Smoking and other forms of bronchial inflammation have, however, been identified as a major cause of hyperreactivity in otherwise healthy subjects which makes it difficult to determine the incidence of latent asthma among chronic bronchitics by this means (van Schayk et al., 1991).

Non-specific bronchial challenge is widely used as a clinical test in Europe, America and Australia but never found great favour except as a research tool in the UK. Its principal use clinically is to identify asthma or other forms of airway inflammation by means of a single test when resting lung function lies within normal limits at the time of attendance. Objective evidence of hyperreactivity may help to clarify symptoms such as cough or breathlessness during litigation following inhalational accidents. The procedure gives essentially similar information in asthmatics to that obtainable from exercise challenge or from measurements of diurnal variation of PEF made by symptomatic patients at home, although $PD_{20}$ varies considerably from day to day in some instances (Josephs et al., 1987). The fact that non-specific bronchial hyperreactivity is commonly found in a number of inflammatory conditions of the airways impairs its usefulness. Exercise testing is easy in children and distinguishes asthma from other forms of chronic airway disease, whereas $PC_{20}$ to methacholine lies below the normal range in the majority of children with non-asthmatic airway disorders (Godfrey et al., 1991). Although exercise tests and home peak flow readings are more time-consuming, the fact that they seem relevant to the patient or parent is helpful and the problem is better understood.

There is substantial evidence confirming that inhaled steroids reduce bronchial sensitivity in asthmatics (e.g. Koeter et al., 1991). This has led to a widespread acceptance of the role of inflammation, as opposed to bronchoconstriction per se, as the underlying cause of asthma. Current guidelines recommend effective inhaled anti-inflammatory agents in all but the mildest cases of bronchial asthma (British Thoracic Society, 1993).

The conclusion is that the demonstration of hyperreactivity may be diagnostic of asthma in

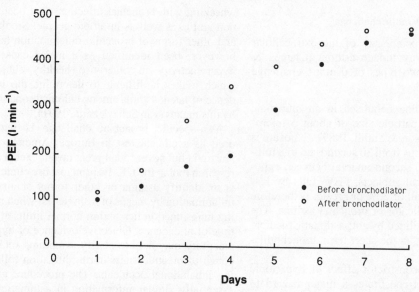

Fig. 7.7. PEF measured at 6 a.m. in a patient recovering from a severe exacerbation of asthma (see text). Filled circles, before nebulised salbutamol; open circles, after nebulised salbutamol.

individuals who have suffered from attacks of breathlessness who are normal at the time of examination, or in groups in which the prevalence of asthma is high. Random challenge testing will generate too many false positive results to make the procedure useful as an epidemiological test for latent asthma (Palmeiro et al., 1992). A negative challenge virtually excludes asthma (Sterk et al., 1993).

### Difficulty of interpreting measurements of reactivity when FEV₁ is low

Provocation tests are difficult to interpret when $FEV_1$ is below normal. The relationship between airway diameter, airway resistance and forced expiratory tests is complex: in a single tube resistance varies with the fourth power of the radius. Therefore, a change of reactivity will not necessarily imply any change of the pharmacological effect of methacholine on the airways.

### Response of airway tests to bronchodilators

The administration of bronchodilators decreases airways resistance by about one half in normal subjects (Higgs, Richardson & Laszlo, 1982).

This can be measured at FRC by body plethysmography or identified by the use of partial flow–volume loops in which the subject breathes in to 60% of TLC and expires forcibly (Zamel, 1984). Peak flow rates and $FEV_1$ increase only marginally in normal subjects (Sourk & Nugent, 1983), because deep inspiration normally causes maximal bronchodilatation for about 15 seconds by the abolition of vagal tone (Nadel & Tierney, 1961). Paradoxically, deep inspiration causes transient bronchoconstriction in many asthmatics (Gayrard et al., 1975; Parhan et al., 1983) which lasts for about 60 seconds and has to be taken into account during challenge studies (Bellegrino et al., 1990).

Bronchodilator response in patients with bronchial asthma depends on the clinical severity of the condition (Fig. 7.7). Patients in complete remission have no capacity for bronchodilatation over the normal range; those with severe, acute or chronic wheezing tend to develop fixed airways obstruction. There may be plugging of the small airways with mucus and inflammatory exudate which clears after a period of time. This may cause obliteration and fibrosis of small airways, in which case it will be irreversible. Some patients show a degree of pharmacological resistance to bronchodilator drugs which may be reversed within a few hours by the use of corticosteroids.

Criteria for reversibility are not generally agreed. Conventionally, improvement of PEF or $FEV_1$ of greater than 20% of the starting value is regarded as unequivocally asthmatic. While this is quite reasonable in the presence of mild or moderate airflow obstruction, it is not useful when $FEV_1$ is below 1.5 litres when the random variation of $FEV_1$ may be as great as 0.3 litre (Sourk & Nugent, 1983). Furthermore, $FEV_1$ may improve consistently by as much as 0.3 litre in non-asthmatic bronchitics. Response of $FEV_1$ to a bronchodilator of more than 0.4 litre or 20%, whichever is greater, indicates a significant asthmatic component to airflow obstruction at all levels of $FEV_1$. In a group of patients with mild or moderate chronic bronchitis without asthma, the mean increase of $FEV_1$ was 6% of the predicted level, or 110% (fig. 4 in Anthonisen et al., 1986). The question is more important for epidemiological studies of hyperreactivity and in the selection of patients for clinical trials than in clinical practice, because the finding of irreversibility or 'fixed airflow obstruction' on a single occasion does not exclude bronchial asthma.

The most commonly used bronchodilators are:

1. Salbutamol (albuterol USA) by pressurised aerosol, 200 micrograms. A 10 minute wait is convenient, but for maximum bronchodilator effect 15 minutes are required.
2. Salbutamol 2.5 mg by nebuliser, 45 minutes.

A greater bronchodilator effect is achieved with nebulisers than with aerosol cans in moderate or severe airflow obstruction. A few laboratories still employ isoprenaline or adrenaline in high doses, and the use of positive pressure machines was commonplace in the USA until fairly recently. The cardiovascular side effects of adrenaline makes this unsuitable for routine administration except in special circumstances, such as prior treatment with a non-cardioselective beta-adrenergic blocking drug. These are poorly reversible to salbutamol in contrast to the bronchoconstriction caused by selective agents (Tattersfield & Harrison, 1983; Dunn et al., 1986).

### Corticosteroid response

Failure to respond to standard bronchodilator drugs in the short or long term does not exclude reversible airflow obstruction. A trial of corticosteroids is usually recommended. Probably all patients with chronic airway obstruction should have such a trial, except perhaps if the history is longer than 5 years, the evidence for emphysema is strong and a history of variable dyspnoea lacking. Most but not all severely obstructed patients, whose lung function subsequently responds to a steroid trial, show a modest improvement after testing with nebulised salbutamol (greater than 0.2 litre and 15%).

Steroid responsiveness may be assessed by means of inhaled corticosteroids in the great majority of patients whose $FEV_1$ is 1.3 litres or more (after salbutamol, if necessary) and in a small proportion whose airway obstruction is more severe than this. For most patients with an $FEV_1$ less than 1.3 litres, however, it is better to prescribe oral prednisolone and to change to an inhaled steroid when the pulmonary function has improved. Prednisolone is often given in a dose of 30 or 40 mg for 2 weeks, but unacceptable side effects are less common if 15 mg is given. This may require up to 6 weeks, but it is wise to repeat the tests after 2 weeks in case a more rapid response occurs, because many patients will discontinue or reduce the dose of steroids. The measurement of peak flow, $FEV_1$ and vital capacity after treatment with steroid is a valuable guide to management of later exacerbations, because it provides a measurement of the patient's best state. Home readings of PEF throughout the day and a record of symptoms such as nocturnal waking and bronchodilator requirement are included in the trial.

After a steroid trial, the drug may be withdrawn gradually over a period which need not be longer than 1–2 weeks. If there is no improvement, this should be recorded prominently.

The failure of a steroid trial in a chronically breathless patient does not preclude a further attempt to improve an acutely deteriorating situation, if there is evidence that an asthmatic element is present or if the deterioration has occurred recently, and other measures such as physiotherapy and antibiotics have failed to restore the clinical state to that noted to be the patient's 'best'. In this situation, the measurements made at the time of the steroid trial provide a target at which to aim in intensive efforts to restore reasonable function.

Patients with steroid-resistant airflow obstruction may obtain relief from high doses of nebulised bronchodilator drugs. Symptomatic benefit has to be judged subjectively and with home peak flow readings which should improve by 15%, because laboratory measurements of $FEV_1$ do not predict clinical response (Goldman, Teale & Muers, 1992; Morrison, Jones & Muers, 1992).

When there is unequivocal improvement of either $FEV_1$, VC or PEF, there is usually an improvement in symptoms of shortness of breath on effort or coughing. Exercise-induced wheezing responds fully to corticosteroids in a proportion of patients; they may still require treatment with beta-adrenergic drugs, but these are usually more effective. The improvement is nearly always present in the baseline as well as the test after bronchodilator: occasionally the steroid drug seems to restore bronchodilator responsiveness but to leave the lowest readings unaltered. When this improvement occurs, the oral steroid may be withdrawn while continuing inhaled steroids.

Some patients with non-asthmatic airflow obstruction respond marginally to corticosteroids (Weir *et al.*, 1990*a*,*b*). In addition, some asthmatics improve symptomatically with very little change of the ventilatory tests in the clinic. There are several possible explanations:

1. Improvement may be caused by a reduction of the diurnal variation of peak flow, particularly the severity of the nocturnal fall, without any change in the readings obtained at the patient's best time of day. This may be resolved by examining home recordings of peak flow and diary card entries recording nocturnal waking. Observations are made while oral steroids are withdrawn: inhaled steroids may be substituted. Any deterioration is usually accompanied by a return of the variability of the readings and fall of the average PEF.
2. There may be an improvement of an acute deterioration of chronic asthma with reduction of lung volumes, notably FRC and RV, but without significant change of PEF and $FEV_1$ (Woolcock & Read, 1965). VC usually improves. This change may be inferred sometimes from a change in the configuration of the chest X-ray and from an obvious reduction of the chest diameter and shape: the shoulders may appear to slope downwards rather than upwards from the neck. This type of steroid response is not common, and therefore it is unusual for the subdivision of lung volumes to be measured. In addition, blood gases sometimes improve rather slowly after an acute attack (Smith, 1981).
3. The patient may experience less coughing and functional hyperventilation because there is less bronchial irritation, in spite of there being little change in the chronic airway obstruction. This situation causes no serious dilemma because the improvement is usually maintained when inhaled steroids are substituted.
4. The patient's outlook on life may improve because of the euphoriant effect of prednisolone, without improving either ventilatory function or effort tolerance. When this occurs, the drug can be reduced very gradually over a period of several weeks, while the keeping a record of peak flow rate at home. In this way, the pharmacological effects of rapid steroid withdrawal may be avoided, while the patient observes that there is no physical deterioration.

## Vital capacity and lung volumes

### Vital capacity and forced vital capacity

VC and FVC vary with clinical state and tend to correlate with arterial $Po_2$. VC varies less than $FEV_1$ and PEF during diurnal and exercise-induced wheezing, but is affected over longer periods by the degree of small airway disease that is present. Thus, during a severe attack, VC may fall so low that $FEV_1/VC$ is higher than when the patient is well (Fig. 2.8). In general, the changes of VC and FVC mirror those of RV.

### Lung volumes

End-expiratory volume ('FRC') and RV are almost always increased during attacks of asthma and may remain so when spirometric indices have returned to normal. The respiratory muscles are not at rest at the end of inspiration (Martin *et al.*, 1980). Lung volumes often return to normal slowly, several days or weeks after a prolonged attack (Woolcock & Read, 1965). Sometimes RV remains increased in remission, while in some patients symptomatic response is delayed until the lung volumes have returned to normal, even though $FEV_1$ and VC are normal.

The lungs appear hyperinflated in full inspiration. Increases of total lung capacity have been described in a number of papers, some using foreign gas methods which can give falsely low results (Woolcock & Read, 1966) (Chapter 2). Body plethysmography has shown similar results in exercise-induced asthma (Freedman, Tattersfield & Pride, 1975). Unfortunately, measurements of lung volumes made by the standard plethysmographic technique of panting against a closed shutter have been shown to overestimate lung volumes in patients with severe airway closure because the oscillations of pressure recorded at the mouth do not reflect changes of alveolar pressure during compression of the thorax (Shore et al., 1983). This problem will probably be overcome in the future by slow panting near TLC. Measurements of lung volumes in patients with chronic airflow obstructions published before 1982 are inaccurate. Blackie et al. (1990) measured radiographic lung volume during acute attacks of spontaneous asthma and found reversible increases of up to 2 litres in the most hyperinflated, but generally the changes were less than had been described.

For the moment it is generally accepted that TLC increases during prolonged episodes of asthma, but short-term changes during exercise are uncertain and probably do not occur during experimentally induced asthma. The mechanism is uncertain, but it is likely to be caused by relaxation of the fibrous tissues of the lungs as a result of stretching (in a manner similar to hair, which can elongate when wet and spring back rapidly). The process can be induced experimentally in animals by inducing chronic hyperinflation with a tracheal valve. Alterations in chest wall compliance may be important. An alternative explanation invokes a change in the surface properties of the lungs, but there is no evidence that this occurs (Cade et al., 1971; Peress, Sybrecht & Macklem, 1976; Holmes, Campbell & Barter, 1978).

Pulmonary fibrosis may reduce TLC and when this is extensive counteracts the hyperinflation. In obese, steroid-treated asthmatics, FRC and TLC may be low without definite evidence of lung fibrosis.

### Pattern of breathing

Studies using magnetometers applied to the chest confirm the clinical observation that there is incoordination between the antero-posterior and lateral chest wall movements which varies with the severity of the attack. The relationship between respiratory effort and inspiratory flow is predictable in that during moderate obstruction inspiratory flow is more rapid than normal but in severe asthma it diminishes. There is tonic activity of the inspiratory muscles throughout the breathing cycle, the expiratory muscles are recruited as the obstruction deteriorates and the increased swings of intrathoracic pressure contribute to the pulsus paradoxus of severe asthma. Inspiratory time is reduced to allow maximum time for expiration, but the respiratory rate is unpredictable (Hillman, Prentice & Finucane, 1986).

### Carbon monoxide transfer

CO transfer tends to be normal in bronchial asthma. Young patients in remission have high normal values. $TLCO/V_A$ remains high (above 4 $ml·min^{-1}·mmHg^{-1}·l^{-1}$ (1.4 $mmol·min^{-1}·kPa^{-1}·l^{-1}$) even when TLCO falls during an episode of asthma. The test is mainly of importance in the assessment of patients with chronic diffuse airway obstruction. A normal value of $TLCO/V_A$ points towards bronchial asthma, rather than emphysema or chronic bronchitis (Knudson, Kattenborn & Burrows, 1990; see also Chapter 6). When TLCO is relatively better preserved than $FEV_1$ it is worth pursuing treatment for some time to try to reverse the obstruction, bearing in mind that polycythaemia or pulmonary plethora due to heart failure or left-to-right intracardiac shunt may also cause an unexpectedly high TL.

### Arterial blood $PO_2$ and $PCO_2$: respiratory failure and oxygen therapy

Blood gases are relatively well preserved in patients with mild bronchial asthma. In most patients it is possible to demonstrate slight abnormalities of alveolar–arterial $PO_2$ difference; in other cases there

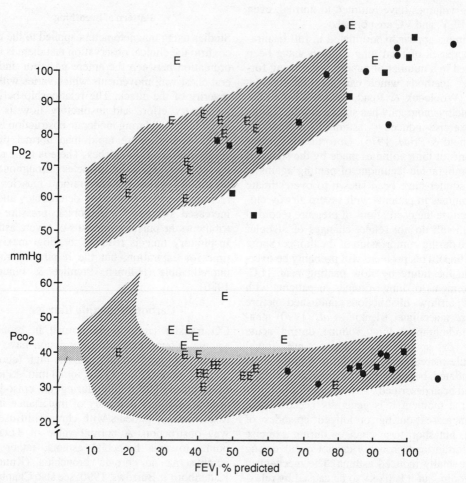

Fig. 7.8. Shaded areas: relationship between ventilatory function and arterial blood gases in patients with bronchial asthma. (Redrawn from McFadden & Lyons, 1968, with permission.) The symbols demonstrate a similar relationship in stable patients with chronic bronchitis (black squares), asthma (black circles), and advanced emphysema (E) (Nicholson, 1980: chapter 6).

are a number of poorly ventilated alveoli. These may be ventilated by collateral airflow because of obstruction of bronchioles. Single breath nitrogen tests (Chapter 4) generally show uneven distribution of inspired gas and ventilation–perfusion inequality, even in remission (Wagner et al., 1977; Rodriguez-Roisin et al., 1991).

In more severe asthma, $P_{CO_2}$ is low: hyperventilation (low $P_{CO_2}$), is an almost inevitable component of moderate bronchial asthma (McFadden & Lyons, 1968). Arterial $P_{O_2}$, breathing air, becomes progressively more abnormal with increasing obstruction (Fig. 7.8).

As $FEV_1$ falls to below 1.0 litre, with increasingly severe asthma, $P_{CO_2}$ rises to become 'normal' or high. Below 0.5 litre, ventilatory failure is the rule. In cases of severe asthma, a normal $P_{CO_2}$ shows incipient ventilatory failure. Generous oxygenation is the rule in such instances, with masks able to deliver up to 40% $O_2$ at least in the initial stage of treatment. It is now recognised that restlessness and anxiety are manifestations of respiratory distress in asthma and not usually part of the cause of the attack. Sedation is likely to be dangerous when $P_{CO_2}$ is high or rising. However, both restlessness and anxiety can make matters worse by two mechanisms:

1. Increasing $O_2$ consumption and $CO_2$ output and therefore ventilatory demand.
2. Triggering a degree of exercise-induced bronchoconstriction.

For these reasons, an attack may appear to settle before treatment can have had any effect. This form of reassurance is of the utmost importance in the emergency treatment of an asthmatic attack, by reducing the need for increased ventilation. Sedative drugs are not a safe substitute for good nursing and calm treatment, but there may be situations when it is felt that undue anxiety is responsible for excessive hyperventilation. The use of sedatives may therefore be justified in exceptional anxiety or uncontrollable behaviour, provided that all of the following criteria are satisfied:

1. PEF after bronchodilators is above 100 l/min.
2. $P_{O_2}$ is normal, breathing air or $O_2$ and $P_{CO_2}$ is low (below 36 mmHg, 4.8 kPa).
3. The patient is under skilled observation and can be ventilated artificially at short notice.

$P_{O_2}$ may fall after the administration of beta-adrenergic bronchodilator drugs or aminophylline (Tai & Read, 1967). The effect is variable, depending on the balance of improved distribution of ventilation (when the asthma is mild and readily reversible) and the loss of control of the pulmonary vasoconstrictor response to local hypoxia which causes a wider distribution of ventilation–perfusion ratios within the lung. Severe reduction of $P_{O_2}$ in response to nebulised salbutamol is exceptional partly because cardiac output increases (Chapter 3). However, significant falls of arterial $P_{O_2}$ to levels which may impair arterial function do occur in some patients with life-threatening asthma. This problem may be overcome by administering oxygen with bronchodilators in severe asthma. The majority of deaths following the intravenous administration of aminophylline appear to occur when the drug is given rapidly, but in a few cases even slow administration has been accompanied by sudden death. Individual experience is limited; probably most of these deaths occurred in patients who were not well oxygenated or who had impaired cardiac function. Intravenous aminophylline has been given quite regularly outside hospitals, usually without harm. At present it is uncertain whether, when the patient is unconscious, it is safer to give aminophylline before the arrival of the ambulance or to withhold it until adequate $O_2$ can be given and ventilation assured. Physicians who treat asthma at home in rural areas carry oxygen.

## Variants of bronchial asthma

In some cases, notably older patients, variant forms of bronchial asthma may present with coughing alone or with shortness of breath unaccompanied by other symptoms (McFadden 1975). These patients do not always wheeze; sometimes the only abnormality on auscultation is a degree of harshness of the expiratory lung sounds. They usually have reduced VC with rather less reduction of the PEF than is associated with the degree of shortness of breath. Readings may remain as high as 300 l/min even when dyspnoea is quite severe. $FEV_1/VC$ ratios are usually low and response to salbutamol is often trivial. Inhaled corticosteroids often relieve the cough and hyperventilation without any very dramatic improvement in the ventilatory function tests. This syndrome is well recognised but not very well documented. The diagnosis of asthma rests on the diurnal variation of PEF, increased airways resistance, the variability of the symptoms, the presence of supporting evidence such as eosinophilia, the absence of demonstrable heart disease and the response to treatment.

A rather similar situation may complicate chronic asthma. After a period of severe chronic airways obstruction, with the usual hyperinflation of the lungs, the patient is seen with an acute illness causing severe dyspnoea and perhaps a cough. Sometimes there is clear evidence of acute bronchitis, pneumonia or left ventricular failure; quite often no very good evidence for any of these is present and an exacerbation of asthma is diagnosed. Dyspnoea, initially at rest and later on effort, is now out of proportion to the trivial or absent wheeze and the breath sounds are harsh. VC and TLC are now much lower than before, and this may be evident from the loss of radiological lung volume. $FEV_1$ is relatively unchanged and PEF may be greater than before. Diurnal variation usually persists. These changes are very similar to those described when heart failure complicates chronic airways obstruction, when an increase of elastic recoil would be expected to have these consequences. These patients are often found to be on very high doses of corticosteroids, partly because the persistent dyspnoea is attributed to intractable asthma and partly because they are very intolerant of even slight deterioration of the underlying bronchial asthma. Obesity makes matters worse, and some such patients improve with reduction of the high doses of steroids, perhaps because there is a fall of the total and therefore the central blood volume. Treatment should be as conservative as possible. Steroid doses should be reduced promptly to normal maintenance doses (prednisolone 10–15 mg daily) and boosted only if there is clear evidence that they are preventing attacks which cannot be prevented by the use of bronchodilators (such as salbutamol by nebuliser). The normal pattern of wheezing and bronchodilator responsiveness is usually restored in 6–8 weeks, but occasionally a long convalescence is required.

# Site of airflow obstruction in bronchial asthma

Bronchoconstriction occurs throughout the length of the lower respiratory tract, which accounts for the lability of all the tests of airway calibre.

Laryngeal narrowing can be demonstrated photographically in asthma (Lisboa *et al.*, 1980; Higenbottam & Payne, 1982; Shidoh *et al.*, 1985). In some stridor is marked. A few asthmatics present from time to time with attacks of transient laryngeal stridor, detectable by the sound, and poorly reproducible lung function tests. Low arterial $Po_2$ usually indicates the extent of the intrapulmonary disease, although a few individuals with recurrent laryngeal wheezing are found on occasion to be hypoxaemic (Chapter 6).

The distinction between central and peripheral airway obstruction can be made by tests of forced expiratory flow–volume curves, breathing air and breathing helium, a gas of low density. In normal subjects maximal expiratory flow increases during forced expiration, while in individuals with chronic airflow obstruction flow rates at low lung volumes are unaltered. Theoretically, breathing gases of low density should result in increased flow in passages where flow is turbulent; laminar flow being affected by viscosity but not density. Laminar flow is thought to occur in small airways, so lack of density dependence should signify limitation of flow in peripheral airways. This occurs in a proportion of more severely affected asthmatics, while in others flow limitation is in proximal airways (Despas, Leroux & Macklem, 1972; Antic & Macklem, 1976; McFadden *et al.*, 1977; Fairshter & Wilson, 1980).

The relative importance of tracheobronchial and bronchiolar constriction varies among asthmatics. The clinical significance of these observations and their relationship to the effectiveness of oral and inhaled therapy remains uncertain.

# Perception of breathlessness and symptoms of asthma

Asthmatics vary in their ability to detect changes in bronchial calibre and in the importance they attach to these. This has been investigated in the laboratory during challenge studies and using ambient peak flow and symptom monitoring. Symptoms have been assessed using visual analogue and category rating scales (Chapter 12). Some investigators have asked the subjects to record breathlessness while others have attempted to obtain a global view of the severity of the asthma. There is general agreement that about 15 to 20% of asthmatics deny having asthma until it is very severe: some are unable to detect bronchoconstriction throughout a methacholine challenge. (Rubinfeld & Pain, 1977; Orehek *et al.*, 1982; Burdon *et al.*, 1982). Exercise, histamine and immediate reactions to allergens produce sensations of a similar magnitude but late reactions possibly cause less severe symptoms in relation to lung function changes perhaps because they occur in more peripheral airways (Turcotte, Corbeil & Boulet, 1990).

In patients recruited through specialist clinics there is a reasonable correlation between the severity of the symptoms and peak flow recordings, though this is less good if the true value of PEF is concealed from the subject by electronic coding or by storing the readings without displaying them in electronic memory (Higgs *et al.*, 1986). Patients who give very low symptom scores to severe falls of PEF deny emotional problems also and appear to be psychologically distinct (Steiner *et al.*, 1987). Treatment with inhaled steroids may reduce perception of asthma independently of any effect on lung function (Higgs & Laszlo, 1984). There is no important difference between the ability of asthmatics and others to detect resistances added to a respiratory circuit.

Nearly all asthmatics in Britain describe a sensation of tightness of the chest during attacks, with 90% describing breathlessness, 70% wheezing and 30% pain in the chest. The symptoms used to identify deterioration differ slightly (Higgs *et al.*, 1985). Exercise ventilation is sensed normally if bronchoconstriction is avoided (Mahler *et al.*, 1991).

## Prognosis

The prognosis of childhood asthma remains uncertain. Less than 50% of those who experience asthma, or an increased bronchial reactivity, in adult life will remit completely when the initial stimulus is withdrawn. Wheezing and dyspnoea developing after sensitisation to isocyanate or other allergens may often require continuous treatment long after the exposure has ceased (Yeung & Grzybowski, 1985). Moreover, a single episode of bronchoconstriction caused by an irritant such as chlorine or sulphur dioxide may precipitate lifelong asthma, as shown by variable lung function tests.

There is ample evidence that the quality of life experienced by asthmatics improves if the condition is diagnosed and treated carefully along conventional lines (British Thoracic Society and others, 1990*a*, *b*; Vermeire, 1992). The distressing cases of sudden death are not all preventable, but many who die or narrowly miss doing so have,

with hindsight, paid too little heed to warning symptoms or have not taken appropriate remedies (Molfino *et al.*, 1992).

## References

Abramson, M.J., Saunders, N.A. & Hensley, M.J. (1990). Analysis of bronchial reactivity in epidemiology studies. *Thorax*, **45**, 924–929.

Allegra, L. & Bianco, S. (1980). Nonspecific bronchoreactivity obtained with an ultrasonic aerosol of distilled water. *European Journal of Respiratory Disease*, **61**, 41–49.

Anderson, S.D. (1988). Exercise-induced asthma. In *Allergy: Principles & Practice*, 3rd edn, ed. C.E. Reed, E. Ellis, N. F. Adkinson, J.W. Yungiger, pp. 1156–1175. St Louis: Mosby.

Anderson, S.D. (1989). Exercise-induced asthma: a difference of opinion regarding the stimulus. *Allergy Proceedings*, **10**, 215–223.

Anderson, S.D., Seale, J.P., Rozea, P., Bandler, L. & Theobald, G. (1976). Inhaled and oral salbutamol in exercise-induced asthma. *American Review of Respiratory Disease*, **114**, 493–500.

Anderson, S.D., Silverman, M., Konig, P. & Godfrey, S. (1975). Exercise-induced asthma. *British Journal of Diseases of the Chest*, **69**, 1–39.

Anderson, S.D. & Smith, C.M. (1989). The use of nonisotonic aerosols for evaluating bronchial hyperresponsiveness. In *Provocative Challenge Procedures: Background and Methodology*, ed. J.L. Spector, New York: Futura.

Anthonisen, N.R., Wright, E.C. & VIPPB Trial Group (1986). Bronchodilator response in chronic asthma. *American Review of Respiratory Disease*, **133**, 814–819.

Antic, R. & Macklem, P.T. (1976). The influence of clinical factors on the site of airway obstruction in asthma. *American Review of Respiratory Disease*, **114**, 851–859.

Barnes, P.J. & Holgate, S.T. (1990). Asthma: Pathogenesis and hyperreactivity. In *Respiratory Medicine*, ed. R.A.L. Brewis, G.T. Gibson & D.M. Geddes, pp. 558–603. London: Baillière Tindall.

Bellegrino, R., Violante, B., Crimi, E. & Brusasco, V. (1990). Effects of deep inhalation during early and late asthmatic reactions to allergen. *American Review of Respiratory Disease*, **142**, 822–825.

Blackie, S.P., Al-Majed, S., Staples, C.A., Hilliam, C. & Paré, P.D. (1990). Changes in total lung capacity during acute spontaneous asthma. *American Review of Respiratory Disease*, **142**, 79–83.

British Thoracic Society and others (1993). Guidelines on the management of asthma. *Thorax*, **48**, S1–S24.

Britton, J., Mortagy, A. & Tattersfield, A. (1986). Histamine challenge testing: comparison of three methods. *Thorax*, **41**, 128–132.

Brooks, M.S. (1982). The evaluation of occupational airways disease in the laboratory or workplace. *Journal of Allergy and Clinical Immunology*, **70**, 56–66.

Burdon, J.G.W., Juniper, E.F., Killian, K.J., Hargreave, F.E. & Campbell, E.J.M. (1982). The perception of breathlessness in asthma. *American Review of Respiratory Disease*, **126**, 825–828.

Cade, J.F. & Pain, M.C.F. (1973). Pulmonary function during clinical remission of asthma: how reversible is asthma? *Australia and New Zealand Journal of Medicine*, **3**, 545–551.

Cade, J.F., Woolcock, A.J., Rebuck, A.S. & Pain, M.C.F. (1971). Lung mechanics during provocation of asthma. *Clinical Science*, **40**, 381–391.

Chai, H., Farr, R.S., Froelick, L.A., Mathison, D.A., McLean, J.A., Rosenthal, R.R., Sheffer, A.L., Spector, S.L. & Townley, R.G. (1975). Standardisation of bronchial inhalation challenge procedures. *Journal of Allergy and Clinical Immunology*, **56**, 323–337.

Cheney, F.W. & Butler, J. (1968). The effects of intrasonically- produced aerosols on airway resistance in man. *Anaesthesiology*, **29**, 1099–1106.

Connolly, C.K. (1979). Diurnal rhythms in airway obstruction. *British Journal of Diseases of the Chest*, **73**, 357–366.

Deal, E.C., McFadden, E.R., Ingram, R.H. & Jaeger, J.J. (1979a). Hyperpnoea and heat flux: initial reaction sequence in exercise-induced asthma. *Journal of Applied Physiology*, **46**, 476–483.

Deal, E.C., McFadden, E.R., Ingram, R.H., Strauss, R.H. & Jaeger, J.J. (1979b). Role of respiratory heat exchange in production of exercise-induced asthma. *Journal of Applied Physiology*, **46**, 467–475.

Deal, E.C., McFadden, E.R., Ingram, R.H., Breslin, F.J. & Jaeger, J.J. (1980). Airway responsiveness to cold air and hyperpnoea in normal subjects and those with lung fever and asthma. *American Review of Respiratory Disease*, **121**, 621–628.

Despas, P.J., Leroux, M. & Macklem, P.T. (1972). Site of airway obstruction in asthma as determined by measuring maximal expiratory flow breathing air and a helium oxygen mixture. *Journal of Clinical Investigation*, **51**, 3235–3243.

Dunn, T.L., Gerber, M.J., Shen, A.S., Fernandez, E., Iseman, M. & Cherniack, R.N. (1986). Effect of topical ophthalmic instillation of timolol and betaxolol on lung function in asthmatic subjects. *American Review of Respiratory Disease*, **133**, 264–268.

Edmunds, A.T., Tooley, M. & Godfrey, S. (1978). The refractory period after exercise-induced asthma: its duration and relation to the severity of exercise. *American Review of Respiratory Disease*, **117**, 247–254.

Eggleston, P.A. & Guerrant, J.L.A. (1978). Standardised method of evaluating exercise-induced asthma. *Journal of Allergy and Clinical Immunology*, **58**, 414–425.

Fairshter, R.D. & Wilson, A.F. (1980). Relationship between the site of airflow limitation and localization of the bronchodilator response in asthma. *American Review of Respiratory Disease*, **172**, 27–32.

Fitch, A.D. & Morton, A.R. (1971). Specificity of exercise in exercise-induced asthma. *British Medical Journal*, **iv**, 577–581.

Freedman, S., Tattersfield, A.E. & Pride, N.B. (1975). Changes in lung mechanics during asthma induced by exercise. *Journal of Applied Physiology*, **38**, 974–982.

Garfinkel, S.K., Kesten, S., Chapman, K.R. & Rebuck, A.S. (1992). Physiologic and non-physiologic determinants of aerobic fitness in mild and moderate asthma. *American Review of Respiratory Disease*, **145**, 741–745.

Gayrard, P., Orehek, J.O., Grimaud, C. & Charpin, J. (1975). Bronchoconstrictor effects of deep inspiration in patients with asthma. *American Review of Respiratory Disease*, **111**, 433–440.

Godfrey, S., Springer, C., Novister, N., Maayan, Ch. & Avital, R. (1991). Exercise but not methacholine differentiates asthma from chronic lung disease in children. *Thorax*, **46**, 488–492.

Goldman, J.M., Teale, C. & Muers, M.F. (1992). Simplifying the assessment of patients with chronic airflow obstruction for home nebuliser therapy. *Respiratory Medicine*, **86**, 33–38.

Hargreave, F.E., Ryan, G. & Thompson, N.C. (1981). Bronchial responsiveness to histamine or methacholine in asthma: measurement and clinical significance. *Journal of Allergy and Clinical Immunology*, **68**, 347–355.

Hartley, J.P.R., Charles, T.J. & Seaton, A. (1977). Betamethasone valerate inhalation and exercise-induced asthma in adults. *British Journal of Diseases of the Chest*, **71**, 253–258.

Heaton, R.W., Henderson, A.F. & Costello, J.F. (1984). Cold air as a bronchial provocation technique. *Chest*, **86**, 810–814.

Henneberger, P.K., Stanbury, M.J., Trimbath, L.S. & Kipen, H.M. (1992). The use of portable peak flowmeters in the surveillance of occupational asthma. *Chest*, **100**, 1515–1521.

Henriksen, J.M. & Dahl, R. (1983). Effects of inhaled budesomide alone and in combination with low dose terbutaline in children with exercise-induced asthma. *American Review of Respiratory Medicine*, **128**, 993–997.

Hetzel, M.R. (1981). The pulmonary clock (editorial). *Thorax*, **36**, 481–486.

Hetzel, M.R. & Clark, T.J.H. (1979). Does sleep cause nocturnal asthma? *Thorax*, **34**, 749–754.

Hetzel, M.R. & Clark, T.J.H. (1980). Comparison of normal and asthmatic circadian rhythms in peak expiratory flow rate. *Thorax*, **35**, 732–738.

Higenbottam, T. & Payne, J. (1982). Glottis narrowing in lung disease. *American Review of Respiratory Disease*, **125**, 746–750.

Higgs, C.M.B., Jones, P., Tanser, A.R. & Laszlo, G. (1985). What are the symptoms of asthma and their importance? (abstract). *Thorax*, **40**, 688.

Higgs, C.M.B., Laszlo, G. (1983). Duration of action of salbutamol and reproterol in the prevention of exercise-induced asthma. *British Journal of Diseases of the Chest*, **77**, 262–269.

Higgs, C.M.B. & Laszlo, G. (1984). Effect of treatment and the perception of asthma (abstract). *Medical Journal of Australia and New Zealand*, **14**, 530.

Higgs, C.M.B., Richardson, R.B. & Laszlo, G. (1982). The effect of regular inhaled salbutamol on the airway responsiveness of normal subjects. *Clinical Science*, **63**, 513–517.

Higgs, C.M.B., Richardson, R.B., Lea, D.A., Lewis, G.T.R. & Laszlo, G. (1986). Influence of knowledge of peak flow on self-assessment of asthma: studies with a coder peak flow meter. *Thorax*, **41**, 671–675.

Hillman, D.R., Prentice, L. & Finucane, K.E. (1986). The pattern of breathing in acute severe asthma. *American Review of Respiratory Disease*, **133**, 587–592.

Holmes, P.W., Campbell, A.H. & Barter, C.E. (1978). Acute changes of lung volume and lung mechanics in asthma and normal subjects. *Thorax*, **33**, 394–410.

Josephs, L.K., Gregory, I., Bain, D.J.G. & Holgate, S.T. (1987). A longitudinal study of non-specific bronchial responsiveness in asthma. *Thorax*, **42**, 711.

Juniper, E.F., Guyatt, G.H., Epstein, R.S., Ferrie, P.J., Jaeschke, R. & Hillier, T. (1992). Evaluation of impairment of health-related quality of life in asthma: development of a questionnaire for use in clinical trials. *Thorax*, **47**, 76–83.

Knudson, R.J., Kattenborn, W.T. & Burrows, B. (1990). Single break carbon monoxide transfer factor in different forms of chronic airflow obstruction in a general population sample. *Thorax*, **45**, 514–519.

Koeter, G.H., Krouwels, F.H., van Aalderen, W.M.C. & Knol, K. (1991). Budesonide and terbutaline or terbutaline alone in children with mild asthma:

effects on bronchial hyperresponsiveness and diurnal variation of peak flow. *Thorax*, **46**, 419–503.

Lisboa, C., Jardim, J., Angus, E. & Macklem, P.T. (1980). Is extrathoracic obstruction important in asthma? *American Review of Respiratory Disease*, **122**, 115–121.

McFadden, E.R. (1975). Exertional dyspnoea and cough as preludes to attacks of asthma. *New England Journal of Medicine*, **292**, 555–559.

McFadden, E.R. (1990). Hypothesis: exercise-induced asthma as a vascular phenomenon. *Lancet*, **335**, 880–883.

McFadden, E.R., Ingram, R.H., Haynes, R.L. & Wellmann, J.J. (1977). Predominent site of flow limitation and mechanisms of post-exertional asthma. *Journal of Applied Physiology*, **42**, 746–752.

McFadden, E.R. & Lyons, H.A. (1968). Arterial blood gas tensions in asthma. *New England Journal of Medicine*, **278**, 1027–1032.

Mahler, D.A., Faryniarz, K., Lentene, T., Ward, J., Olmstead, E.M. & O'Connor, G.T. (1991). Measurement of breathlessness during exercise in asthmatics. *American Review of Respiratory Disease*, **144**, 39–44.

Malo, J-L, Cartier, A., Pineau, L., Gagnon, G. & Martin, R.R. (1985). Slope of the dose–response curve to inhaled histamine and methacholine and PC20 in subjects with symptoms of airway hyperexcitability and normal subjects. *American Review of Respiratory Disease*, **132**, 644–647.

Martin, F., Powell, S., Shore, S., Emrich, J. & Engel, L.A. (1980). The role of the respiratory muscles in the hyperinflation of bronchial asthma. *American Review of Respiratory Disease*, **121**, 441–447.

Molfino, N.A., Nannini, L.J., Rebuck, A.S. & Slutsky, A.S. (1992). The fatality-prone asthmatic patient: follow-up study after a near-fatal attack. *Chest*, **101**, 621–623.

Moreno, R.H., Hogg, J.C., Paré, P.D. (1986). Mechanics of airway narrowing. *American Review of Respiratory Disease*, **133**, 1171–1180.

Morrison, J.F.J., Jones, P.C. & Muers, M.F. (1992). Assessing physiological benefit from domiciliary nebulised bronchodilators in severe airflow limitation. *European Respiratory Journal*, **5**, 424–429.

Nadel J.A. & Tierney, D.F. (1961). Effect of a previous deep inspiration on airway resistance in man. *Journal of Applied Physiology*, **16**, 717–719.

Newman Taylor, A.J. (1986). Inhalation challenge with sensitising and occupational agents. *European Journal of Respiratory Disease*, 68 (suppl.), **143**, 35–38.

Newman Taylor, A.J. & Davies, R.J. (1982). Inhalation challenge testing. In *Occupational Lung Diseases:*

*Research Approach and Methods* ed. H. Weill & M. Turner-Warwick, pp. 143–167. New York: Marcel Dekker.

O'Byrne, P.M., Ryan, G., Morris, M., McCormack, D., Jones, N.L., Morse, J.L.C. & Hargreave, F.E. (1982). Asthma induced by cold air and its relation to non-specific bronchial responsiveness to methacholine. *American Review of Respiratory Disease*, **125**, 281–285.

Orehek, J., Beaupré, A., Badier, M, Nicoli, M.M. & Delpierre, S. (1982). Perception of airway tone by asthamatic patients. *Bulletin Européen Physiopathologie Respiratoire*, **18**, 601–607.

Orehek, J., Gayrard, P., Smith, A.P., Grimaud, C. & Charpin, J. (1976). Airway responses to carbachol in allergic and non-allergic subjects. *American Review of Respiratory Disease*, **113**, 579–586.

Orehek, J., Nicoli, M.M., Delpierre, S. & Beaupré, A. (1981). Influence of the previous deep inspiration on spirometric measurement of provoked bronchocon-striction in asthma. *American Review of Respiratory Disease*, **123**, 269–272.

Palmeiro, E.M., Hopp, R.J., Biven, R.E., Bewtra, A.K., Nair, N.N., Townley, R.G. (1992). Probability of asthma based on methacholine challenge. *Chest*, **101**, 630–633.

Parhan, W.M., Shepard, K.H., Norman, P.S. & Fish, J.E. (1983). Analysis of the course and magnitude of lung inflation effects on airway tone: relation to air-way reactivity. *American Review of Respiratory Disease*, **128**, 240–245.

Pattemore, P.K., Asher, M.I., Harrison, A.C., Mitchell, E.A., Rea, H.H. & Stewart, A.W. (1990). The inter-relationship among bronchial hyperresponsiveness, the diagnosis of asthma and asthma symptoms. *American Review of Respiratory Disease*, **142**, 549–551.

Peiffer, C., Marsac, J. & Lockhart, A. (1989). Chronobiological study of the relationship between dyspnoea and airway obstruction in symptomatic asthma subjects. *Clinical Science*, **77**, 237–244.

Peress, L., Sybrecht, G. & Macklem, P.T. (1976). The mechanism of increase in total lung capacity during acute asthma. *American Journal of Medicine*, **61**, 165–169.

Perrin, B., Lagier, F., L'Archevêque, J., Cartier, A., Boulet, L-P, Lôte, J. & Malo, J.L. (1992). Occupational asthma: validity of monitoring of peak expiratory flow rates and non-allergic bronchial challenge as compared to specific inhalation chal-lenge. *European Respiratory Journal*, **5**, 40–48.

Philips, Y.Y., Jaeger, J.J., Lambe, B.L. & Rosenthal, R.R. (1985). Eucapnic voluntary hyperventilation of compressed gas mixture. A simple system for bronchial challenge by respiratory heat loss. *American Review of Respiratory Disease*, **131**, 31–35.

Rodriguez-Roisin, R., Ferrer, A., Navajas, D., Augusti, A.G.N., Wagner, P.D. & Roca, J. (1991). Ventilation–perfusion mismatch after methacholine challenge in patients with mild bronchial asthma. *American Review of Respiratory Disease*, **144**, 89–94.

Rosenman, K.D. (1992). Asthma and work: how do you diagnose the association? *Chest*, **100**, 1481–1482.

Rubinfeld, A.R. & Pain, M.C.F. (1977). Perception of asthma. *Lancet*, **i**, 882–883.

Ruff, D.B., Choudry, N.B., Pride, N.B. & Ind, P. (1989). The effect of prolonged submaximal warm-up exercise on exercise-induced asthma. *American Review of Respiratory Disease*, **139**, 479–484.

Ryan, G., Dolovitch, N.B., Roberts, R.S., Frith, P.A., Juniper, E.F. & Hargreave, F.E. (1981). Standardisation of inhalation provocation tests. *American Review of Respiratory Disease*, **123**, 195–199.

Ryan, G., Latimer, K.M., Dolovich, J. & Hargreave, F.E. (1982). Bronchial responsiveness to histane, relationship to diurnal variation of peak flow rate, improvement after bronchodilator and airway cali-bre. *Thorax*, **37**, 423–429.

Schachter, E.N., Doyle, C.A. & Beck, G.J. (1984). A prospective study of asthma in a rural community. *Chest*, **85**, 623–630.

Sekizawa, K., Sasaki, H., Shimuzu, Y. & Takishima, T. (1986). Dose–response effects of methacholine in normal and in asthmatic patients. *American Review of Respiratory Disease*, **133**, 593–599.

Shidoh, C., Sekizawa, K., Hida, W., Sasaki, H. & Takashima, T. (1985). Upper airway response during bronchoprovocation and asthma attack. *American Review of Respiratory Disease*, **132**, 671–678.

Shore, S.A., Huk, O., Mannix, S. & Martin, J.G. (1983). Effect of panting frequency on the plethys-mographic determination of thoracic gas volume in chronic obstructive pulmonary disease. *American Review of Respiratory Disease*, **128**, 54–59.

Silverman, M. & Anderson, S.D. (1972). Standardisation of exercise tests in asthmatic chil-dren. *Archives of Disease in Childhood*, **47**, 882–889.

Smith, A.P. (1981). Patterns of recovery for acute severe asthma. *British Journal of Diseases of the Chest*, **75**, 132–140.

Smith, E.C., Clark, R.A., Dhillon, P. & Laszlo, G. (1990). The effect of salbutamol controlled release on exercise-induced asthma (abstract). *Thorax*, **45**, 796.

Sourk, R.L. & Nugent, K.M. (1983). Bronchodilator testing: confidence intervals derived from placebo inhalations. *American Review of Respiratory Disease*, **128**, 153–157.

Stanescu, D., Rodenstein, D., Cauberghs, G. & van der Woestijne, K.P. (1982). Failure of body plethysmography in bronchial asthma. *Journal of Applied Physiology*, **52**, 939–948.

Steiner, H., Higgs, C.M.B., Fritz, G.K., Laszlo, G. & Harvey, J.E. (1987). Defense style and the perception of asthma. *Journal of Psychosomatic Medicine*, **49**, 35–44.

Sterk, P.J., Fabbri, L.M., Quanjer, Ph.H., Cockcroft, D.W., O'Byrne, P.M., Anderson S.D., Juniper, E.F. & Malo, J.-L. Airway responsiveness. *European Respiratory Journal*, **6**, (Suppl. 16), 53–83.

Strauss, R.H., McFadden, E.R., Ingram, R.H., Deal, E.C. & Jaeger, J.J. (1978). Influence of heat and humidity on the airway obstruction induced by asthma in exercise. *Journal of Clinical Investigation*, **61**, 433–440.

Tai, E. & Read, J. (1967). Response of blood gas tensions to aminophyline and isoprenoline in patients with asthma. *Thorax*, **22**, 534–539.

Tattersfield, A.E. & Harrison, R.N. (1983). Effect of beta-blocker therapy on airway function. *Drugs*, **25**, (suppl. 2), 227–231.

Tollerud, D.J., O'Connor, G.T., Sparrow, D. & Weiss, S.T. (1991). Asthma, hay fever and phlegm production associated with distinct patterns of allergy, skin test reactivity, eosinophilia and serum IgG levels. *American Review of Respiratory Disease*, **144**, 716–781.

Trigg, C.J., Bennett, J.B., Tooley, M., Sibbald, B. D'Souza, M.F. & Davies, R.J. (1990). A general practice based survey of bronchial hyperresponsiveness and its relation to symptoms, sex, age, atopy and smoking. *Thorax*, **45**, 866–872.

Turcotte, H., Corbeil, F. & Boulet, L-P. (1990). Perception of breathlessness induced by antigen, exercise and histamine challenge. *Thorax*, **45**, 914–918.

Turner-Warwick, M. (1977). On observing patterns of airflow obstruction in chronic asthma. *British Journal of Diseases of the Chest*, **71**, 73–86.

Vanethen, A.S., Knox, A.J., Wisniewski, A & Tattersfield, A.E. (1991). Effect of inhaled budesomide in bronchial reactivity and histamine, exercise and euapnic dry air hyperventilation in patients with asthma. *Thorax*, **46**, 811–816.

van Noord, J.A., Clement, J., van de Woestijne, K.P. & Demets, D. (1989). Total respiratory resistance and reactance as a measuring response to bronchial challenge with histamine. *American Review of Respiratory Disease*, **131**, 921–926.

van Schayk, C.P., Dompeling, E., van Herwaarden, C.L.A., Wever, A.M.J. & van Weel, C. (1991). Interacting effects of atopy and bronchial hyperresponsiveness on the annual decline in lung function and the exacerbation rate in asthma. *American Review of Respiratory Disease*, **144**, 1297–1301.

Vermeire, P. (1992). Growing consensus in asthma? *European Respiratory Journal*, **5**, 509–511.

Wagner, P.D., Dantzker, D.R., Iacovoni, V.E., Tomlin, W.R. & West, J.B. (1977). Ventilation–perfusion inequality in asymptomatic asthma. *American Review of Respiratory Disease*, **118**, 511–524.

Weir, D.C., Grove, R.I., Robertson, A.S. & Burge, P.S. (1990a). Corticosteroid trials in non-asthmatic chronic airflow obstruction: a comparison of oral prednisolone and inhaled beclomethasone diproprionate. *Thorax*, **45**, 112–117.

Weir, D.C., Robertson, A.S., Grove, R.I. & Burge, P.S. (1990b). Time course of response to oral and inhaled corticosteroid in non-asthamic airflow obstruction. *Thorax*, **45**, 118–121.

Weiss, S.T., Tager, I.B., Munoz, A. & Speizer, F.G. (1985). The relationship of respiratory infections in early childhood to the occurrence of increased levels of bronchial responsiveness and atopy. *American Review of Respiratory Disease*, **131**, 573–578.

Woolcock, A. & Read, J. (1965). Improvement in bronchial asthma not reflected in forced expiratory volume. *Lancet,* **ii**, 1323–1324.

Woolcock, A. & Read, J. (1966). Lung volumes in exacerbations of asthma. *American Journal of Medicine*, **41**, 259–273.

Woolcock, A.J., Salome, C.M. & Yan, K. (1984). The shape of the dose–response curve to histamine in asthmatic and normal subjects. *American Review of Respiratory Disease*, **130**, 71–75.

Yan, K., Salome, C. & Woolcock, A.J. (1983). Rapid method for measurement of bronchial responsiveness. *Thorax*, **38**, 760–765.

Yeung, M. & Grzybowski, S. (1985). Prognosis in occupational asthma. *Thorax*, **40**, 241–243.

Zamel, N. (1984). Partial flow-volume loops. *Bulletin Européen Physiopathologie Respiratoire*, **20**, 471–476.

Zhong, N.S., Chen, R.C., O-yang, M., Wu, J.Y., Fu, W.X. & Shi, L.J. (1990). Bronchial hyperresponsiveness in young students of Southern China: relation to respiratory symptoms, diagnosed asthma and risk factors. *Thorax*, **45**, 860–865.

# 8 Diffuse interstitial lung disorders

The diffuse interstitial lung disorders described in this chapter are non-infectious inflammatory disorders mostly of unknown cause. They have in common widespread or patchy oedema, cellular infiltration, smooth muscle proliferation, fibrosis or calcification of the alveolar space, the alveolar walls or the lobular septa. The main sites of pathological abnormality are distal to the terminal bronchiole. Peripheral airways may be involved in the inflammatory process or they may be distorted by traction from the adjacent fibrotic areas. The alveolar damage is not distributed uniformly, except in the most florid examples. In practice, the most common causes of diffuse non-obstructive disease referred for assessment are the pneumoconioses, sarcoidosis, cryptogenic fibrosing alveolitis, allergic alveolitis, disseminated malignancy, systemic sclerosis, pulmonary vasculitis associated with the rheumatoid and collagen vascular diseases and radiation pneumonia. Organising exudate can affect lung function in the same way in patients who have recovered from uraemia, respiratory distress syndrome, viral pneumonia, lung haemorrhage and cardiogenic pulmonary oedema.

The pulmonary function laboratory has an important contribution to make in the assessment of patients suffering from these disorders. The diagnosis of diffuse interstitial lung disease is often made on the basis of the pattern of abnormality found. Published accounts of these conditions often cause confusion for several reasons. Their classification and nomenclature are not generally agreed; the interpretation of pulmonary function studies is often oversimplified and the descriptions by physiologists of the ways in which diffuse alveolar disease causes pulmonary insufficiency have changed frequently.

## Pathophysiology of the diffuse interstitial lung diseases

The presentation of these diseases may be acute, or, more commonly, insidious. Inflammation and oedema ('alveolitis') are followed by fibrosis, the severity of which may depend on the duration of the inflammatory phase. There is a reduction of the gas exchanging capacity of parts of the lungs, affecting both $TL_{CO}$ and arterial $P_{O_2}$. Inflammation, oedema and fibrosis of the alveoli usually results in loss of lung volume, all the subdivisions of TLC being reduced. The elastic recoil of these parts of the lung is increased, causing reduction of lung compliance. There is an increase of expiratory flow rates relative to lung volumes, resulting in a high ratio of PEF to $FEV_1$ and TLC. Concomitant airway disease or emphysema causes the opposite effects and may mask the presence of diffuse interstitial fibrosis.

Airflow obstruction occurs when there is complicating infection, and when the process is caused by hypersensitivity to inhaled material affecting bronchioles as well as alveolar walls.

In 1951 Austrian et al. introduced the term 'alveolar capillary block' to describe the physiological and pathological disturbance, implying that the reduction of alveolar–arterial $P_{O_2}$ difference found in many of these patients was caused by a structural barrier to the diffusion of oxygen between the alveoli and the pulmonary capillaries. It is currently believed that ventilation–perfusion mismatching accounts for 80% of the desaturation noted in exercise, approximately 20% being due to additional factors such as a possible diffusion barrier. The subject is pursued in more depth later.

The low lung volumes and vital capacity found in breathless patients with diffuse interstitial lung diseases were described by the term 'restrictive ventilatory defect' (Baldwin, Cournand & Richards, 1948, 1949). This described the group of diseases in which reduction of VC is associated with low static lung volumes. In contrast, obstructive disease reduces VC by airway closure, TLC is not reduced and there is an increase in the residual lung volume (Chapter 2). These distinctions may be made clinically or by estimation of lung volumes from the chest radiograph as well as by lung function tests.

In their mildest form diffuse fibrosing diseases of alveoli are patchy, and suspected only because of the presence of a few characteristic crackles at the bases of the lungs or radiographic changes. Lung function may be within normal limits or it may only be possible to demonstrate very subtle abnormalities such as widening of the alveolar–arterial $Po_2$ difference at submaximal exercise.

At the other extreme, the whole lung may be involved with extensive fibrosis and the appearance of 'honeycombing' on radiographs and computed tomographs: this is caused by the development of cystic spaces, possibly dilated terminal bronchioles, lined with respiratory epithelium and sometimes smooth muscle. They are probably the result of traction on the respiratory bronchioles by local fibrosis. These air spaces are ventilated, but poorly perfused. Lung scans which somewhat resemble those of pulmonary embolism are seen in over 50% of these patients.

The interpretation of published data on the disorder of physiology in these diseases depends on whether substantial numbers of patients with this most severe form were included. These patients have mainly irreversible changes and symptomatic improvement can only be achieved by treatment of associated disorders which may make lung function worse, such as fluid retention and infection.

## Plan of investigation

The diffuse interstitial lung diseases are relatively uncommon, and there is no general agreement

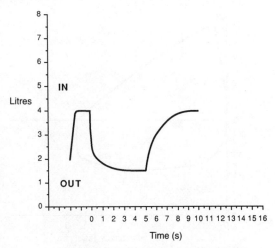

Fig. 8.1. Timed forced expiration in a patient with diffuse lung fibrosis. $FEV_1 = 2.3$ litres, FVC = 3.0 litres, $FEV_1/FVC = 77\%$, $FIV_1 = 2.0$ litres. Forced inspiratory flow is usually reduced because of the increased elastic work of breathing.

about the cause, prognosis and treatment of many of them. For this reason, full investigation at the outset is highly desirable, especially if a form of therapy which is experimental or hazardous is planned. It is neither possible nor necessary to repeat every procedure frequently. Some tests tend to improve more strikingly than others when clinical improvement occurs. Full physiological investigation of an ambulant patient includes lung volumes, spirometry, peak flow rate, CO transfer and a standard exercise test with direct or indirect measurement of blood gases. Acutely ill, nervous and elderly patients will need sensible modification of the tests, as will many who are disabled by other conditions.

### Forced expiration

The shape of the forced expired trace is normal. Sometimes it is exceptionally steep, with a correspondingly high peak flow (Figs. 8.1, 8.2). This implies dense, diffuse fibrosis. $FEV_1/VC$ is normal or high unless there is associated airflow obstruction.

### Lung volumes

In severe cases, all the subdivisions of lung volume are reduced. FRC is low because the

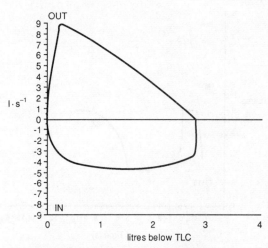

Fig. 8.2. As Fig. 8.1, expressed as a flow–volume plot. Maximum expiratory flow = 9 l·s⁻¹ (540 l·min⁻¹), maximum inspiratory flow =.4.2 l·s⁻¹ (252 l·min⁻¹), maximum flow at 50% VC (MEF₅₀) = 4.8 l·s⁻¹ (288 l·min⁻¹), MEF₅₀/MEF = 46% (normally 40—60%).

increased retractile force of the fibrosed lung holds the chest at a relatively low volume when there is no respiratory effort. When the disease is mild and vital capacity is not reduced, FRC and RV are often reduced but may sometimes be normal.

### Lung compliance and airways resistance

The elastic recoil pressure of the lung is increased. Loss of distensibility of individual alveoli may in part be responsible, because of the fibrosis within their walls. Obliteration of alveoli can also contribute to increased lung elasticity, because the remaining alveoli have to be stretched further (Gibson & Pride 1977; Chapter 2). Conversely, smoking decreases lung elasticity in patients with cryptogenic fibrosing alveolitis and sarcoidosis. The influence of these changes on symptoms is unknown. Because lung compliance is not as easy to measure as the static lung volumes and provides very little extra information in the individual case, this measurement is not very useful in routine practice unless some associated neurological disorder is suspected, when maximal recoil pressure will be lower than expected for the lung volume.

Airways resistance is normal in uncomplicated cases when the disease is confined to the distal air spaces.

### Carbon monoxide transfer factor

The CO transfer factor is the most sensitive of the simple tests of pulmonary function for the detection of fibrosing lung conditions. Abnormalities of this test tend to correlate with the presence of infiltration of the alveolar walls with inflammatory cells or extensive fibrosis. Granulomatous and nodular fibrotic lesions situated focally in relation to terminal bronchioles are found to have a minor effect on resting pulmonary function: TLco is often normal in the presence of quite marked X-ray changes. Such lesions are found in sarcoidosis and coal-workers' pneumoconiosis.

TLco/$V_A$ is reduced in only a small proportion of patients with fibrosing lung disorders. There is an inverse relationship between the distensibility of the whole lung and TLco/$V_A$ such that if TLC is severely reduced TLco/$V_A$ is usually normal. There are other patients in whom the fibrotic areas coexist with regions of normally distensible lung. These overinflate in full inspiration and receive a high proportion of the inspired gas, In addition they show the normal tendency for TLco/$V_A$ to fall with increasing lung volume, because the pulmonary vascularity does not increase in proportion to lung volume during inspiration. In individuals with this type of abnormality, TLco/$V_A$ is markedly reduced and TLC relatively well preserved.

### Arterial blood gases

$Pco_2$ is normal or low until terminal respiratory failure occurs. Alveolar–arterial $Po_2$ difference is abnormal at rest in the presence of extensive alveolar wall disease; dead space is increased.

### Exercise ventilation and gas exchange

Breathless patients with fibrosing lung conditions have an increased minute ventilation, usually because of increased dead space. Breathing tends to be shallow and rapid, consuming very little excess energy (Javaheri & Sicilian, 1992). Abnormal alveolar–arterial $Po_2$ difference is a hallmark of cryptogenic fibrosing alveolitis and severe forms of diffuse interstitial pulmonary fibrosis, but it is not, as is sometimes stated, invariably wider in exercise than at rest. A wide alveolar–arterial $Po_2$ difference is not invariably accompanied by desaturation: sometimes there is such severe hyperventilation that the oxyhaemoglobin level is maintained at the cost of a severe fall of arterial $Pco_2$ (Chapter 3).

When reading earlier papers, it is important to notice whether the arterial blood was sampled during exercise or after a period of stepping or leg raising. $Po_2$ falls after a period of hyperventilation at rest. Calculation suggests that if hyperventilation and exercise cease at the same time there may be a transient fall of $Po_2$, though this is not necessarily accompanied by an increase of alveolar–arterial difference. Post-hyperventilation states are easily recognised by low values of R, the respiratory exchange ratio, but this information is not always available. Arterial sampling after exercise does not, therefore, provide the same information as sampling during exercise.

### Respiratory muscle power

Allowing for lung volume abnormalities, maximal inspiratory and expiratory pressures are generally normal (de Troyer & Yernault, 1980).

### Distribution of ventilation and perfusion

Typically the whole alveolar volume is rapidly accessible to inspired gas except where there is concomitant emphysema. Measurements of residual volume and total lung capacity made during single breath tests of $TLco$ are on average the same as equilibration values or those obtained by body plethysmography (range $\pm 0.7$ litre).

## Extrinsic allergic alveolitis

Inhalation of antigenic organic dusts into the alveoli can cause allergic alveolitis. Farmer's lung is the best known, but there is a growing list of other hazards, notably avian proteins. Classically, dyspnoea, chest tightness, coughing and crackles are accompanied by a febrile response with a polymorphonuclear leucocytosis 8–48 hours after exposure, with spontaneous resolution. Precipitating IgG antibody to the offending agent adds weight to the diagnosis in some, but not all

of these syndromes, with frequent false positive and false negative findings.

The first few attacks may be followed by complete recovery, hastened by oral steroids (Kokkarinen, Tukainen & Terbo, 1992) Eventually some permanent bronchial or pulmonary damage usually develops. The presentation of sensitised domestic budgerigar owners and smallholders who are continually exposed to small amounts of faecal antigenic material is different, there being a tendency for the lung damage to progress insidiously without any dramatic episodes. Again, some permanent damage is the rule, but even after several months or years of symptoms, improvement may occur after removal of the source of the antigen.

Investigation of this problem consists of a baseline study, followed by a period of stabilisation of environment, until reasonably reproducible values for VC are obtained. Another series of detailed measurements is then made. If the patient recovers satisfactorily and is content to avoid the suspected hazard, it may be as well to let matters rest there. Steroids are usually given in this phase, and their withdrawal can be monitored in the same way. A further deliberate environmental challenge may be justified if the patient's recovery was rapid and complete when the offending agent was first withdrawn. Patients usually request this if they are sceptical of the suggested cause of their symptoms, or if there are pressing financial reasons for establishing the diagnosis beyond doubt. Otherwise, they may prefer to accept the diagnosis proposed and avoid the sensitising agent. The demonstration of antibodies, or the knowledge of other similar patients, may add weight to the diagnosis and reduce the need for further investigation.

Occasionally, the physician may ask the patient to submit to an environmental or laboratory challenge. This is justified when a previously unknown hazard is under investigation or when, by fractionation or purification of the antigen, there is a possibility that improvement of a manufacturing process might reduce the hazard to the working population and possibly to the users of the product. Such studies should be undertaken only by those who have studied challenge procedures in detail. Choosing appropriate measurements is important; paramount is the need to study only those subjects who have recovered virtually normal function and who are asymptomatic.

Challenges always carry some risk, although the likelihood of a reaction being significantly more severe than the previous one is much less for late or delayed reactions than for anaphylactoid reactions or bronchial asthma. Most referral centres do not undertake laboratory challenge at the request of either party solely for medico-legal reasons.

Acute attacks of extrinsic alveolitis are generally characterised by reduction of VC and TLC. $FEV_1/VC$ ratios of 75% or less are found, a high ratio being unusual. Alveolar–arterial $Po_2$ difference is widened, $Pco_2$ usually normal or low, $TLco$ reduced.

Inhalation challenge results in similar findings, the most useful test being VC, which is reduced by 15% or more in 95% of cases, accompanied by pyrexia (>37.2°C), leucocytosis (a rise of more than 2.5/fl) and a 15% decrease of maximal exercise ventilation. $TLco$ and lung volume changes are less sensitive (Hendrick *et al.*, 1980).

After several attacks, or long continued exposure, infection becomes the rule, with exacerbation of sputum and evidence of airflow obstruction superimposed on reduction of lung volume. Treatment directed against infection and residual alveolitis may produce modest improvements in sputum volume, VC and arterial oxygenation, often without significant effects on lung volumes and CO transfer.

## Cryptogenic fibrosing alveolitis

### Nomenclature

The first account of diffuse interstitial pulmonary fibrosis was by Hamman & Rich (1935, 1944). They described four patients with advanced, rapidly progressive disease who had severe dyspnoea, clubbing, cyanosis and fine rales. At postmortem, the lungs were severely fibrosed. Later, it was recognised that the disease could present in a chronic or insidious way. The appearances on lung biopsy were those of diffuse alveolar obliteration by fibrosis, but in some areas the alveoli appeared to be thickened by the presence of inflammatory cells as well as by fibrous tissue. The histological appearance varied from one part of the lung to another, but in general steroid responsiveness was related to the cellularity of the alveoli: as might be expected, the fibrosis was irreversible. Response to corticosteroids was found to be variable and difficult to predict, with a minority of patients appearing to improve. The overall prognosis is poor, with a mortality of about 50% at 5 years (Turner-Warwick, Burrows & Johnson, 1980; Rudd, Haslam & Turner-Warwick, 1981).

In 1965, Liebow, Steer & Billingsley described a condition which they called 'desquamative interstitial pneumonia' (DIP). This presented as a relatively acute illness with a dry cough, dyspnoea at rest or on exertion and numerous rales similar to those of diffuse pulmonary fibrosis. Chest radiographs, which were not always abnormal, showed the condition to be diffuse. The lungs histologically showed little fibrosis, the characteristic appearance being intra-alveolar exudation (erroneously called 'desquamation') of macrophages as well as an increase of type II alveolar cells within alveolar walls. Although it was recognised that this condition was in many ways similar to the Hamman-Rich type of diffuse interstitial pulmonary fibrosis, some clinicians in the USA found it convenient to retain Liebow's nomenclature, recognising two conditions – desquamative interstitial pneumonia (DIP), and 'usual' interstitial pneumonia (UIP). Bronchiolitis obliterans with organising pneumonia (BOOP), sometimes called cryptogenic organising pneumonia (COP), is also thought to be in this group of diseases. DIP and COP have a good prognosis, respond to steroids in many instances and may remit with little loss of function.

In the UK, many patients suffering from diffuse interstitial pulmonary fibrosis were referred to the Brompton Hospital where open lung biopsy was carried out. On the basis of these studies, Scadding concluded that all these histological appearances could coexist, forming a spectrum of disease of unknown cause which ranged from an active inflammatory process, with or without desquamation, to dense fibrosis (Scadding & Hinson, 1967). He proposed the widely accepted term 'fibrosing alveolitis' to describe this spectrum of disease. Since then, there have been numerous attempts at broadening the classification to take account of all the histological features of the condition.

### Similar disorders

Classical 'cryptogenic' fibrosing alveolitis may occur in association with a number of other immunological disorders, including chronic active hepatitis, renal tubular acidosis, mixed connective tissue disease and occasionally systemic lupus erythematosus. At least 5% of men with rheumatoid arthritis have a pulmonary condition which is indistinguishable histologically from the chronic form of the disease. This is similar histologically to rheumatoid alveolitis, but weakness and impairment of mobility changes the relationship between symptoms, clinical findings and lung function (Gorini *et al.*, 1990). Systemic sclerosis causes basal lung fibrosis which is histologically similar to the cryptogenic form (Harrison *et al.*, 1991), but presents with rather different symptoms. Asbestosis affects a proportion of those exposed to the fibres of asbestos, causing dense basal pulmonary fibrosis. This is described later; it resembles the cryptogenic variety, but with a typical dense pleural fibrosis which is unique to asbestosis.

### Presentation

Cryptogenic fibrosing alveolitis affects mainly men aged 40 to 70 years. The majority have smoked at some time. It presents typically with dyspnoea on exertion and a dry cough, usually arising insidiously but occasionally following a febrile illness resembling influenza. Fine basal crackles are heard at the end of inspiration in almost all cases. Clubbing of the fingers occurs in 60% of chronic cases. The chest X-ray shows changes which progress, but lung function cannot be predicted from the X-ray appearance. There may be no abnormality in as many as one case in three (Epler, McLoud & Gaensler, 1978). The earliest abnormality is loss of alveolar aeration, amounting to a ground glass shadowing usually concentrated at the bases. Later, these changes are covered by a reticulo-nodular or reticular pattern which suggests that the interlobular septa and

Table 8.1. *Lung function in cryptogenic fibrosing alveolitis*

| | |
|---|---|
| VC and TLC | Low |
| FRC | Low |
| RV | Low, except in smokers or with airflow obstruction |
| Static lung compliance | Reduced |
| TLco and TL/$V_A$ | Low |
| Alveolar–arterial $P_{O_2}$ difference | Wide: increases in exercise |
| $P_{CO_2}$ | Normal or low |
| Physiological dead space | Increased |
| Ventilatory requirement in exercise | Increased |
| Exercise tolerance | Usually limited by breathlessness at submaximal $O_2$ uptake |

areas of the lung are developing dense fibrosis. This may give way to generalised honeycombing – the development of cyst-like spaces 0.5–1 cm in diameter within the fibrotic regions. Multiple small nodules resembling sarcoidosis and changes concentrated in the upper zones are seen less frequently.

Histologically, the appearances are of inflammation and fibrosis without granuloma formation or vasculitis. The cellular component contains polymorphs, eosinophils and plasma cells as invariable features as well as macrophages and a few lymphocytes within the alveolar wall. Type II alveolar cells proliferate. There is an apparent increase of fibrillary collagen and sometimes of smooth muscle. Muscular pulmonary arteries are thickened in about 70% of cases.

### Relationship between lung function and pathology

The characteristic abnormalities of lung function found in this condition have been described on pp. 115–117 and in Table 8.1. Physiological tests are helpful in diagnosis as lung volumes, TLco and alveolar arterial $P_{O_2}$ in exercise are abnormal in the great majority of patients (Wright *et al.*, 1981; Risk, Epler & Gaensler 1984). Current

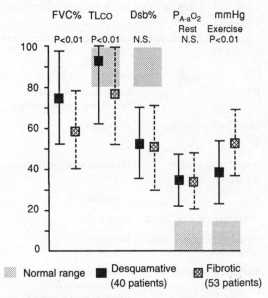

Fig. 8.3. Lung function at presentation in patients subsequently undergoing lung biopsy with a principally 'fibrotic' pattern of alveolitis and with 'desquamative' histology. Vital capacity was significantly lower in the patients with extensive fibrosis. (Redrawn from Carrington *et al.*, 1978, by permission of the *New England Journal of Medicine* (vol. 298, pp. 801–8, 1978).

smokers have similar low values of $FEV_1$, VC and TLco, but RV and TLC are increased. Ex-smokers differ very little from non-smokers (Schwartz *et al.*, 1991).

The clinical and pathological significance of abnormal pulmonary function studies have been studied over many years by Carrington and his colleagues (1978). They performed open lung biopsies and classified the patients into those with 'usual' (mural) and 'desquamative' interstitial pneumonia, according to the amount of intra-alveolar abnormality. Those cases severe enough to have progressed to the stage of honeycomb lung were excluded, if a pathological diagnosis of the underlying disease was impossible. As a result, the series contains useful information about the investigation of milder cases. Fig. 8.3 shows the range of abnormalities found at the first test performed on presentation.

Patients with desquamative histology were more likely to have normal FVC and TLC than those with a mural pattern. Airway obstruction, shown by $FEV_1/VC$ of less than 70%, occurred mainly in smokers with chronic bronchitis.

Single breath and steady state CO transfer and alveolar–arterial $Po_2$ difference, both at rest and in exercise, were always abnormal and were affected equally in the two types of disease. Deterioration of alveolar–arterial $Po_2$ difference after exercise was more likely to occur in usual than in desquamative disease. $Po_2$ and alveolar–arterial $Po_2$ difference do not invariably deteriorate during exercise in patients with fibrosing alveolitis, although they are more likely to do so in fibrotic cases. Patients with desquamative disease who improved markedly tended to be less hypoxaemic but nearly all desaturated during exercise. There was no correlation between prognosis and desaturation. This finding was probably influenced by the exclusion of patients with 'honeycomb lung' and contrasts with the claim made in an important contemporary review that arterial $Po_2$ always falls after exercise to an extent which correlates with the degree of fibrosis and with prognosis (Crystal *et al.*, 1976; Fulmer *et al.*, 1979) In fact some patients breathe inefficiently at rest, and a few patients hyperventilate during exercise to such an extent that the fall of $Pco_2$ and gross increase in ventilation limit exercise tolerance and the severity of the desaturation found.

It is possible to guess at loss of lung volume, fibrosis and overall likely functional impairment from large biopsy specimens. Exercise $Po_2$ and alveolar–arterial $Po_2$ difference correlated best with the pathologists' impressions. Loss of lung volume was predicted well by the pathologists in mural, but not in desquamative, disease. The likely explanation is that the areas of the lung which are less severely affected are more distensible when desquamative changes predominate (Carrington *et al.*, 1976; Fulmer *et al.*, 1979). In a smaller series, Chinet *et al.* (1990) confirmed that there was an overall correlation between their pathological scores and TLco, lung volumes and exercise gas exchange, but they were unable to distinguish between fibrosis and inflammation by means of physiological tests.

Cystic spaces are often present which resemble emphysema. They are lined with alveolar respiratory epithelium. These regions are visible on CT scans. They are accessible to inspired gas and do not constitute a poorly ventilated space, in contrast to the emphysema of smokers. Thus RV or alveolar volume measurements made during single breath tests give the same result as those during rebreathing and these spaces appear ventilated on radioactive scans. They may sometimes be poorly perfused, with an appearance of an unmatched defect mimicking pulmonary embolism.

It is difficult to assess patients over a long period of time because the clinical, radiological and physiological changes evolve separately. Combined scoring systems may help to evaluate the progress of the disorder during clinical trials (for example, Walters *et al.*, 1986).

## Sarcoidosis

Sarcoidosis is a multi-system disease. Pulmonary involvement may present with a non-productive cough, vague chest pains or shortness of breath, or may be discovered on a radiograph of the chest. There are non-caseating granulomata which, though concentrated in the upper zones, are widespread throughout the lungs and hilar nodes. The lesions are seen at biopsy and involve the bronchi, as well as the tissues more closely related to the alveoli and blood vessels. This accounts for the ease with which characteristic lesions are obtained from bronchial and lung biopsy.

Sarcoid granulomata heal either by resolution or by hyalinisation and scarring. In the lung, this process usually starts between 1 and 2 years after the development of the acute lesions (Colp, Park & Williams, 1976; Hillerdal *et al.*, 1984). Rapid progression to right heart failure is rare, probably occurring only in patients with pulmonary angiitis.

As well as granuloma formation and resolution, some tissue damage is mediated by T lymphocyte infiltration of the intercapillary portions of the alveolar walls. T lymphocytes constitute an abnormally high proportion of the cellular material obtained from alveolar lavage.

The lack of relationship between the density of the radiographic opacification and the degree of disability or pulmonary function disturbance makes assessment difficult. Carrington *et al.* (1976) suggested that the widespread granulomata are situated in the peribronchial zones in such a way as to cause little interference with gas exchange or with the mechanical properties of the lungs. There is a definite, though not close, correlation between functional disturbance and the degree of interstitial round cell inflammatory involvement of the alveolar walls. Extensive angiitis occurs infrequently and may be a cause of pulmonary hypertension. Huang *et al.* (1979) also showed the finding of normal lung function tests predicted that there would be little histological change, but in general the relationship between breathing tests and the severity of pathological changes in their samples was poor.

Conventional staging of the chest X-ray is helpful (Table 8.2; Miller *et al.*, 1980; Deremee, 1983). In addition, numerous tests including gallium scanning, magnetic resonance imaging, biopsy and cytological material obtained from broncho-alveolar lavage show that a significant number of patients without radiographic evidence of lung damage have evidence of alveolitis and of fibrosis (Keogh *et al.*, 1983) These too bear only a loose relationship to lung function results (Valeyre *et al.*, 1982).

### Pulmonary function tests

Abnormalities of pulmonary function are characteristically mild and overlap with the normal range. Severe disturbances are unusual and general caused by:

1. Severe fibrosis or honeycomb lung with cor pulmonale.
2. Pulmonary angiitis and pulmonary hypertension (Rizatto *et al.*, 1980).
3. Emphysema (about 15% develop extensive areas of 'vanishing lung', usually after some years, which is not invariably related to smoking: Sahetya *et al.*, 1980).
4. Stenosing fibrosis of the airways (Hadfield *et al.*, 1982).

In patients with diffuse lung changes, the most commonly demonstrable disturbances are

Table 8.2. *Pulmonary sarcoidosis*

| Radiological stage | Definition | Clinical syndromes |
|---|---|---|
| I | Hilar adenopathy | (a) *Acute hilar adenopathy with erythema nodosum*<br>Associated with circulating immune complexes. Arthralgia and systemic symptoms respond to anti-inflammatory agents. Good prognosis: 90–95% remit spontaneously |
|  |  | (b) *Asymptomatic*<br>Usually only found if a chest X-ray is taken as part of the investigation of non-pulmonary manifestation |
| II | Adenopathy + pulmonary infiltrates | (a) *Acute*<br>Chest illness, with cough and dyspnoea at rest or in exertion, sometimes simulating pneumonia. More common in black races |
|  |  | (b) *Subacute*<br>Insidious onset of exertional dyspnoea, sometimes with dry cough at rest or after exertion |
|  |  | (c) *Asymptomatic* |
| III | Pulmonary infiltrates ± fibrosis without adenopathy | (a) *Symptomatic*<br>These stages represent chronic sarcoidosis. Symptoms may be caused either by inflammation within the lungs, by bronchial obstruction or by irreversible fibrotic change |
| IV | Fibrosis | (b) *Asymptomatic*<br>Diagnosed radiologically, these stages may have caused insufficient damage to result in symptoms. Continued activity of the granulomatous process is difficult to determine |

- low VC;
- low TLC;
- low RV;
- FEV$_1$/VC ratio normal or reduced to about 60% when there is bronchial obstruction;
- low TLCO;
- normal or high TLCO/$V_A$;
- static lung compliance within the normal range;
- abnormal exercise ventilation and gas exchange.

Reduction of lung compliance or capillary blood volume (the oxygen-dependent portion of the single breath CO transfer) are regarded as signs of severe and probably irreversible pulmonary damage (Saumon *et al.*, 1976). Alveolar–arterial Po$_2$ difference is normal or only slightly widened at rest and usually remains constant during exercise (Sears 1980; Risk *et al.*, 1984). There is a poor correlation between TLCO and blood gases in sarcoidosis. A few patients with normal values of TLCO at rest have low exercise transfer factor, presumably because of damage to pulmonary capillaries which prevents them from dilating sufficiently to accommodate the increased blood flow. Increased exercise ventilation is the rule in dyspnoeic patients with sarcoidosis and occurs in some in some asymptomatic subjects (unpublished observations).

There is, as might be expected, a gradual decline of all measurements of pulmonary function when patients are classified according to radiological stage. The percentage of 'abnormal' cases also increases, but many patients with radi-

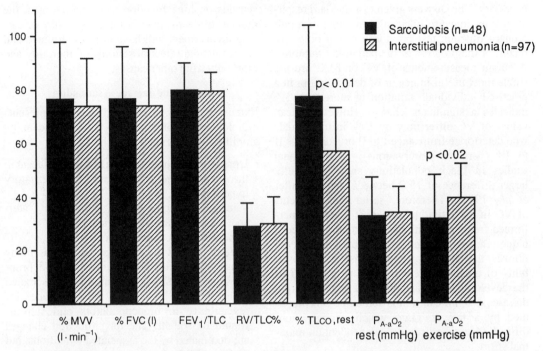

Fig. 8.4. Lung function at presentation in patients with histologically proven sarcoidosis and fibrosing alveolitis, excluding those with very severe fibrosis (honeycomb lung). In general, the functional impairment is greater in fibrosing alveolitis. (Data from Carrington *et al.*, 1976.)

ologically advanced diseases have only minor physiological abnormalities (Winterbauer & Hutchison 1980). The disturbance of pulmonary gas exchange in fibrotic sarcoidosis is less marked than in cryptogenic fibrosing alveolitis of comparable radiographic severity (Fig. 8.4).

### Monitoring of lung function

Although VC, TLco and lung volumes are often within normal limits in stage II sarcoidosis, on average these measurements are reduced by about 10–20%. In young patients, the tests often improve by a corresponding amount to values which are at the upper end of the normal range during remission.

Pulmonary function studies performed at presentation do not predict the outcome of treatment or of observation. Symptoms, radiographic

changes and reduction of lung volumes and gas transfer may be mild, moderate or severe in any combination. An exercise test is valuable when symptoms are out of proportion to the results of resting pulmonary function studies.

Having established, for an individual patient, the relationship between dyspnoea, radiographic change and pulmonary dysfunction at the outset, it is possible to obtain objective evidence of deterioration. When dyspnoea increases as a result of advancing pulmonary sarcoidosis, there is usually some deterioration in the appearances on radiograph, a fall of VC or TLco or combinations of all of these.

The most impressive manifestation of asymptomatic or mild stage II pulmonary sarcoidosis is the radiographic appearance, but it can be very difficult to assess progress on the chest X-ray. There may be considerable disagreement over the degree of change in a very densely affected film, or over the presence or absence of minor abnormalities. When fibrosis replaces extensive granulomatosis, the shadows become less dense and may appear to be improving when function is deteriorating. Other indicators are therefore necessary. The answers given to a standard respiratory questionnaire filled in at the time of a pulmonary function test provide a useful objective record of the progress of the patient's symptoms. Accurate measurements of VC or FVC are the single most useful indicator of deterioration: in a practised individual, variation of more than 5% indicates a significant change. However, mean values of VC differ only by 10% in individuals who deteriorate from stage I to II or from stage II to III (personal observations); cross-sectional studies in black populations show a slightly larger difference of 15% between stages (Miller et al., 1980). Therefore, serial measurements of VC in an individual are most helpful if performed frequently with careful attention to technique. Before any fall is attributed to sarcoid fibrosis, the physician should consider the possibility of an intercurrent respiratory infection or the development of asthma or seasonal allergic disease. A significant fall is sometimes accompanied by a fall of TLco which, though more difficult to standardise, is not dependent on maximal effort.

Objective measurement of the results of treatment needing a trial of corticosteroids because of dyspnoea is usually straightforward. Normally, there is relief of symptoms accompanied by an improvement in the chest X-ray and the expected increase of VC, TLco and TLC. When steroids are withdrawn, relapses are accompanied by deterioration of all the measurements towards their previous value. It is often supposed that a rise of TLco/$V_A$ or TLco alone is a sufficient indicator of improvement, but corticosteroids, which cause an increase of central blood volume, may perhaps cause a spurious increase of CO uptake; this requires investigation.

Whether or not to treat asymptomatic or irreversible sarcoidosis with corticosteroids remains uncertain because no prospective long-term controlled trials have been completed. Steroids suppress the inflammatory process, but there is no evidence to show that they prevent progression of the fibrosis in the lungs or elsewhere. Frequent, carefully performed measurements of VC and TLco, with occasional estimations of blood gases and exercise ventilation and gas exchange, will provide information about the possible benefits of

steroids on lung function. Any reduction in the number of deaths from respiratory failure or cardiac involvement will have to be determined and set against the effect of steroids on mortality and morbidity from other causes.

### Severe lung damage in sarcoidosis

Extensive, irreversible sarcoid (stage IV) presents radiologically in a number of ways. CT scanning amplifies the information on chest X-rays:

- Upper lobe contraction with fibrosis, adjacent to the upper mediastinum and compensatory hyperinflation.
- Widespread emphysema, sometimes interspersed with sheets of fibrotic tissue.
- Aspergillosis in a scarred area.
- Chronic airflow obstruction, which has many causes. These include emphysema and bronchostenosis. Asthma is commonly associated with sarcoid, however, and evidence for reversibility to bronchodilators and steroids should be sought. The lung function changes are dominated by the associated conditions, but TLC and FRC are usually lower than in uncomplicated asthma or emphysema because of the associated fibrosis.

Patients with chronic sarcoidosis tend to die at about 60 years of age (Wurm & Rosner, 1976). The short-term mortality was 4% in a series with a high number of black patients, who tend to suffer from aggressive forms of the disease. In Europe benign forms of the disease are seen and the population under study needs to be appreciated when reviewing the literature (Huang et al., 1980).

## Pneumoconioses: diseases caused by the inhalation of mineral dusts

Particles of 1–5 micrometres in diameter are deposited in the bronchi and lungs. Smaller particles mostly remain suspended in the air and are exhaled, while larger particles are deposited in the upper airways. Particles deposited in the bronchi are engulfed in mucus and moved outwards by the cilia. In the respiratory bronchioles they are phagocytosed by macrophages. Some of these find their way into the bronchi but many are impacted on the walls of the bronchioles, and some pass along the lymphatics to regional lymph nodes. Their fate depends partly on the toxicity of the dust for macrophages. Highly toxic substances such as silica and the silicate mixture, asbestos, cause breakdown of macrophages with liberation of lysozymes capable of invoking a local inflammatory reaction, with eventual dense fibrosis; this determines the fibrogenicity of a dust. Individual variation of immunological reactivity may play a part, as only 10–20% of those exposed are affected. The ease with which deposits of a dust can be detected on a chest X-ray depends also on its radiodensity. Some quite inert dusts, such as tin and iron, cause an impressive amount of radiological shadowing without any important physiological effects. Silicosis and coal-workers' pneumoconiosis are intermediate; multiple nodules may cause little disability in spite of their apparent profusion on the chest X-ray. Asbestos is the most toxic dust known, as well as being carcinogenic. Its fibres, $3 \times 10$ micrometres, are inhaled and deposited according to their narrower diameter, while the long straight fibres of crocidolite (South African blue asbestos, now banned in the UK) readily penetrate as far as the sub-pleural alveoli.

## Asbestosis

Asbestosis is pulmonary fibrosis induced by the inhalation of asbestos fibres. It is one of a group of asbestos-related pulmonary conditions, which comprise:

1. Asbestosis.
2. Recurrent pleural effusion and/or fibrosis (Chapter 9).
3. Pleural plaques (Chapter 9) and pleural pseudotumours.
4. Pleural and peritoneal mesothelioma.

Asbestosis is in many respects similar to cryptogenic fibrosing alveolitis. In its early stages the pulmonary changes are predominantly basal. Clinical and physiological manifestations may be more impressive than the chest X-ray. The latter is often normal, or affected by basal shadows, characteristically but not always with pleural changes (Rosenstock et al., 1988). The appearances in the lungs and pleura are more easily detected by CT. The development of basal crackles precedes clubbing, which is present in about three quarters of established cases, and the reduction of CO transfer.

Many asymptomatic patients have detectable abnormalities. Dyspnoea is initially accompanied by abnormalities of static lung compliance pulmonary gas exchange, with reduced CO transfer, abnormally wide alveolar–arterial $Po_2$ difference, and mild desaturation with increased ventilatory requirement in exercise (Jodoin et al., 1971; Murphy et al., 1978). Small airways are affected, with abnormalities of closing volume, single breath nitrogen slope and maximal expiratory flow–volume curves (Cohen, Adasczik & Cohen, 1984). The changes are much more marked in smokers and allowance must be made for this (Sue et al., 1985). As fibrosis progresses, VC and maximum voluntary ventilation are not greatly reduced (Barnhart et al., 1988).

The pathophysiology of the disease is essentially the same as that of slowly progressive cryptogenic fibrosing alveolitis (Tukiainen et al., 1978). It is usually unresponsive to corticosteroids, although there is evidence of acute inflammatory activity histologically and desquamative disease may occur (Freed et al., 1991). The condition may remain static for many years, but tends to progress even after withdrawal from the hazardous environment, with varying degrees of disability.

Carcinoma of the bronchus is the most common cause of the death of patients with asbestosis, especially among smokers.

Pleural disease is discussed in Chapter 9.

## Coal-workers' pneumoconiosis and silicosis

The pneumoconioses formerly suffered by miners should disappear in civilised countries, but they remain important in many parts of the world. They illustrate the contribution of physiology to epidemiology, to clinical evaluation and to medicolegal practice. Silicosis and coal-workers' pneumoconiosis occur in simple and complicated forms. The main pathological feature of simple coal-workers' pneumoconiosis (CWP) is the coal macule, an aggregate of dust-laden macrophages with surrounding inflammatory tissue and fibrosis, in contact with respiratory bronchioles. Some alveolar wall destruction near the macule is commonly present (Heppleston, 1972). Descriptions of the pathology of the condition have varied from one geographical region to another, perhaps because of the small number of pathologists interested in the minutiae of the condition and perhaps because of variations in the composition of coal dust. Radiologically, these appear as multiple nodules, appearing initially in the middle and upper zones of the plain chest X-ray, but becoming quite profuse. Classification of the lesions according to size and profusion is now standard (International Labour Office, 1980). To simplify, there are three main categories:

1. Limited to part of the lung.
2. Involving the whole lung field.
3. Confluent.

CWP may become complicated by progressive massive fibrosis. Massive confluent lesions 5 cm or more in diameter disfigure the X-ray and are associated with significant dyspnoea. They lead to hypoxaemia, pulmonary hypertension and respiratory failure (Fernie et al., 1983).

Silicosis is a more aggressive condition. The nodules are softer and there is a greater inflammatory component. The hilar nodes are often enlarged and surrounded by a rim of calcification; the pleura may be thickened. Diffuse interstitial pulmonary fibrosis or massive fibrosis may occur. There is an increased risk of pulmonary tuberculosis. Occupations at risk, unless extreme measures to extract dust are taken, include:

- Mining of precious metals, tin, copper, graphite, mica, anthracite.
- Quarrying and dressing of slate, granite, sandstone.
- Road drilling.
- Pottery and ceramics.
- Boiler scaling.
- Grinding (new techniques avoid silica).

Silicosis tends to cause more disability than CWP, but many of the generalisations which follow about respiratory function apply to both conditions.

There is good correlation between the radiographic category of CWP and the measurement of dust and metals within the lung (Rossiter, 1972). Pathologists experienced in looking at lung biopsies of patients with diffuse interstitial pulmonary fibrosis were able to predict the functional status of patients with silicosis remarkable accurately, taking account of the extent of the generalised fibrotic reaction. In contrast, there is remarkably little correlation between radiographic category and impairment of VC and TLco, even when populations exposed to uniform types of dust are studied (Cochrane, 1976; Parkes, 1982). This has led to the supposition in some influential quarters that CWP, at any rate, is a radiographic disease, and that disability when it occurs is caused by airflow obstruction, chronic bronchitis and emphysema (Brooks, 1981). However, the loss of lung density caused by emphysema alters the X-ray appearances, by making the nodules look smaller, and makes the diagnosis of diffuse pulmonary fibrosis more difficult (Cockroft et al., 1982a). There is little doubt that occupational exposure to coal predisposes to emphysema (Seaton 1982a, b; Cockroft et al., 1982b; Ruckley et al., 1984).

The finding of a slightly reduced mean single breath TLco among those with lesions smaller than 1.5 mm and not among those with lesions 1.5–3 mm (Frans, Veriter & Brasseur, 1975) may be due to the presence of paraseptal emphysema. In this study there were no major abnormalities of airways resistance or static compliance but conflicting results have been reported (Legg, Cotes & Bevan, 1983).

The great majority of miners used to smoke, so the incidence of chronic bronchitis and small airways disease attributed to occupation alone is difficult to assess. In a study by the National Coal Board, $FEV_1$ declined in English miners exposed to dust by an average of 0.1 litre per year, greater than expected and slightly greater than the rate attributable to smoking (Rogan et al., 1973). No apparent interaction was found in this study between cigarette smoking and dust exposure. These findings point to a significant contribution of occupational exposure to disturbances of function, but chronic bronchitis of this overall severity is not grossly disabling. The rapid decline of $FEV_1/VC$ among smokers is caused by a few patients with severe disease (Chapter 6). If this were also true of miners, then the frequency of severe respiratory failure from this cause would be considerable. There are theoretical reasons for not extrapolating from one condition to the other, since there are subtle physiological differences which distinguish miners' bronchitis from smokers' bronchitis (Morgan, 1978). There is general agreement that the bronchitis of dusty occupations is independent of radiological category, and occurs in miners without pneumoconiosis to the same extent as those who are eligible for compensation. However, non-smoking miners do not have demonstrable abnormalities of lung volumes and expiratory flow rates (Morgan et al., 1972; Hankinson et al., 1977). It is now appreciated that mucus hypersecretion is not a precursor of chronic airflow obstruction and many environmental factors as well as smoking contribute to ventilatory impairment, which is frequently absent or trivial in simple pneumoconiosis (Parkes, 1982).

Studies of disabled miners have shown that it is usually possible to identify physiological abnormalities which can account for the dypsnoea (Sadoul, 1975). Gaensler et al. (1972) tested a number of patients with varying degrees of disability, drawn from all categories of simple silicosis. Those who were not breathless mostly had normal ventilatory capacity, and breathed normally in exercise. The majority of their breathless patients with silicosis had a reduced ventilatory capacity (MVV), and a correspondingly increased ventilatory requirement. Widening of the alveolar–arterial $Po_2$ difference was almost invariable. Others have confirmed that most breathless patients with CWP and silicosis have reduced ventilatory capacity, but when this is not found, measurements of ventilation and blood gases in exercise may reveal the respiratory abnormality (Ulmer & Reichel, 1972). Applicants for compensation as a group claim to be more breathless in relation to their $FEV_1$ than participants in research studies, but the difference is not great and probably accounted for by a few individuals (Cotes, 1975). In general, ventilatory tests predict maximal oxygen uptake very poorly in these subjects

and exercise testing is helpful (Cotes, Zejda & King, 1988).

As in sarcoidosis, CO transfer factor is very variable in asymptomatic patients with silicosis. In one group of 13 patients who underwent percutaneous lower lobe lung biopsy, transfer defects were found in those with alveolar wall involvement (Tukiainen et al., 1978). In general, normal lower lobe histology or scattered granulomata alone were found when TLco was normal. Reduction of VC was associated with interstitial fibrosis and with pleural involvement. These findings contrasted markedly with those from patients exposed to asbestos, or a mixture containing asbestos, in whom reduction of TLco was the rule, again illustrating the importance of the diffuse nature of the interstitial thickening in causing defects of CO transfer. Such thickening is found in the majority of patients with asbestosis and fibrosing alveolitis and in a minority of patients with silicosis and sarcoidosis. Mean values of VC and TLco in such patients are usually at the lower end of the predicted range, so it is not strictly accurate to say that scattered nodular lesions have no effect on pulmonary function; rather, they have less effect than might be expected from their profusion on the chest X-ray.

In conclusion, a profusion of radiologically dense pulmonary nodules situated near the terminal airways may cause remarkably little loss of pulmonary reserve, although they cause identifiable alterations to sensitive tests designed to detect involvement of the bronchi. When symptoms occur, they may be caused by progressive airways obstruction or by diffuse fibrosis, poorly correlated with the severity of the X-ray changes. These may be detected by the presence of a reduced ventilatory capacity and abnormal blood gases. It is not known whether the presence of pulmonary fibrosis obscures the physiological changes of pulmonary emphysema, but emphysema makes the changes of fibrosis more difficult to see on the X-ray. Detailed studies are required to delineate the nature of the physiological and structural abnormality in any individual patient; it is unwise to report that pulmonary function is normal on the basis of screening tests (spirometry, lung volumes and TLco) alone if the patient complains of dyspnoea.

## Miscellaneous chronic lung diseases affecting the alveoli

### Conditions leading to 'honeycomb lung'

Cryptogenic fibrosing alveolitis and sarcoidosis are the commonest disorders which lead to the end-stage condition characterised radiographically and pathologically by a network of cysts which is aptly described as honeycomb lung. Several rare diseases may lead to the same condition.

#### Eosinophilic granuloma (histiocytosis X, Hand-Schüller-Christian disease)

The lungs may be involved in addition to the more characteristic deposits in bone and elsewhere, or they may be the only site affected. Small airways and lung parenchyma are affected, with severe reduction of TLco (Powers, Askin & Cresson, 1984).

#### Lymphangioleiomyomatosis

Smooth muscle tissue invading and obstructing pulmonary and other lymphatic channels, and thought to arise from uterine rests results in the radiographic appearance of widespread reticulation, sometimes complicated by chylous effusions and ascites (Dishner et al., 1984).

#### Tuberous sclerosis, neurofibromatosis

In these conditions, crackles are often absent. They cause reduction of TLco, and later, reduction of VC. TLC may fall, but in some instances it is normal and RV is high, indicating that some of the cystic spaces may behave like emphysematous bullae. Hypoxaemia is generally mild until a late stage, and desaturation during exercise is variable. In the later stages of their progression, airflow obstruction may predominate. Cor pulmonale generally follows, but these diseases follow a slow and unpredictable course over many years.

#### Imperfect resolution of pneumonia and adult respiratory distress syndrome (ARDS)

Return of VC and lung volumes to normal is the rule, but severe viral pneumonia and ARDS tend to resolve with some impairment of TLco

(Lakshimirayan, Stanford & Petty, 1976; Gea et al., 1988). Previously healthy subjects are not generally limited by these changes, but those with lung disease may experience permanent deterioration of their breathlessness.

### Radiotherapy

Localised radiotherapy to part of the lungs has the same effect. The patient may or may not notice the acute phase of radiation pneumonia, which occurs about 6–12 weeks after treatment. During this phase symptoms and signs of inflammation (crackles, rapid breathing at rest) are present, but these tend to improve with clearing of the chest radiograph. Second courses, whole lung irradiation, higher than conventional doses or the addition of chemotherapeutic regimes which potentiate the effects of irradiation may result in progressive fibrosis with reduction of VC and a striking increase of pulmonary dead space. Hypoxaemia is a late feature but effort tolerance is limited. The symptoms have a rather variable course over the ensuing 5 years, but may be accepted as an inevitable loss of effort tolerance or become apparent because of the development of another respiratory problem such as acute infection.

### Malignant disease

Four types of malignant disease masquerade as diffuse pulmonary damage:

1. Alveolar cell carcinoma of the bronchus.
2. Carcinomatous lymphangitis. Progressive dyspnoea is accompanied by widespread radiographic changes, crackles and cyanosis. Lung volumes are reduced, generally without airflow obstruction, and there is hypoxaemia with hyperventilation.
3. Lymphatic leukaemia, pseudolymphoma, macroglobulinaemia. The alveolar walls and spaces may be infiltrated by malignant cells with impairment of lung volumes, CO transfer and arterial oxygenation.
4. Multiple metastases. Large 'cannonball' metastases have little effect on pulmonary function until they are very large, and then tend to behave as if they had simply replaced lung

tissue, with reduction of VC and little effect on pulmonary gas exchange. Multiple small metastases may mimic the inflammatory or infiltrative disorders or may cause pulmonary vascular occlusion.

### Alveolar proteinosis

This condition is recognised by apparent exudation of PAS-positive, proteinaceous material into the alveolar spaces. The material is probably released by broken-down type II alveolar cells. Progressive dyspnoea is accompanied by dense white confluent shadowing on the chest X-ray. Lung volumes, CO transfer and oxygen saturation deteriorate, with substantial areas of zero ventilation–perfusion ratio (anatomical shunt). The condition responds to alveolar lavage, and partial recovery of pulmonary function may be expected (Rogers *et al.*, 1978).

## Theoretical and historical aspects of the physiology of DIPF

### Reduced 'diffusing capacity for oxygen' and the syndrome of alveolar-capillary block

The concept of alveolar-capillary block was presented in 1951, shortly after the technique of repeated blood gas analysis became available with the introduction of indwelling needles and the measurement of $PCO_2$ and $PO_2$ by Riley's bubble method. It is a classic example of the seductive effect of an imaginative hypothesis presented in elegant prose. The idea was that in mild cases of pulmonary fibrosis there was often no reduction of the maximum breathing capacity. There was also thought to be uniform distribution of inspired gas throughout the alveoli, which in fact is usually not the case. The conclusion was that disease at the alveolar level could be demonstrated by a widening of the alveolar–arterial $PO_2$ difference, caused by imperfect equilibration of alveolar and arterial $PO_2$, because thickening of the alveolar walls constituted a barrier to the diffusion of gases. The finding of a normal $PCO_2$ was explained by the greater solubility, and therefore higher diffusivity, of $CO_2$. The idea was subsequently discredited for reasons which were also based on imperfect knowledge, so a detailed examination of the arguments is rewarding.

Alveolar-capillary block was defined as 'a syndrome of alterations of the pulmonary diffusing surface [causing] . . . a reduction of the oxygen diffusing capacity of the lungs . . . The term "alveolar-capillary block" is tentatively offered as it describes the essential histologic as well as the physiologic features' (Austrian *et al.*, 1951). This classic paper describes twelve patients with a variety of diffuse lung diseases. They were selected because they had in common a reduction of the oxygen diffusing capacity of the lungs (Lilienthal *et al.*, 1946) estimated by a method (described later) in which arterial $PO_2$ is measured while the patient breathes air, and again breathing 12% $O_2$. The majority had normal measurements of maximal breathing capacity. VC and TLC were reduced, and in most RV/TLC was normal. Ventilation–perfusion relationships were abnormal, with an increased venous admixture and physiological dead space in the majority, but $N_2$ wash-out was not grossly impaired; $PCO_2$ was normal or low. It was emphasised that arterial $O_2$ saturation was normal at rest breathing air in most of the patients, but fell in the minute after recovery from exercise to below 90% in all the patients who were able to perform the test. (One patient improved and did not desaturate on a second occasion.) Ventilation was increased at rest and in exercise and ventilatory reserve was reduced.

The concept of defective diffusion as a cause of arterial hypoxaemia in patients with thickened alveolar septa was intellectually satisfying. However, Staub, Bishop & Forster (1962) calculated that the septa would have to be very thick indeed to cause measurable alveolar–arterial $PO_2$ differences at rest and concluded on theoretical grounds that ventilation–perfusion imbalance must be the predominant problem in patients with fibrosing alveolitis. In 1962, Finley, Swensen & Comroe published a series of studies in twelve further patients with diffuse lung fibrosis, in which they identified areas of low ventilation–perfusion ratio of sufficient magnitude to account for the arterial blood gases. Their patients were very similar to those originally described, with almost identical mean values of lung volumes, $PCO_2$, arterial oxygen saturation and dead space. Several had abnormal single breath $N_2$ plateaus, pointing to uneven ventilation. Their interpretation was based mainly, however, on a technique designed to measure the fraction of the cardiac output which perfuses a slowly ventilated compartment (Finley, 1961). Alveolar $P_{O_2}$ and $P_{N_2}$ were measured repeatedly while the subjects breathed pure oxygen. A delay of denitrogenation of the lungs identified a slowly ventilated alveolar space, while any further delay in the rise of arterial $P_{O_2}$ to the level in the alveoli was attributed to the fraction of the cardiac output distributed to the poorly ventilated, rather than the well ventilated portion of the lung. During quiet breathing, the poorly ventilated region occupies about 40% of the normal lung, but its perfusion is appropriately matched. In the patients studied, the perfusion to the poorly ventilated region was 4–8 times what it should have been to achieve perfectly even distribution. Measured arterial $O_2$ saturations matched exactly those predicted from the results of the wash-in curves during oxygen breathing. It was, therefore, concluded that the imperfect distribution of ventilation and perfusion accounted for the arterial hypoxaemia found in these patients. The authors went on to discuss the likely effects of uneven distribution of compliance on pulmonary ventilation, and made the point that theoretically even the most extreme thickening of the alveolar septa would be unlikely to cause a measurable alveolar–arterial $P_{O_2}$ difference attributable to a diffusion disequilibrium at rest.

This analysis was gradually accepted, and for a while textbooks stated that the hypoxaemia of diffuse lung fibrosis was caused by ventilation–perfusion mismatching and not by a barrier to diffusion. Other studies confirmed the presence of uneven ventilation in these patients. In 1976, Wagner, West and their colleagues studied a similar series of patients using multiple inert gas elimination (Chapter 14). They concluded that the hypoxaemia of these subjects at rest was attributable to ventilation–perfusion mismatching, but that $P_{O_2}$ was lower than would be predicted from an analysis of inert gas transfer in some patients during exercise. They concluded that there must be a significant gradient between the alveolar $P_{O_2}$ and the $P_{O_2}$ of the blood leaving the lung, in other words a diffusion defect: about 20% of the total

alveolar–arterial $P_{O_2}$ difference during exercise in patients with fibrosing alveolitis is attributable to a difference between mean alveolar and end-capillary $P_{O_2}$.

Looking back over the arguments which have spanned 40 years it is remarkable that so much confusion has arisen. The patients reported by Austrian *et al.* and by Finley *et al.* are almost identical. In each case, they employed methods published in separate papers and hardly ever used again. The reason for the difference in the interpretation of their findings is simply that Riley's three-compartment analysis is very insensitive to the presence of areas of moderately low ventilation–perfusion ratio, and the resulting 'venous admixture' therefore appeared to be trivial. The two-compartment analysis used by Finley *et al.* is more sensitive to this type of abnormality.

Looking again at the original description of the 'alveolar-capillary block syndrome', its conclusions are not far short of the mark. Emphasis is laid on the lack of resting desaturation in all but the most severe cases. Austrian *et al.* wrote 'The low diffusing capacity may either be due to a reduction of the total area of the alveolar membrane which is available for the diffusion of gases, or to a reduction in permeability of this membrane per unit area, or to both. The observation of rather widespread thickening of the alveolar capillary septa, suggests that the reduction in permeability per unit area is the major reason for the low diffusing capacity'. In the next paragraph the authors pointed out that theoretically, the lowered diffusing capacity would not be expected to cause important arterial hypoxaemia at rest breathing air, and suggested that the presence of arterial desaturation during exercise might be caused by a failure of the area for $O_2$ exchange to increase in the normal manner. These concepts are still standard teaching today.

### Diffusing capacity calculated from alveolar–arterial $P_{O_2}$ difference during hypoxia

The contribution of venous admixture to the alveolar–arterial $P_{O_2}$ difference is calculated from the results of the analysis of gas pressures in blood and expired air analysis sampled during the breathing of room air (Chapter 3). The alveolar–arterial $P_{O_2}$ difference at low inspired $O_2$ should fall if there is no change in the distribution of ventilation–perfusion ratios in the lung, because the dissociation curve for $O_2$ in whole blood is much steeper at low $P_{O_2}$ – in other words, there is a small change of $P_{O_2}$ when considerable volumes of oxygen are added to or removed from the arterial blood. On the other hand, the speed of uptake of oxygen across the alveolar membrane and into the red cells is reduced because the $P_{O_2}$ difference between the alveolar gas and red cells is reduced. Diffusion limitation of oxygen uptake can, theoretically, occur under these conditions, resulting in a difference between $P_{O_2}$ in the alveolar gas and the end of the pulmonary capillary.

The calculation of $O_2$ diffusing capacity is more difficult than that of CO diffusing capacity. The equation

$$\text{Dgas} = \text{uptake of gas/alveolar-mean capillary pressure difference} \quad (8.1)$$

is more easily solved for CO because capillary $P_{CO}$ is assumed to be zero and constant. The mean of the changing $P_{O_2}$ in the capillary was derived in Riley's method by stepwise integration calculating the rise of $P_{O_2}$ along the capillary as with progressive oxygen uptake. This can be solved graphically, but assumptions are needed about the shape of the $O_2$ dissociation curve and mixed venous $O_2$ content.

The $O_2$ diffusing capacity was never measured very much. Apart from the formidable difficulty experienced by those without mathematical training in understanding it, it was not easy for the patient, and required arterial puncture. There were moreover some serious objections to the assumptions on which it was based:

1. Breathing hypoxic gas mixtures would certainly be expected to alter the distribution of ventilation and perfusion in normal lungs, though this would not necessarily be so in patients with severely damaged lungs, in whom measurements of gas transfer are remarkably reproducible.
2. The presence of severe disturbances of ventilation and perfusion affects gas transfer, as does the uneven distribution of diffusion capacity.

Therefore, although estimates of whole lung diffusing capacity give an indication of the maximum capacity of the lung to exchange gas, and are therefore useful, they do not actually measure diffusion limitation at the alveolar membrane. As CO transfer was found to yield the same information as the $O_2$ diffusing capacity, at the price of much less effort, the latter was soon abandoned. Measurements of the '$O_2$ diffusing capacity' were only satisfactory as crude indicators of the whole lung gas transfer analogous to CO transfer factor. Several attempts have been made to extend the approach using isotopes of oxygen, but no analysis of whole lung gas transfer based on simple models stands up to rigorous analysis (Piiper & Scheid, 1980).

## Pathophysiology of the 'restrictive ventilatory defect'

The classification of disturbances of lung mechanics into restrictive and obstructive was introduced by Baldwin, Cournand & Richards (1948, 1949).

It is usually supposed that the thickening of the alveolar walls leads to a reduction of lung compliance, because the stiff lung tissue should, theoretically, need more negative intrathoracic pressure to achieve a given volume expansion. Gibson & Pride (1977) suggested that it is more accurate to consider the lungs of patients with advanced fibrosing alveolitis as 'shrunken'; that is, they consist of a mixture of obliterated alveoli which hardly aerate at all during inspiration, and alveoli which have essentially a normal distensibility but are subjected to abnormally great distending pressures. Expiratory quasi-static pressure–volume curves were obtained in eight patients with reduced TLC. As expected, these curves were flat when volumes were expressed in litres or as a percentage of predicted normal (Fig. 2.7). However, when lung volume was expressed as a percentage of the measured TLC, only three patients fell outside the normal range (Fig. 2.6). Small lungs have a lower static compliance throughout their range of expiration than large lungs: this is reflected in the lower normal values of compliance in children and small animals.

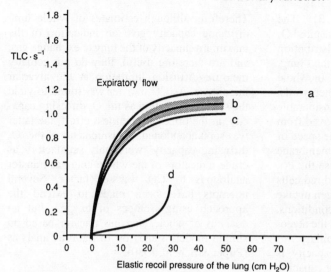

Fig. 8.5. Expiratory airflow (expressed as total lung capacity per second) plotted against elastic recoil pressure. The stippled area describes the relationship in normal subjects. Curve a, fibrosing alveolitis with stiff lungs. Curve b, fibrosing alveolitis: loss of alveoli with preservation of the airways. Curve c, fibrosing alveolitis with loss of airways as well as of alveoli. Curve d, emphysema. Expressing flow as the fraction of the total lung capacity exhaled in one second ($TLC \cdot s^{-1}$) corrects for lung size and provides an index of airway function. At the same recoil pressure, a larger lung should deliver a higher flow rate. (Based on data from Gibson & Pride, 1977.)

The analysis is made more difficult by the fact that inspiratory muscles are at a greater mechanical advantage at mid-inspiration than at full inspiration. At TLC, a normal adult can only suck to a pressure of -30 cm $H_2O$ (-4 kPa), but at 2 litres below TLC, pleural pressures of -70 cm $H_2O$ (-9 kPa) are achieved. The patients with fibrosing alveolitis were able, therefore, to subject their least affected alveoli to about twice the distending force when they inspired fully: consequently, ratio of measured to predicted TLC underestimated the degree of loss of lung volume by shrinkage. Gibson & Pride allowed for this by plotting intrapleural pressure against a theoretical maximal lung volume, obtained by applying an exponential extrapolation to the volume–pressure curves, which corresponds closely to the TLC measured by removing the lung from the chest and pumping it up. This idea is more or less the same as expressing lung volume as a percentage of that expected at any reasonable distending (pleural) pressure, for example, 25 cm $H_2O$ (3.5 kPa); applying this calculation to the results of the compliance curves in normal subjects and patients with fibrosing alveolitis, 4 out of 8 patients lay outside the normal range, though not greatly. The conclusion was that in about one half of patients with advanced fibrosing alveolitis, the restrictive ventilatory defect is explicable by obliteration of alveoli, the remainder of the alveoli having more or less normal distensi-

bility. The true proportion may be higher (Gibson et al., 1979). Some patients have normal lung distensibility and in many such patients large cystic spaces are present, especially in the upper lobes. These may be 'scar emphysema', but radioisotope scanning shows that they are well ventilated and poorly perfused and are the most important single cause of misleading lung scans. Lung volume measurements, especially TLC and FRC, correlate well with compliance measurements. The latter are unlikely to be abnormal in patients with well-preserved VC. Inspired gas is rapidly distributed throughout the lung in patients with diffuse pulmonary fibrosis.

Airway function is also impaired in some patients with diffuse pulmonary fibrosis. High rates of flow are usually found throughout forced expiration (Fig. 8.2), but flow rate is often reduced in relation to elastic recoil pressure (transpulmonary pressure) (Fig. 8.5). This could be caused by:

1. Obliteration of airways.
2. Functional loss of airways in association with fibrosed lung units (Fig. 8.6). This effect can be allowed for by expressing expiratory flow as TLC per second.
3. Concomitant emphysema or airway narrowing.

It may be concluded that there is a distinctive syndrome of disordered physiology which is typi-

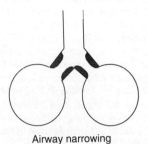

Airway narrowing

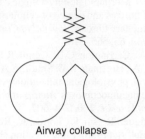

Airway collapse

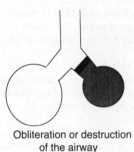

Obliteration or destruction
of the airway

Fig. 8.6. Reasons for reduction of maximum expiratory flow rate in relation to lung recoil (Fig. 8.5). For explanation see text.

fied by advanced cases of cryptogenic fibrosing alveolitis. Lungs are 'stiff', often because of shrinkage rather than because of thickening of alveolar walls. Impairment of gas exchange may sometimes precede abnormalities of lung mechanics. The classical descriptions of this syndrome laid emphasis on the importance of the thickened alveolar walls which were supposed to restrict expansion and impair diffusion between the alveoli and the pulmonary capillaries. These have been superseded: not all patients have a restrictive ventilatory defect and the 'block' between the alveoli and the pulmonary capillaries is unimportant compared with their widespread destruction.

## References

Austrian R., McClement, J.H., Renzetti, A.D., Donald, K.W., Riley, R.L. & Cournand, A. (1951). Clinical and physiological features of some types of pulmonary disease with impairment of pulmonary diffusion: the alveolar capillary block syndrome. *American Journal of Medicine*, **11**, 667–685.

Baldwin, E. de F., Cournand, A. & Richards, D.W. (1948). Pulmonary insufficiency. I. Physiological classification, clinical methods of analysis, standard values in normal subjects. *Medicine*, **27**, 243–278.

Baldwin, E. de F., Cournand, A. & Richards, D.W. (1949). Pulmonary insufficiency. II. A study of 39 cases of pulmonary fibrosis. *Medicine*, **28**, 1–25.

Barnhart, S., Hudson, L.D., Mason, S.E., Pierson, D.J. & Rosenstock, L. (1988). Total lung capacity: an insensitive measure of impairment in patients with asbestosis and COPD. *Chest*, **93**, 299–302.

Becklake, M.R., Fournier Massey, G., McDonald, J.C., Siemiatycki, J. & Rossiter, C.E. (1970). Lung function in relation to chest radiographic changes in Quebec asbestos workers. In *Pneumoconiosis: Proceedings of the 1969 International Conference, Johannesburg*, ed. H.A. Shapiro, Cape Town: O.U.P.

Bellomo, R., Finlay, M., McLaughlin, P & Tai, E. (1991). Clinical spectrum of cryptogenic organising pneumonia. *Thorax*, **46**, 554–558.

Brooks, S.M. (1981). An approach to patients suspected of having an occupational pulmonary disease. *Clinics in Chest Medicine*, **2**, 171–178.

Carrington, C.B., Gaensler, E.A., Coutu, R.E., Fitzgerald, M.X. & Gupta, R.G. (1978). Natural history and treated course of usual and desquamative interstitial pneumonia. *New England Journal of Medicine*, **298**, 801–808.

Carrington, C.B., Gaensler, E.A., Mikos, J.P., Schachter, A.W., Burke, G.W. & Goff, A.M. (1976). Structure and function in sarcoidosis. *Annals of the New York Academy of Sciences*, **278**, 265–282.

Chinet, T., Joubert, F., Dusser, D., Danel, C., Chrétien, J. & Huchon, G.J. (1990). Effects of inflammation and fibrosis on pulmonary function in diffuse lung fibrosis. *Thorax*, **45**, 675–678.

Cochrane, A.L. (1976). An epidemiologist's view of

the relationship between simple pneumoconiosis and morbidity and mortality. *Proceedings of the Royal Society of Medicine*, **69**, 12–14.

Cockroft, A., Berry, G., Cotes, J.E. & Lyons, J.P. (1982*a*). The shape of small opacities and lung function in coalworkers. *Thorax*, **37**, 765–769.

Cockroft, A., Wagner, J.C., Ryder, R., Seal, R.M.E., Lyons, J.P. & Andersson, N. (1982*b*). Post mortem study of emphysema in coalworkers and non-coalworkers. *Lancet,* **ii**, 600–603.

Cohen, B.M., Adasczik, A & Cohen, E.M. (1984). Small airways changes in workers exposed to asbestos. *Respiration*, **45**, 296–302.

Colp, C., Park, S.S. & Williams, M.H. (1976). Pulmonary function follow-up of 120 patients with sarcoidosis. *Annals of the New York Academy of Sciences*, **278**, 301–307.

Cotes, J.E. (1975). Assessment of disablement due to impaired respiratory function. *Bulletin Européen Physiopathologie Respiratoire*, **11**, 210P-217P.

Cotes, J.E., Zejda, J., & King, B. (1988). Lung function impairment as a guide to exercise limitation in work-related lung disorders. *American Review of Respiratory Disease*, **137**, 1089–1093.

Crystal, R.G., Fulmer, J.D., Roberts, W.C., Moss, M.L., Line, B.R. & Reynolds, H.Y. (1976). Idiopathic pulmonary fibrosis: clinical, histiologic, radiographic, physiologic, scintigraphic, cytologic and biochemical aspects. *Annals of Internal Medicine*, **85**, 769–788.

Deremee, R.A. (1983). The roentgenographic staging of sarcoidosis. *Chest*, **83**, 128–133.

de Troyer, A. & Yernault, J-C. (1980). Inspiratory muscle force in normal subjects and patients with interstitial lung disease. *Thorax*, **35**, 92–100.

Dishner, W., Cordasco, E.M., Blackburn, J., Demeter, S., Levin, H. & Carey, W.D. (1984). Pulmonary lymphangioleiomyomatosis. *Chest*, **85**, 796–799.

Epler, G.R., McLoud, T.C., Gaensler, E.A., Mikos, J.P. & Carrington, C.B. (1978). Normal chest roentgenograms in chronic diffuse infiltrative lung disease. *New England Journal of Medicine*, **298**, 934–939.

Epler, G.R., Saber, F.A. & Gaensler, E.A. (1980). Determination of severe impairment (disability) in interstitial lung disease. *American Review of Respiratory Disease*, **121**, 647–659.

Fernie, J.M., Douglas, A.N., Lamb, D. & Ruckley, V.A. (1983). Right ventricular hypertrophy in a . group of coalworkers. *Thorax*, **38**, 436–442.

Finley, T.R. (1961). The determination of uneven pulmonary blood flow from the arterial oxygen tension during nitrogen washout. *Journal of Clinical Investigation*, **40**, 1727–1734.

Finley, T.R., Swenson, E.W. & Comroe, J.H. (1982).

The causes of arterial hypoxaemia at rest in patients with 'alveolar-capillary block syndrome'. *Journal of Clinical Investigation*, **41**, 618–622.

Frans, A., Veriter, C. & Brasseur, L. (1975). Pulmonary diffusing capacity for carbon monoxide in simple coalworkers' pneumoconiosis. *Bulletin Européen Pathophysiologie Respiratoire*, **11**, 479–502.

Freed, J.A., Miller, A., Gordon, R.E., Fischbein, A., Kleinerman, J. & Langer, A.M. (1991). Desquamative interstitial pneumonia associated with chrysotile asbestos. *British Journal of Industrial Medicine*, **48**, 332–337.

Fulmer, J.D., Roberts, W.C., von Gal, E.R. & Crystal, R.G. (1979). Morphologic-physiologic correlates of severity of fibrosis and degree of cellularity in idiopathic pulmonary fibrosis. *Journal of Clinical Investigation*, **63**, 665–676.

Gaensler, E.A., Carrington, C.B., Coutu, R.E., Tomasian, A., Hoffman, L. & Smith, A.A. (1972). Pathological, physiological and radiological correlations in the pneumoconioses. *Annals of the New York Academy of Science*, **200**, 574–607.

Gea, J., Rodriguez-Roisin, R., Torres, A., Roca, J. & Agusti-Vidal, A. (1988). Lung function changes following Legionnaire's disease. *European Respiratory Journal*, **1**, 109–114.

Gibson, G.J. & Pride, N.B. (1977). Pulmonary mechanics in fibrosing alveolitis: the effects of lung shrinkage. *American Review of Respiratory Disease*, **116**, 637–637.

Gibson, G.J., Pride, N.B., Davis, J. & Schroter, R.C. (1979). Exponential description of the static pressure–volume curve of normal and diseased lung. *American Review of Respiratory Disease*, **120**, 799–811.

Gorini, M., Ginanni, R., Spinelli, A., Duranti, R., Andreotti, L. & Scano, G. (1990). Inspiratory muscle strength and respiratory drive in patients with rheumatoid arthritis. *American Review of Respiratory Disease*, **142**, 289–294.

Hadfield, J.W., Page, R.L., Flower, C.D. & Stark, J.E. (1982). Localised airway narrowing in sarcoidosis. *Thorax*, **37**, 443–447.

Hamman, L. & Rich, A.R. (1935). Fulminating diffuse interstitial fibrosis of the lungs. *Transactions of the American Clinical Climatological Association*, **51**, 154–163.

Hamman, L. & Rich, A.R. (1944). Acute diffuse interstitial fibrosis of the lungs. *Bulletin of The Johns Hopkins Hospital*, **74**, 177–212.

Hankinson, J.L., Reger, R.B., Fairman, R.P., Lapp, N.L. & Morgan, W.K.C. (1977). Maximal expiratory flow in coal miners. *American Review of Respiratory Disease*, **116**, 175–186.

Hanley, M.E., King, T.E., Schwartz, M.I., Walters, L.C., Shen, A.S., Cherniack, R.M. (1991). The impact of smoking on mechanical properties of the lung in idiopathic pulmonary fibrosis and sarcoidosis. *American Review of Respiratory Disease*, **144**, 1102–1106.

Harrison, N.K., Myers, A.R., Corrin, B., Sooray, G., Dewar, A., Black, C.M., Dubois, R.M. & Turner-Warwick, M. (1991). Structural features of interstitial lung disease in systemic sclerosis. *American Review of Respiratory Disease*, **144**, 706–713.

Hendrick, D.J., Marshall, R., Faux, J.A. & Krall, J.M. (1980). Positive 'alveolar' responses to inhaled antigen inhalation provocational tests: their validity and recognition. *Thorax*, **35**, 415–427.

Heppleston, A.G. (1972). The pathological recognition and pathogenesis of emphysema and fibrocystic disease of the lung with special reference to coal workers. *Annals of the New York Academy of Sciences*, **200**, 347–369.

Hillerdal, G., Nou, E., Osterman, K. & Schmekel, B. (1984). Sarcoidosis: epidemiology and prognosis. *American Review of Respiratory Disease*, **130**, 29–32.

Huang, C.T., Henrich, A.E., Rosen, Y., Moon, S.A. & Lyons, H.A. (1979). Pulmonary sarcoidosis: roentgenographic, functional and pathologic changes. *Respiration*, **37**, 337–345.

Huang, C.T., Henrich, A.E., Sutton, A.L., Rosen, Y. & Lyons, H.A. (1980). Mortality in sarcoidosis. In *Eighth International Conference on Sarcoidosis and Other Granulomatous Diseases*, ed. W. Jones Williams & B.H. Davies, pp. 522–531. Cardiff: Alpha Omega.

International Labour Office (1980). Guidelines for the use of ILO international classification of radiographs of pneumoconioses. *Occupational Safety and Health*, series 22 (Rev 80). Geneva: ILO.

Javaheri, S. & Sicilian, L. (1992). Lung function, breathing pattern and gas exchange in interstitial lung disease. *Thorax*, **47**, 93–97.

Jodoin, G., Gibbs, G.W., Macklem, P.T., McDonald, J.C. & Becklake, M.R. (1971). Early effects of asbestos exposure on lung function. *American Review of Respiratory Disease*, **104**, 525–535.

Keogh, B.A., Hunninghake, G.W., Leric, B.R. & Crystal, R.G. (1983). The alveolitis of pulmonary sarcoidosis. *American Review of Respiratory Disease*, **128**, 256–265.

Kilburn, K.H., Warshaw, R.H. (1991). Abnormal lung function associated with asbestos disease of the pleura, the lung and both: a comparative analysis. *Thorax*, **46**, 33–38.

Kokkarinen, J.I., Tukiainen, H.O. & Terho, E.O.

(1992). Effect of corticosteroid treatment on the recovery of pulmonary function in farmer's lung. *American Review of Respiratory Disease*, **145**, 3–5.

Lakshimirayan, S., Stanford, R.F. & Petty, T.L. (1976). Prognosis after recovery from adult respiratory distress syndrome. *American Review of Respiratory Disease*, **113**, 7–16.

Legg, S.J., Cotes, J.E., & Bevan. C. (1983). Lung mechanics in relation to radiographic category of coal miners' simple pneumoconiosis. *British Journal of Industrial Medicine*, **40**, 28–33.

Liebow, A.A., Steer, A. & Billingsley, J.G. (1965). Desquamative interstitial pneumonia. *American Journal of Medicine*, **39**, 369–404.

Lilienthal, J.L., Riley, R.L., Proemmel, D.D. & Franke, R.E. (1946). An experimental analysis in man of the $O_2$ pressure gradient from alveolar to arterial blood during rest and exercise at sea level and at altitude. *American Journal of Physiology*, **147**, 199–216.

Miller, A., Einstein, K., Thornton, J., Teirstein, A.S. & Siltzbach, L.E. (1980). Physiologic classification and staging of intrathoracic sarcoidosis. In *Eighth International Conference on Sarcoidosis and Other Granulomatous Disorders*, ed. W. Jones Williams & B.H. Davies, pp. 331–336. Cardiff: Alpha Omega.

Morgan, W.K.C. (1978). Industrial bronchitis. *British Journal of Industrial Medicine*, **35**, 285–291.

Morgan, W.K.C., Seaton, A., Burgess, D.B., Lapp, N.L. & Reger, R. (1972). Lung volumes in working coal miners. *Annals of the New York Academy of Science*, **200**, 478–493.

Murphy, R.L.H., Gaensler, E.A., Ferris, B.G., Fitzgerald, M., Solliday, N., Morrisey, W. (1978). Diagnosis of asbestos: observations from a longitudinal study of shipyard pipe coverers. *American Journal of Medicine*, **65**, 488–498.

Parkes, W.R. (1982). *Occupational Lung Disorders*. London: Butterworth & Co.

Piiper, J. & Scheid, P. (1980). Blood gas equilibration in lungs. In *Pulmonary Gas Exchange*, vol. 1, ed. J.B. West, pp. 152–161. New York: Academic Press.

Powers, M.A., Askin, F.B. & Cresson, D.H. (1984). Pulmonary eosinophilic granuloma: 25–year follow up. *American Review of Respiratory Disease*, **129**, 503–507.

Pride, N.B. & Macklem, P.T. (1986). Lung mechanics in disease. In *Handbook of Physiology*, section 3, vol.II, part 2, ed. P.T. Macklem & J. Mead, pp. 665–683. Bethesda: APS.

Rienmuller, R.K., Behr, J., Kalender, W.A., Schatzl, N., Altmann, I., Merin, M. & Beinert, T. (1991). Standardised quantitative high resolution CT in lung diseases. *Journal of Computer Assisted Tomography*, **15**, 742–749.

Risk, C., Epler, G.R. & Gaensler, E.A. (1984). Exercise alveolar–arterial oxygen pressure difference in interstitial lung disease. *Chest*, **85**, 69–74.

Rizzatto, G., Bramvilla, I., Bertoli, L., Conti, F., Merlini, R. & Mantero, O. (1980). Impaired airway function and pulmonary haemodynamics in sarcoidosis. In *Eighth International Conference on Sarcoidosis and Other Granulomatous Disorders*, ed. W. Jones Williams & B.H. Davies, pp. 349–360. Cardiff: Alpha Omega.

Rogan, J.M., Attfield, M.D., Jacobson, M., Rae, S., Walter, D.D. & Walton, W.A. (1973). Role of dust in the working environment in the development of chronic bronchitis in British coal miners. *British Journal of Industrial Medicine*, **30**, 217–226.

Rogers, R.M., Levin. D.C., Gray, B.A. & Moseley, L.W. (1978). Physiologic effects of bronchopulmonary lavage in alveolar proteinosis. *American Review of Respiratory Disease*, **118**, 255–264.

Rosenstock, L., Barnhart, S., Hujer, N.J., Pierson, D.J. & Hudson, L.D. (1988). The relation among pulmonary function, chest roentgenographic abnormalities and smoking status on an asbestos-exposed cohort. *American Review of Respiratory Disease*, **138**, 272–277.

Rossiter, C.E. (1972). Relation between content and composition of coalworkers' lungs and radiological appearance. *British Journal of Industrial Medicine*, **29**, 31–44.

Ruckley, V.A., Gauld, S.J., Chapman, J.S., Davis, J.M.G., Douglas, A.N., Fernie, J.M., Jacobsen, M. & Lamb, D. (1984). Emphysema and dust exposure in a group of coal workers. *American Review of Respiratory Disease*, **129**, 528–532.

Rudd, R.M., Haslam, P.L. & Turner-Warwick, M. (1981). Cryptogenic fibrosing alveolitis: relationships of pulmonary physiology and bronchoalveolar lavage to response to treatment and prognosis. *American Review of Respiratory Disease*, **124**, 1–9.

Scadding, J.G. & Hinson, K.W.F. (1967). Diffuse fibrosing alveolitis (diffuse interstitial fibrosis of the lungs). *Thorax*, **22**, 291–304.

Sadoul, P. (1975). Fonctions respiratoires et pneumoconioses. *Bulletin Européen Physiopathologie Respiratoire*, **11**, 403–414.

Sahetya, G.K., Cobb, W.B., Facen, H.T., Hassan, S.N., Kumar, B. & Young, R.C. (1980). Pulmonary sarcoidosis: a significant cause of chronic airways obstruction. In *Eighth International Conference on Sarcoidosis and Other Granulomatous Disorders*, ed. W. Jones Williams & B.H. Davies, pp. 361–367. Cardiff: Alpha Omega.

Saumon, G., Georges, R., Loiseau, A. & Turiaf, J. (1976). Membrane diffusing capacity and pulmonary capillary blood volume in pulmonary sarcoidosis. *Annals of the New York Academy of Science*, **278**, 284–291.

Schwartz, D.A., Merchant, R.K., Helmers, R.A., Gilbert, J.R., Dayton, C.S. & Hunninghake, G.W. (1991). Influence of cigarette smoking on lung function in patients with idiopathic pulmonary fibrosis. *American Review of Respiratory Disease*, **144**, 504–506.

Sears, M.R. (1980). Pulmonary gas transfer and alveolar–arterial oxygen difference in sarcoidosis. In *Eighth International Conference on Sarcoidosis and Other Granulomatous Disorders*, ed. W. Jones Williams & B.H. Davies, pp. 343–348. Cardiff: Alpha Omega.

Seaton, A. (1982a). Coal and the lung (editorial). *Thorax*, **38**, 241–243.

Seaton, A. (1982b). Coal and the lung (letter). *Thorax*, **38**, 878–879.

Smith, D.D. & Agostini, P.G. (1989). The discriminatory value of $PA-aO_2$ during exercise in the detection of asbestos in asbestos-exposed workers. *Chest*, **95**, 52–55.

Staub, N.C., Bishop, J.M. & Forster, R.E. (1962). Importance of diffusion and chemical reaction rates in $O_2$ uptake in the lung. *Journal of Applied Physiology*, **17**, 21–27.

Sue, D.Y., Oren, A., Hansen, J. & Wasserman, K. (1985). Lung function and exercise performance in smoking and non-smoking asbestos-exposed workers. *American Review of Respiratory Disease*, **132**, 612–618.

Tukiainen, P., Taskinen, E., Korhola, O. & Valle, M. (1978). Trucut needle biopsy in asbestosis and silicosis: correlation of histological changes with radiographic changes and pulmonary function in 41 patients. *British Journal of Industrial Medicine*, **35**, 292–304.

Turner-Warwick, M. (1968). Fibrosing alveolitis and chronic lung disease. *American Journal of Medicine*, **37**, 133–149.

Turner-Warwick, M., Burrows, B. & Johnson, A. (1980). Cryptogenic fibrosing alveolitis: response to corticosteroid treatment and its effect on survival. *Thorax*, **35**, 593–599.

Ulmer, W.T. & Reichel, G. (1972). Functional impairment in coalworkers' pneumoconiosis. *Annals of the New York Academy of Science*, **200**, 405–412.

Valeyre, D., Saumon, G., Bladier, D., Amouroux, J., Pre, J. Battesti, J.P. & Georges, R. (1982). The relationships between non-invasive explorations in sarcoidosis of recent origin, as shown in bronchoalveolar lavage, serum and pulmonary functions tests. *American Review of Respiratory Disease*, **126**, 41–45.

Wagner, P.D., Dantzker, D.R., Dueck, R., de Polo, J.L., Wasserman, K. & West, J.B. (1976). Distribution of ventilation–perfusion ratios in patients with interstitial lung disease. *Chest*, **69** (Suppl.), 256–257.

Walters, L.C., King, T.E., Schwarz, M.I., Waldron, J.A., Stanford, R.E. & Cherniack, R.M. (1986). A clinical radiographic and physiologic scoring system for the longitudinal assessment of patients with idiopathic pulmonary fibrosis. *American Review of Respiratory Disease*, **133**, 97–103.

Williams, R. & Hugh Jones, P. (1960). The significance of lung function changes in asbestosis. *Thorax*, **15**, 109–119.

Winterbauer, R.H. & Hutchison, J.F. (1980). Clinical significance of pulmonary function tests: use of pulmonary function tests in the management of sarcoidosis. *Chest*, **78**, 640–647.

Wright, P.H., Heard, B.E., Steel, S.J. & Turner-Warwick, M. (1981). Cryptogenic fibrosing alveolitis: assessment by graded trephine lung biopsy compared with clinical radiographic and physiological features. *British Journal of Diseases of the Chest*, **75**, 61–70.

Wurm, K. & Rosner, R. (1976). The prognosis of chronic sarcoidosis. *Annals of the New York Academy of Sciences*, **278**, 732–735.

# 9 Miscellaneous conditions causing breathlessness

## Cardiac disorders

Cardiac diseases impair effort tolerance, often cause dyspnoea and may affect lung function in characteristic ways. Patients whose effort tolerance is reduced because of cardiac disease give similar answers to questions on dyspnoea as those with respiratory disorders who are disabled to the same degree (Warley *et al.*, 1987).

### Hypertension and ischaemic heart disease

Hypertension and ischaemic heart disease have no measurable effects *per se* on pulmonary function. Patients who are dyspnoeic on exertion generally have impaired pulmonary function, with reduced VC and TLC. This may be due to incipient or previous pulmonary oedema and pleural effusion. Treatment with beta-adrenergic blockade may cause exacerbations of bronchial asthma or a progressive shortness of breath because of airflow obstruction which reverses over some weeks when the drug is withdrawn. Response to beta-adrenergic bronchodilators is usually lost when non-selective agents are used and preserved when selective agents are employed. Even the latter may cause dangerous bronchoconstriction, however, and in the rare instances when they have to be given lung function has to be monitored.

#### Heart failure

The pulmonary changes of heart failure are caused by pulmonary oedema which occurs when the ability of the pulmonary lymphatics to clear transuded fluid is overwhelmed (Snashall, 1980; Laine *et al.*, 1986). The changes depend on the severirty of the rise of left atrial pressure. They usually occur in the following sequence:

1. Increased pulmonary blood volume.
2. Peribronchial oedema.
3. Alveolar flooding.
4. Pleural effusion.

Increasing enlargement of the heart may also affect measurements of lung volume. Tests show:

1. Reduction of VC, TLC and dynamic compliance (Christie & Meakins, 1934); generally $FEV_1/VC$ and PEF are well preserved.
2. Airway closure with normal or high RV (Collins, Clark & Brown, 1975).
3. A biphasic effect on TLco, and $TLco/V_A$ which may be raised when blood volume is increased, and tends to fall with progressive pulmonary oedema.
4. Wide alveolar–arterial $Po_2$ difference. Cyanosis and severe desaturation occur only in the most severe forms of alveolar flooding. There is a large true shunt, with persistence of the wide alveolar–arterial $Po_2$ difference (Al-Bazzaz & Kazemi, 1972).
5. Dead space is variable. There is abnormal filling of apical blood vessels in the upright position which results in a reduction of physiological dead space in some individuals (Saunders, 1966).
6. Arterial $Pco_2$ depends on the severity of the condition. It is reduced in mildly hypoxic patients with disturbed gas exchange but may rise if alveolar flooding is sufficiently severe, or if opiates and high concentrations of oxygen are administered injudiciously to individuals with associated chronic airflow obstruction (Avery, Samet & Sackner, 1970). The very old and the very young

138

are particularly affected. Metabolic acidosis may compound the respiratory problem, because excess $CO_2$ is generated by reaction of hydrogen ions with plasma bicarbonate.

7. Associated airflow obstruction. Bronchial responsiveness to methacholine is increased during attacks (Pison et al., 1989). Asthmatics and chronic bronchitics generally wheeze if they develop left ventricular failure (cardiac asthma). Increases of closing volume and high RV/TLC are features of pulmonary congestion but $FEV_1$/VC is generally above 60% and PEF above 200 l·min$^{-1}$. The mixing time for inert gases is not more delayed than would be accounted for by airway closure (Hales & Kazemi, 1974; Collins, Clark & Brown, 1975). The classic paper by von Basch (1887) described stiffness and decreased aeration of engorged lungs. Similar effects occur when the blood volume of normal subjects is increased experimentally (Collins et al., 1973). Generalised oedema causes abdominal distension which impairs chest wall movement. Other forms of abdominal distension may have the same effect (Mutoh et al., 1992).

8. Impaired effort tolerance. Breathlessness and fatigue limit walking in patients with heart failure. This is mediated by low cardiac output and impaired skeletal muscle performance. Aerobic working capacity is reduced (Chapter 13) (Moore et al., 1992). Nevertheless, many patients with severely impaired left ventricular function achieve good levels of exercise. A number of compensatory mechanisms exist in patients with left ventricular dilation of which the most important is probably the ability to tolerate elevated pulmonary venous pressures of up to 35 mmHg without dyspnoea. Cardiac output may be maintained within near-normal limits at the cost of elevating plasma noradrenaline levels (Litchfield et al., 1982). It follows that cardiac performance cannot be determined from measurements of cardiac output in exercise: isotopes give the most accurate non-invasive estimates.

## Mitral valve disease

Mitral stenosis has been studied intensively because it impairs pulmonary function in a characteristic way and it causes dyspnoea which should theoretically be due both to circulatory impairment and to loss of pulmonary reserve (Rhodes et al., 1982). The changes of pulmonary function are analogous to those of chronic heart failure and histologically resemble them. There is excessive alveolar fibrosis, sometimes with haemosiderosis, and there may be bronchial narrowing. The pulmonary circulation is affected by a chronic rise in left atrial and pulmonary arterial pressure and by recurrent pulmonary infarction. Respiratory muscle weakness is a common finding (de Troyer, Estenne & Yernault, 1980). Cardiac enlargement causes loss of lung volume. The respiratory abnormalities, which are related to both the severity and the duration of the condition, mirror these findings. They include:

1. Low VC.
2. Low TLC and FRC.
3. Normal or high RV, high RV/TLC ratio.
4. Normal or slightly reduced $FEV_1$/VC.
5. Normal 10–second helium distribution.
6. Increased apical perfusion in the upright position, with an increase of dead space in exercise (Dawson, Rozamora & Morgan, 1976; McEvoy, Drew & Mahar, 1986).
7. Reduced static compliance (Fig. 9.1).
8. TLco occasionally high at first but later low, mirroring pulmonary hypertension and smoking habit (Aber & Campbell, 1965; Bates, Macklem & Christie, 1972).
9. Low maximum inspiratory and expiratory pressures.

Atrial fibrillation is an important determinant of dyspnoea, which otherwise is mirrored closely by VC but not by intracardiac pressures. The relationship between VC and MRC dyspnoea grade is identical in mild mitral stenosis and chronic airflow obstruction (Fig. 9.2).

When mitral valve disease and chronic airflow obstruction are found together, it may be helpful to determine which is the major cause of disability. $FEV_1$/VC ratio below 60% and an unventilated space greater than 0.7 litre point to significant emphysema. A characteristic diurnal variation of PEF suggests bronchial asthma, as does an improvement of $FEV_1$ after nebulised salbutamol but these may be found in association with increased bronchial responsiveness in a

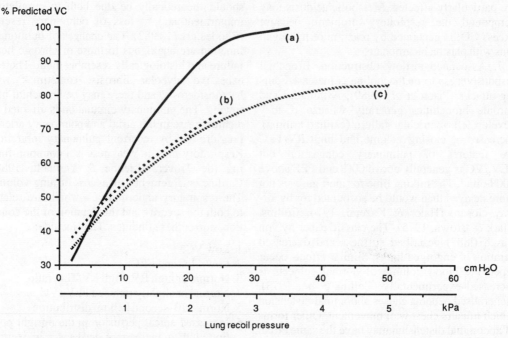

Fig. 9.1. Pressure–volume diagram of the lungs: (a) normal, (b) mitral stenosis, (c) pulmonary fibrosis. The lung recoil pressure–volume curve in mitral stenosis differs from that of pulmonary fibrosis because of the low maximal pressures caused by reduction of respiratory muscle power.

number of patients with mitral stenosis (Rolla *et al.*, 1992). Patients with both asthma and significant mitral valve disease who suffer episodes of dyspnoea unrelieved by regular bronchodilators and inhaled steroids generally improve after mitral valve surgery.

The benefits of mitral valve surgery on exercise tolerance relate mainly to the improved efficiency of oxygen delivery during exercise and to reduction of exercise-induced fatigue. VC and exercise MVV change only marginally, so maximum oxygen uptake measured in tests of short duration cannot be expected to improve very much (Gilmour *et al.*, 1976; Mustaf *et al.*, 1984; Rhodes *et al.*, 1985).

## Aortic valve disease

Aortic stenosis and incompetence may occasionally be difficult to diagnose clinically. The dimensions of the heart on the chest X-ray may not be

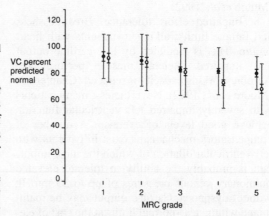

Fig. 9.2. Relationship between effort tolerance, as judged by the MRC five-point dyspnoea scale, and VC. Patients with chronic bronchitis and emphysema (open circles) compared with patients with mitral stenosis (filled circles), from the author's laboratory. Disability in the early stages of mitral stenosis occurs in proportion to the airway and lung disease that it causes. The most important determinant of severe dyspnoea in patients with mitral stenosis appears to be the development of atrial fibrillation. Other indices of the severity of the stenosis, such as left atrial and pulmonary arterial pressures, do not correlate with the degree of effort dyspnoea.

out of the ordinary. Patients with these conditions are occasionally referred for respiratory investigation. The cardiac origin of the problem is generally evident in patients with breathlessness solely from this cause, but from time to time patients with mild airflow obstruction are investigated whose disability seems out of proportion to the ventilatory impairment. Auscultation and ultrasound cardiography are the ways in which functionally significant aortic valve disease is diagnosed and both are technically more difficult when hyperinflated lungs separate the heart anteriorly from the chest wall.

Severe breathlessness is associated with progressive reduction of VC, lung volumes and TLco (Fig. 9.3). These changes are thought to be related to incipient heart failure and generally occur when left atrial pressure rises (Yernault & de Troyer, 1980).

### Left ventricular dysfunction

Patients with left heart disease may be able to maintain a normal cardiac output in exercise but do so at the loss of raised left atrial pressure. Exercise is limited by breathlessness, unless angina pectoris occurs to prevent this (Chapter 13). Changes in lung mechanics are transient, but pulmonary blood volume is increased. Patients vary widely in the extent to which they are distressed by rises of pulmonary venous pressure (Benge, Litchfield & Marcus, 1980; Litchfield et al.., 1982). Exercise testing in cardiac disease is discussed in Chapter 13.

### Septal defects

Left-to-right shunting is associated with a considerable increase in pulmonary blood volume, which causes a rise of TLco. TLco/$V_A$ (Bedell & Adams, 1962) may be twice normal. TLco/$V_A$ correlates with the magnitude of the shunt. The lung volumes and TLco fall with progressive pulmonary hypertension which develops with advancing years.

### Cyanotic congenital heart disease

Right-to-left shunting causes:

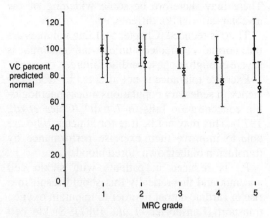

Fig. 9.3. As Fig. 9.2, for aortic stenosis (filled circles). There is more disability for a given loss of respiratory reserve than is seen in patients with pure respiratory disorders. This is explored further in Chapter 12.

1. Arterial $O_2$ desaturation, not reversed by breathing 100% $O_2$ but improving after squatting or lying down because these positions increase venous saturation and therefore less reduced haemoglobin is shunted (Lurie, 1953).
2. Worsening of hypoxaemia in exercise with blunting of the ventilatory response to hypoxia (Edelman et al., 1970).
3. A normal level of Pco$_2$ at rest, which generally rises in exercise. Lung volumes are reduced, sometimes with mild airflow obstruction. Intrapulmonary gas mixing is normal. Isotope injected during lung scanning fills the abdominal viscera.

### Anaemia

Anaemia affects cardiorespiratory function directly by reducing the oxygen carrying capacity of the blood. For a given Po$_2$, the oxygen content is reduced. The oxygen saturation, which is the ratio of oxyhaemoglobin concentration to total reduced and oxygenated haemoglobin, is unimpaired (Chapter 3). Cardiac output increases at rest and in exercise to compensate in part for the reduction of oxygen carrying capacity of each unit of blood volume. Because this compensation cannot be complete, mixed venous Po$_2$ is low.

There may therefore be some widening of the alveolar–arterial $Po_2$ difference.

TLco is reduced (Chapter 5). Lung volumes are not normally affected, unless the anaemia is severe enough to cause cardiac failure.

Exercise tolerance is not affected by iron deficiency in sedentary populations unless haemoglobin concentration falls to 7 $g \cdot dl^{-1}$ (Cotes *et al.*, 1972). This may not be true for athletes, who are able to improve their exercise performance by transfusion of their own stored blood.

$P_{50}$ is reduced in patients with sickle cell anaemia and theoretically this should result in a rise of cardiac output in order to maintain oxygen transport (Lansdorfer *et al.*, 1987). Sickle cell anaemia causes a number of pulmonary and systemic disorders and hampers growth: these problems dominate the lung function findings.

Treatment of patients receiving haemodialysis with erythropoietin to achieve a modest improvement in haemoglobin increased maximal oxygen uptake and exercise endurance time. As heart size also diminished and TLco improved even when corrected for haemoglobin, it seems likely that this agent reduced pulmonary oedema in some of the patients (McDougall *et al.*, 1990).

### Myelocytic leukaemia

Various lung diseases complicate the myeloproliferative disorders. Blood containing very large numbers of granulocytes may have a falsely low $Po_2$ because of oxygen consumption by the white cells.

## Pneumonectomy and lobectomy

The volume of the right lung is about 60% of TLC.

Removal of one lung leads over some months to over-inflation of the remaining lung. VC and TLC are greater than 50% of predicted normal. Residual volume is about twice that expected for one lung. TLco changes are explicable by the elastic recoil of the thorax acting on the remaining lung, together with some unexplained increase in distensibility, similar to that which occurs during an asthmatic attack (Schilling, 1965).

Lobectomy appears to have very little effect on basic lung function tests although compensatory hyperinflation can be identified on the chest X-ray as separation of the main vessels (Berend, Woolcock & Martin, 1980). Thoracoplasty was used as a treatment for tuberculosis and is still employed to remove aspergillomas attached to the chest wall. In addition to the problems caused by the underlying disease on the remaining lung, the collapsed chest wall is sucked in during inspiration further dissipating the work of breathing. Respiratory failure is common. The cardiorespiratory response to exercise is severely impaired in proportion to the reduction of $FEV_1$, pulmonary hypertension, hypoxaemia and a rapid, shallow breathing pattern (Phillips *et al.*, 1989).

## Neuromuscular disease

The respiratory muscles are usually affected when there is generalised muscular weakness or wasting. Dyspnoea of effort can occur but is an uncommon presenting feature, because of generally impaired mobility. Respiratory impairment becomes important in the presence of associated respiratory disease, and when lung function has deteriorated to the point where there is difficulty in coughing, inadequacy of tidal volume, nocturnal hypoventilation, shortness of breath at rest or overt respiratory failure.

Measurement of VC and estimates of arterial $Po_2$ and $Pco_2$ provide information about impending respiratory failure. $Pco_2$ is usually low until VC falls to 1.5 litres or less; if maximum expiratory pressure is less than 40 cm $H_2O$ and VC below 1.0 litre, there is substantial likelihood of ventilatory failure. Measurements should be made daily, or more often when there is rapidly progressive and potentially reversible respiratory failure in conditions such as polyneuritis or poliomyelitis.

Chronic neuromuscular diseases such as the proximal myopathies, motor neurone diseases and rarer neuromyopathies usually involve the respiratory muscles (Kreitzer *et al.*, 1978; Serisier, Mastaglia & Gibson, 1982; Braun, Arora & Rochester, 1983). They tend to be progressive and from time to time recurrent infections, or respiratory embarrassment, will lead to a referral for investigation. Standard lung function tests may need modification because of difficulties with mouthpieces experienced by patients with oro-facial weakness. Mechanical changes reflect the balance of inspiratory and expiratory muscle power as well as the degree of preservation of activity. In most instances, VC is reduced, a large RV (loss of expiratory reserve) being an earlier finding than low TLC (loss of inspiratory reserve). Because only half of the inspiratory muscle strength is required to inflate normal lungs to 80% of VC, this falls rather late in the disease (de Troyer, Borenstein & Cordier, 1980). FRC may be low because of loss of stability or recoil of the chest wall, or it may be high because of loss of expiratory muscle tone. Maximal expiratory and inspiratory airflow is reduced at all lung volumes. TLco is normal, unless there is failure to achieve a satisfactory inspiration, when TLco is low and TLco/$V_A$ high.

## Ataxia

Parkinson's disease causes apparent weakness of respiratory muscles, with marked reduction of PEFR, $FEV_1$ and MVV which improve after l-dopa incoordination impaired spirometry (Neu et al., 1967). Cerebellar ataxia may also reduce MVV.

## Myasthenia gravis

In myasthenia gravis, the abnormalities are similar to those of other chronic neuromuscular diseases, but vary in severity and may improve after administration of anticholinesterases (de Troyer & Borenstein, 1980; Radwan, Strugalska & Koziorowski, 1988). These may occasionally cause asthma, or increased airways resistance, in susceptible subjects (Ringqvist & Ringqvist, 1971). In theory, MVV should be lower than the figure predicted from $FEV_1$, but in practice this is not a reliable indicator of myasthenia.

## Diaphragm weakness

Impaired conduction through the phrenic nerves is generally caused by C3–4 root lesions or by damage to the phrenic nerves. The common causes are herpes zoster, isolated neuropathy, trauma or thoracotomy. The phrenic nerves may be involved in brachial plexus neuritis and occasionally in chronic central neuropathies, notably Charcot-Marie-Tooth disease. Respiratory muscle failure has been described in the Lambert-Eaton syndrome (Green & Laroche, 1990).

Isolated bilateral diaphragmatic weakness is generally suspected when there is elevation of one or both domes on the radiograph. It causes dyspnoea of effort and may come to light after an episode of respiratory failure when adequate spontaneous respiration is not restored after recovery from the pulmonary infection. The specific test for this condition is the measurement of transdiaphragmatic pressure, best performed during sniffing. A fall of VC in the supine position of greater than 25% is virtually diagnostic (Chapter 2). VC in the upright position may be as high as 70% of predicted. Studies of regional ventilation suggest that basal expansion may be impaired. Sleep apnoea or respiratory failure are not usual unless there is associated lung disease or disorders of other muscles, but there may be hypoxaemia during REM sleep (Newsom Davis et al., 1976). Operations in the neck intended to release the C3–4 nerve roots put the patient at risk of respiratory failure because of interference with the accessory muscles of respiration, especially the scalenus anterior.

Unilateral weakness may go unnoticed, but causes symptoms if it occurs suddenly. If there is already some ventilatory impairment or if ventilatory control is critical, as in singing or public speaking, it produces similar effects but they are less marked, VC and TLC being 80–100% of predicted normal. The change of VC on recumbency is greatest when the right side is involved because of the weight of the liver (Clague & Hall, 1979; Easton et al., 1983).

## Quadriplegia, with preservation of the diaphragm

Under normal conditions action of the diaphragm accounts for 60–70% of VC. In quadriplegia, VC is reduced to a lower percentage of normal than this, especially in the upright position because expiratory reserve is lost and because of the alterations of volume–pressure relationship caused by loss of intercostal tone. Paradoxical inspiratory indrawing in seen in the upper chest. Muscle power is reduced. The changes may improve with time (Mortolo & Sant'Ambrogio, 1978; de Troyer & Heilporn, 1980).

## Plan of investigation

Investigation of respiratory function in patients with neuromuscular disorders helps to identify involvement of respiratory muscles (Chapter 2) and any associated lung disease.

1. Maximal inspiratory and expiratory mouth pressures screen for the presence of global weakness, but do not always detect clinical disorders characterised by fatiguability of muscles. Maximal sniff oesophageal pressure is more reliable when facial weakness makes mouthpieces difficult to use. Diaphragm tests are indicated in all neurological disorders as the phrenic nerve and diaphragm are involved in a wide variety of pathological states. The phrenic nerve may be stimulated by surface electrodes to localise the lesion in cases of diaphragm weakness, though this requires neurophysiological expertise.
2. Lung volumes and $TLCO/V_A$ help to identify associated bronchopulmonary disease. Response to anticholinesterases may be estimated by measuring $FEV_1$ and VC.
3. $PCO_2$ is low in patients with mild respiratory impairment, when VC is below 2 litres. A 'normal' $PCO_2$ is a sign of incipient respiratory failure in patients with impaired ventilatory function. Low $PO_2$ and high $PCO_2$ call for assisted ventilation when the condition is reversible or when prolongation of life is justified.
4. As patients with chronic neuromuscular disorders frequently hypoventilate during sleep, their health may be improved by nocturnal ventilatory support: sleep studies will identify these individuals (Chapter 15).

## Alcoholism and cirrhosis of the liver

Alcoholics are often heavy smokers and suffer the expected consequences. They often have exertional dyspnoea which seems out of proportion to the degree of airflow obstruction present, perhaps because of an associated respiratory muscle weakness or cardiomyopathy. A seemingly intelligent patient who appears incomprehensibly incapable of performing the necessary respiratory gymnastics for measurement of single breath TLCO and lung volumes is probably alcoholic.

Basal mottling on chest X-ray and intrapulmonary shunting are surprising features of chronic liver disease (Stanley & Woodgate, 1972; Stanley et al., 1977). The lesions are intrapulmonary arteriovenous anastomoses (Seidman & Mark, 1992). They are responsible for shunting a substantial fraction of the pulmonary blood flow. They may cause finger clubbing. Polycythaemia is often more marked than that found in patients with uncomplicated chronic bronchitis. 'True shunt' is demonstrable and hypoxaemia found during 100% $O_2$ breathing. TLCO and $TLCO/V_A$ are reduced in a proportion of these patients, unlike the findings in other forms of arteriovenous malformation, possibly because of uneven distribution of diffusing capacity or structural changes to pulmonary arterioles. There may be minor abnormalities of lung function caused by fluid retention secondary to hypoalbuminaemia, especially reversible hypoxaemia, low TLCO and increased airway closure. Ventilation–perfusion mismatching accounts for most of the hypoxaemia in uncomplicated cases (Ruff et al., 1971; Agusti et al., 1989; Melot et al., 1989; Rodriguez-Roisin, Agusti & Roca, 1992).

A few patients with autoimmune hepatitis and primary biliary cirrhosis also have a lung condition similar to fibrosing alveolitis. One or two patients have presented initially with budgerigar-fancier's lung (personal observation).

## Uraemia

'Uraemic lung' is a form of exudative pulmonary oedema, characterised by low lung volumes and TLCO (Lee, Stretton & Barnes, 1975). Patients with chronic renal failure with normal chest X-rays tend to have impaired CO uptake, even allowing for anaemia.

Haemodialysis worsens hypoxaemia, probably because of $CO_2$ excretion into the dialysis fluid with consequent alveolar hypoventilation: this can have important consequences in the presence of ventilatory impairment (Patterson *et al.*, 1981).

## Pulmonary haemorrhage: monitoring in Goodpasture's syndrome

Intra-alveolar red cells which have recently been extravasated take up CO. If a baseline value for $TL_{CO}$ can be established, further haemorrhage can be identified by a rising value which must be corrected for circulating haemoglobin concentration because this falls during significant pulmonary haemorrhage. Changes of $TL_{CO}$ precede frank haemoptysis.

A standard bedside test for measuring $TL_{CO}$ by rebreathing has proved valuable in this context (Chapter 5).

CO is taken up by stagnant red cells. This was demonstrated by measurement of thoracic radioactive $^{15}CO$, which is taken up after inhalation and remains in the thorax for a surprisingly long time. Lung haemorrhage causes a high uptake of CO during a single breath or rebreathing test. Studies employing a cyclotron have shown that low thoracic clearance of $^{15}CO$ is slow.

## Thyroid disease

### Hyperthyroidism

Thyrotoxicosis may present with breathlessness or angina pectoris. Slight reduction of VC is associated with respiratory muscle weakness and with increased lung recoil at TLC (Freedman, 1971), perhaps related to vascular congestion. $TL_{CO}$ and its subdivisions are normal. Ventilation and respiratory frequency are excessive in relation to muscular work, probably because of increased oxygen uptake in relation to workload. This, combined with the occasional finding of alveolar hyperventilation, probably accounts for the dyspnoea commonly encountered in this condition. There are anecdotal accounts of an association between the development of thyrotoxicosis and the onset of bronchial asthma, but this could not be reproduced experimentally. Increased non-specific bronchial reactivity is not a cause of impaired exercise performance (Irwin *et al.*, 1985; Kendrick, O'Reilly & Laszlo, 1988).

Interestingly, an increased ventilatory response to $CO_2$ is also associated with excessive frequency and low tidal volume (Engel & Ritchie, 1971). This is in contrast to left ventricular insufficiency where the tidal volume is low in exercise and normal during $CO_2$ stimulation, again suggesting that pulmonary vascular engorgement may be present at rest, in spite of the normal $TL_{CO}$.

Lung function changes currently being reported are fairly subtle and not grossly different from normal. They tend to recover with treatment. Earlier researchers who relied on less sensitive indices reported more florid abnormalities. Hyperthyroidism has to be remembered as a cause of 'functional hyperventilation' or 'unexplained dyspnoea'.

### Hypothyroidism

Myxoedema causes respiratory muscle weakness, anaemia, obstructive sleep apnoea, cardiac failure and respiratory failure (Freedman, 1971; Skatrud *et al.*, 1981).

## Acromegaly

The lungs enlarge in acromegaly, as do other viscera, and high levels of TLC are found. This is normal. Obstructive sleep apnoea is a common feature of this condition (Toppel, Atkinson & Whitcomb, 1973; Evans, Hipkin & Murray, 1977; Perks *et al.*, 1980).

## Obesity

Quite modest weight gain can impair exercise performance on hills and stairs because of the increased work involved. Truncal weight is supported on a stationary ergometer, but excessive weight on the thighs can impair performance.

Spirometry is usually within normal limits; nevertheless, VC varies as weight is gained and lost. Static lung volume measurements show a reduction of FRC and experimental reserve volume, FRC being close to RV. The basal airways are closed. Mild basal underventilation results in modest hypoxaemia, with $Po_2$ around 70 mmHg (9 kPa). Grossly obese patients develop arterial oxygen desaturation during sleep and in recumbency. The chest wall is poorly compliant, and if this is allowed for, ventilatory effort response to $CO_2$ inhalation is not impaired (Ray et al., 1983; Burki & Baker, 1984).

Obesity is an important determinant of obstructive sleep apnoea (Lopata & Önal, 1982).

Obesity causes:

1. Normal $FEV_1$ and VC.
2. Normal TLC.
3. Low FRC.
4. Low ERV.
5. Normal TLco.
6. Normal or high $TLco/V_A$.
7. Wide alveolar–arterial $Po_2$ difference.

## Systemic lupus erythematosus

A wide variety of pathological changes are found in systemic lupus erythematosus, including pleural effusions, pulmonary infarction, pulmonary hypertension and occasionally pneumonia, bronchiolitis or lung fibrosis. A characteristic X-ray change is 'shrinking lung', with high, fairly mobile diaphragms. These are thought to be paralysed or weakened because low maximal lung recoil pressures and low trans-diaphragmatic pressures are found. Previous pleural effusions may be responsible but the severity of the paresis may reflect activity of the disease and therefore be part of a myopathy (Gibson, Edmonds & Hughes, 1977; Silberstein et al., 1980; Thompson et al., 1985; Miller, Greenberg & McLarty, 1985). Systemic lupus erythematosus causes:

1. Low VC.
2. Low TLco.
3. Low maximal inspiratory and expiratory pressures.
4. Normal lung perfusion scan when the chest X-ray is clear.
5. Reduced exercise tolerance.

## Thoracic cage disease

### Kyphosis and scoliosis

Severe distortion of the thoracic cage in childhood causes impairment of lung growth. There is reduction of inspiratory reserve and proportional hypoxaemia and impairment of effort tolerance. Regional ventilation is impaired on the side of the concavity (Littler, Brown & Roaf, 1972). Chest wall compliance may be impaired (Kafer, 1975), but this is not always the case (Cooper et al., 1984) and there may be impaired lung growth, atelectasis and respiratory muscle weakness in addition (Jones et al., 1981). Kyphoscoliosis leads to respiratory failure in middle age especially if there is associated weakness of respiratory muscles, or if the onset of the condition occurs in childhood rather than in adolescence.

Spinal deformity prevents the development of expected height, so predicted values are usually related to arm span as this corresponds closely to height (Linderholm & Lindgren, 1978).

The degree of angulation determines the reduction of VC and TLC, and the latter is a good predictor of hypoxaemia (Kafer, 1975).

$TLco/V_A$ is high and TLco reduced, but not in proportion to VC. Exercise is limited by reduced ventilatory capacity (Kafer, 1975; Shneerson, 1978a). Pulmonary artery pressure is elevated in proportion to the degree of hypoxaemia and rises further in exercise (Shneerson, 1978b). It has been suggested that there may in addition be outflow obstruction caused by kinking of the main pulmonary vessels (Bergofsky, Turino & Fishman, 1959). Respiratory failure may present with heart failure: the development of congestive changes and peripheral oedema precede dyspnoea. The lungs become oedematous. Normally the ventilatory response to $CO_2$ is reduced. A breathless cyanosed patient treated with diuretics and $O_2$ may develop $CO_2$ retention unexpectedly, because resolution of pulmonary oedema causes improvement of lung function and increased arterial oxygenation, thus depressing ventilation.

Surgical correction has little immediate effect on lung function but may prevent deterioration.

The effects of kyphoscoliosis are:

1. Low VC with normal or high $FEV_1$/VC ratio.
2. Low TLC.
3. Low maximal inspiratory and expiratory pressures.
4. Hypoxaemia.
5. (later) Raised $PCO_2$.

## Ankylosing spondylitis

In the presence of complete ankylosis of the spine and ribs, respiration depends on the diaphragm. This moves normally: $PCO_2$ is normal and $O_2$ exchange is minimally impaired except when there is interference with abdominal relaxation, for example after laparotomy. Apical ventilation is impaired (Stewart, Ridyeard & Pearson, 1978). Some patients develop bilateral apical fibrosis which has an additional effect on lung volumes.

As in scoliosis, reference data have to allow for loss of height.

## Pectus excavatum

Pectus excavatum is regarded by many as unsightly but it rarely has any functional significance. Severe cases affect effort tolerance in a number of ways:

1. By reducing the stroke volume of the heart.
2. By restricting expansion.
3. By imposing a rapid, shallow breathing pattern during exercise, as a result of both these phenomena.

Detailed cardiopulmonary evaluation is needed before any surgery is contemplated (Beiser *et al.*, 1972; Castile, Staats & Westbrook, 1982; Mead *et al.*, 1985).

## Pleural thickening

Dense pleural thickening may occur after resolution of inflammatory pleural effusions and is found as a result of asbestos exposure. The severity of the changes correlate with VC. Loss of

inspiratory capacity results in a high elastic recoil at TLC. TLCO may be below normal, but $TLCO/V_A$ is high when measured correctly at TLC (Wright *et al.*, 1980). It is difficult to identify minor degrees of alveolar disease in pleural fibrosis by means of pulmonary function tests.

It has generally been held that pleural disease has no functional significance in patients exposed to asbestos. A recent study of large numbers of men with asbestos exposure demonstrated minor degrees of airflow obstruction, with reduced values of $FEV_1$ and mid-expiratory flow rates but without reduction of TLC. These men had similar lung function to those with minor changes of asbestosis on chest X-ray. The changes are likely to represent bronchiolar deposition of asbestos and may be the earliest manifestations of asbestos-related disease (Kilburn & Warshaw, 1991). Falls of VC and $FEV_1$ have been described in patients developing dense pleural fibrosis ('lung en cuirasse'), but this situation is relatively unusual (Britton, 1982). $PO_2$ is often abnormal with quite mild pleural involvement (Hillerdal, Malmberg & Hemingsson, 1990). The significance of pleural disease needs to be evaluated further.

## Rejection of transplanted heart and lungs

Donor lungs function well in the absence of rejection after transplantation. If a good match is found, static lung volumes lie within normal limits and TLCO is approximately 80% of predicted. Serial measurements of $FEV_1$ help to identify episodes of rejection and infection, with a mean fall of 1 litre of $FEV_1$, FVC and TLC, about 33% of baseline. TLCO also falls by about 30% on average, but the coefficient of variation of this test approaches 6% while that of VC is 2.5% among patients measuring their own spirometric indices on a portable electronic device (Otulana *et al.*, 1990). Bronchial lavage and transbronchial biopsy are performed when these tests deteriorate and are not needed at other times.

After retraining, heart–lung recipients breathe at a normal rate with normal tidal volumes. This applies also to exercise. Those recipients who

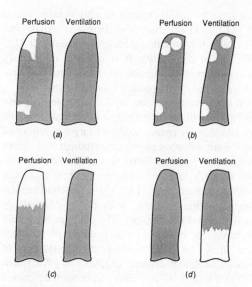

Fig. 9.4. Ventilation–perfusion lung scans (diagrammatic). (*a*) Perfusion defects with uniform ventilation. The wedged segmental defects indicate pulmonary vascular occlusion. (*b*) Matched perfusion and ventilation defect: the poorly perfused areas found in the lungs of patients with chronic airflow obstruction are caused by or associated with reduced ventilation. (*c*) Mismatched defects of perfusion in a patient with fibrosing alveolitis and extensive cystic change. These cysts are well ventilated. (*d*) Unventilated lung in a patient with a pleural effusion. The bases appear well perfused because the isotope was injected with the patient lying down, but ventilation is absent in the seated position when the fluid gravitates towards the base of the lung.

develop obliterative bronchiolitis breathe more rapidly and shallowly but maintain normal blood gases at rest and during exercise (Sciurba *et al.*, 1991). It appears, therefore, that an intact pulmonary vagal innervation is not needed to control the rate and depth of breathing.

## Pulmonary thrombo-embolism

Until recently, a diagnostic pulmonary angiograph was regarded as the 'gold standard' on which research into this topic had to be based, emboli being identified by the presence of filling defects within the lumen of major vessels or by a 'sawn

off' appearance indicating total occlusion (Goodman, 1984). Pulmonary angiography is hazardous in the presence of pulmonary hypertension. It has been replaced by ventilation–perfusion scanning as the basis of clinical diagnosis. Moreover the sensitivity and specificity of angiography are not as great as was formerly thought, since small emboli are missed by both angiography and scanning, while the appearances of both emphysema and primary pulmonary hypertension may be mistaken for embolic vascular occlusion. Combined ventilation and perfusion scanning carried out to a high standard, are therefore generally used as the confirmatory diagnostic procedure in life (Polak & McNeil, 1984) (Fig. 9.4).

The typical appearance is of one or more perfusion defects with uniformly good ventilation to that site. When the appearances are classical the diagnosis can usually be made with confidence, with one caution: that cystic areas of lung in patients with fibrosing alveolitis are well ventilated and may be very poorly perfused at rest (Chapter 8).

Pulmonary emboli present in three ways, according to the size and distribution of the occluded vessels and the severity of any associated lung or heart disease.

1. Occlusion of a major vessel or several segmental vessels causes severe obstruction to right ventricular outflow. The manifestations include:
   severe dyspnoea;
   anginal chest pain;
   hypotension;
   signs of right ventricular failure, including a loud delayed pulmonary second sound and a third heart sound over the right ventricle. In a shocked patient, an important distinguishing feature of myocardial infarction is the presence of a raised jugular venous pressure which suggests pulmonary embolism or, more rarely, pericardial tamponade or tension pneumothorax;
   electrocardiographic changes of right ventricular preponderance.
2. Occlusion of segmental vessels results in shortness of breath, on exertion or possibly at rest.
3. Infarction causes haemoptysis, pleuritic pain

and sometimes pleural effusion though this is rarely greater than half the height of the chest. Radiographic shadows may be characteristic in shape, or there may be elevation of one or both diaphragms.

The development of infarction depends partly on the size of the occluded vessel, which (*a*) has to be distal to the distribution of the bronchial vessels and (*b*) has to be large enough to be an end-artery. Poorly ventilated lung segments are more likely to infarct.

Infarcted segments resorb, leaving a little fibrosis. Otherwise emboli tend to dissolve by clot lysis, with restoration of lung function. Residual defects are probably the exception.

Pulmonary oedema may be occasionally demonstrated on chest X-ray (Manier *et al.*, 1984). It is probably caused by high pressure in the perfused areas of lung when there is extensive vascular obstruction. Pulmonary oedema worsens the clinical state of the patient and may cause diagnostic confusion. Pulmonary oedema is also a feature of pulmonary veno-occlusive disease, a rare cause of pulmonary hypertension which may develop acutely or gradually.

Persistent perfusion defects cause permanent impairment of effort tolerance. Thrombo-embolic pulmonary hypertension occurs when recurrent minor embolic episodes which may pass unnoticed or undiagnosed except with hindsight, may be responsible; there may be no history attributable to pulmonary embolisation (Huisman *et al.*, 1989). It is a disabling condition, leading to severe dyspnoea and exhaustion on slight effort with signs of right ventricular failure. The disease is then impossible to distinguish from the idiopathic or 'primary' form except at lung biopsy or post-mortem. It will be suspected if there is an identifiable venous thrombosis, usually in the thigh or pelvis but occasionally axillary.

Lung mechanics are typically affected only if there is infarction or pleural effusion (Williams, Adler & Colp, 1969). There are anecdotal accounts of asthma imitated or precipitated by a major embolic episode, and asthmatics may wheeze at the onset of an attack (hypothetically because of platelet alteration and the release of serotonin and other mediators).

### Gas exchange in pulmonary embolism

There are invariably disturbances of pulmonary gas exchange. Small emboli, which cause transient dyspnoea lasting few hours, result in a low $P_{CO_2}$ with a wide alveolar–arterial $P_{O_2}$ difference. Medium-sized emboli, affecting lobar or segmental vessels, typically cause abnormalities on lung isotope emission scans. Ventilation is uniform, while embolised areas show defects in perfusion. The diagnosis is difficult to make in patients with airflow obstruction who supposedly have matched defects of both ventilation and perfusion, because exact matching cannot be demonstrated by present techniques. Dead space is increased in these areas. Measurements of $V_D/V_T$ in the emergency room are abnormal in virtually all patients subsequently shown to have abnormal lung scans (Burki, 1986). A similar technique employs analysis of the difference between arterial $P_{CO_2}$ and rapid analysis of $P_{CO_2}$ at the end of expiration (end-tidal $P_{CO_2}$), which is widened when dead space is increased. This technique may distinguish patients with airflow obstruction because they show a different pattern of $CO_2$ excretion similar to the steep slope of Phase III of the nitrogen excretion test (Chapter 4) (Huisman *et al.*, 1989). Unfortunately this is not completely reliable and fails to distinguish pulmonary embolism from heart failure, which shows a similar pattern.

$P_{CO_2}$ is low. $P_{O_2}$ is also low, in proportion to the severity of the pulmonary vascular obstruction: when hyperventilation is extreme, $P_{O_2}$ may be within the normal range unless $P_{CO_2}$ is allowed for by the calculations of alveolar–arterial $P_{O_2}$ difference (Critanic & Marino, 1989). It seems likely that the introduction of simultaneous arterial and mixed expired $P_{O_2}$ and $P_{CO_2}$ in emergency rooms would help to distinguish pulmonary embolism from psychogenic hyperventilation in patients with normal airway tests and normal chest X-rays, because very few other disorders cause these abnormalities of gas exchange in the absence of bronchial or alveolar disease. Some information may be gleaned from blood gases alone (Chapter 3, p. 45).

Inert gas studies (Chapter 14) suggest that the reasons for the low $P_{O_2}$ may be complex:

1. There is 'true' shunting, thus perhaps as a result of high pulmonary artery pressure the flow through the foramen ovale or other defect.
2. Although $PCO_2$ is low, there may be sufficient $CO_2$ exchange in the embolised zones to compensate for a modest degree of underventilation in those areas of lung which have an intact pulmonary circulation. This may be because occlusion of one pulmonary artery causes total abolition of oxygen uptake but not of $CO_2$ output because $CO_2$ is excreted into the ventilated lung from the bronchial circulation (Langley *et al.*, 1975).
3. In major pulmonary embolism, a low cardiac output and therefore low mixed venous $PO_2$ aggravates the effects of ventilation–perfusion mismatching.

The disturbances of gas exchange persist for several days after acute embolisation (D'Alonzo *et al.*, 1983; D'Alonzo & Dantzker, 1984; Manier, Castaing & Guenard, 1985; Kapitan *et al.*, 1989; Manier & Castaing, 1992).

TLco gives no consistent diagnostic information. It is often normal, and if it is less than 50% of expected normal, lung disease is probably present. Quite severe perfusion defects and pulmonary hypertension may be accompanied by only modest reduction of TLco (70% of expected normal being average) (Williams, Adler & Colp, 1969).

'Membrane' diffusing capacity is more strikingly reduced than the capillary blood volume, as judged by the oxygen-dependent and oxygen-independent components of TLco. These changes reflect the increased dead space and diversion of pulmonary blood to healthy areas of lung. There is very little useful information on this topic (Fennerty, Gunarwardene & Smith, 1988; Wimalaratna, Farrell & Lee, 1990).

## Strategy for investigation

It is important to establish the diagnosis of pulmonary embolism with documentary evidence whenever possible. Anticoagulants provide effective prophylaxis and may be given long term. A single episode occurring post-operatively or because of some identifiable, temporary and preventable period of high risk needs anticoagulant prophylaxis only for a short period. It seems sensible to reassess each patient to determine the likelihood of future recurrence and the likely severity of respiratory impairment. This leads to lifelong anticoagulation for those with chronic venous insufficiency, and for most of those in whom the reason for the occurrence was not apparent. Lifelong anticoagulation is given to patients with persistent perfusion defects or reduced TLco, in whom another episode might be crippling. The majority of the latter have chronic lung disease.

The plan of the investigation will depend on the clinical presentation.

### Pulmonary thromboembolism presenting with acute dyspnoea

1. $PO_2$ and $PCO_2$ are measured to confirm hyperventilation with an abnormal alveolar–arterial $PO_2$ difference. The approximate calculation of this (described in Chapter 3) is useful. Normal dead space is found in normal hyperventilating subjects but not invariably in heart failure.
2. $FEV_1$ and PEF are usually normal.
3. Ventilation–perfusion scanning is performed as soon as possible. Immediate scanning theoretically provides the highest yield, but it is not always feasible and its value has not been demonstrated.
4. The ECG may show right ventricular predominance or a characteristic pattern described as S1 Q3 T3 (s waves in lead 1, q wave and inverted t wave in lead 3).

### Severe dyspnoea with circulatory failure

This is usually associated with the following findings:

1. Arterial $PO_2$ is profoundly reduced.
2. Arterial $PCO_2$ is low.
3. Peak flow is normal.
4. Spirometry is usually impracticable.
5. ECG changes are described above.

Pulmonary angiography has generally been employed before surgery or thrombolytic therapy.

### Chronic dyspnoea

Lung function tests show:

1. Normal spirometry.
2. Normal lung volumes or mild restriction (Horn *et al.*, 1983).

3. Variable TLco.
4. Ventilation and perfusion lung scans show mismatched defects in patients with multiple or unresolved emboli. Lung scans often show apparently uniform perfusion when thromboembolic pulmonary hypertension develops after recurrent small infarcts. In this situation the diagnosis is difficult to distinguish from cryptogenic (primary) pulmonary hypertension.
5. $Pco_2$ is normal or low at rest, with increased dead space tidal volume ratio.
6. Pulmonary artery pressure, when measured, is raised in severe disease and rises further with moderate exercise.
7. Exercise testing shows high ventilation, failure of dead space/tidal volume to fall from resting values and wide alveolar–arterial $Po_2$ difference, normal $O_2$ saturation.

Deaths occurring after exercise testing in patients with severe pulmonary hypertensive disorders have been reported, although cause and effect have not been established.

Chronic thrombo-embolic disease should be suspected in breathless patients with normal lungs, normal spirometry, right ventricular prominence with a loud pulmonary second sound, the appearances of a large pulmonary arterial trunk on the chest X-ray and electrocardiographic change of right ventricular strain or enlargement.

**Acute pleurisy**

When pulmonary embolism presents with acute pleurisy, $Po_2$ is low, and alveolar–arterial $Po_2$ difference wide. The changes are generally similar to those of pneumonia with consolidation, so blood gas measurements help to determine the need for oxygen therapy but have no diagnostic value.

Spirometry is unhelpful in the presence of pleuritic chest pain.

## Pregnancy

Pregnancy affects breathing in three ways:

1. Increased circulating blood volume and low haemoglobin concentration.
2. Abdominal distension.
3. Stimulation of ventilation by circulating progesterone.

Dyspnoea is a common symptom which starts in early pregnancy. Because there is little mechanical interference with breathing during the first trimester, the sensation is thought to be related to the awareness of the increased ventilatory requirement due to the abnormal drive and to the alterations in pulmonary haemodynamics. Most studies of gas exchange have shown very little other abnormality, but measurements of TLco made before 1985 have generally not been corrected for anaemia (Chapter 5). The mechanical changes which occur during late pregnancy are similar to those of obesity. The topic has been reviewed in detail by Weinberger et al. (1980).

## References

Aber, C.P. & Campbell, J.A. (1965). Significance of the changes in the pulmonary diffusing capacity in mitral stenosis. *Thorax*, **20**, 134–145.

Agusti, A.G., Roca, J., Rodriguez-Roisin, R., Morstar, R., Wagner, P.D. & Bosch, J. (1989). Pulmonary haemodynamics and gas exchange during exercise in liver cirrhosis. *American Review of Respiratory Disease*, **139**, 485–491.

Al-Bazzaz, F. & Kazemi, H. (1972). Arterial hypoxaemia and distribution of pulmonary perfusion after uncomplicated myocardial infarction. *American Review of Respiratory Disease*, **116**, 919–943.

Amis, T.C., Crofetta, G., Hughes, J.M.B. & Loh, L. (1980). Regional lung function: bilateral diaphragmatic paralysis. *Clinical Science*, **59**, 485–492.

Avery, W.G., Samet, P. & Sackner, M.A. (1970). The acidosis of pulmonary edema. *American Journal of Medicine*, **48**, 320–324.

Bates, D.V., Macklem, P.T. & Christie, R.V. (1972). *Respiratory Function in Disease*, 2nd edn. Philadelphia; Saunders.

Bedell, G.N. & Adams, R.W. (1962). Pulmonary diffusing capacity at rest and in exercise: a study of normal persons and persons with atrial septal defect frequency and pulmonary disease. *Journal of Clinical Investigation*, **41**, 1908–1914.

Beiser, G.D., Epstein, S.E., Stampfer, N., Goldstein, R.E., Noland, S.P. & Levitsky, S. (1972). Improvement of cardiac function in patients with pectus excavatum after operative correction. *New England Journal of Medicine*, **287**, 267–272.

Benge, W., Litchfield, R.L. & Marcus, M.L. (1980). Exercise capacity in patients with severe left ventricular dysfunction. *Circulation*, **61**, 955–959.

Berend, N., Woolcock, A.J. & Marlin, G.E. (1980). Effects of lobectomy on lung function. *Thorax*, **35**, 145–150.

Bergofsky, E.H., Turino, G.M. & Fishman, A.P. (1958). Cardiorespiratory failure in kyphoscoliosis. *Medicine*, **38**, 263–317.

Braun, N.M.T., Arora, N.S. & Rochester, D.F. (1983). Respiratory muscle and pulmonary function in polymyositis and other proximal myopathies. *Thorax*, **38**, 616–623.

Britton, M.G. (1982). Asbestos pleural disease. *British Journal of Diseases of the Chest*, **76**, 1–10.

Burki, N.K. (1986). The dead space to tidal volume ratio in the diagnosis of pulmonary embolism. *American Review of Respiratory Disease*, **133**, 679–685.

Burki, N.K. & Baker, R.W. (1984). Ventilatory regulation in eucapnic morbid obesity. *American Review of Respiratory Disease*, **129**, 538–543.

Castile, R.G., Staats, B.A. & Westbrook, P.R. (1982). Symptomatic pectus deformities of the chest. *American Review of Respiratory Disease*, **126**, 564–568.

Christie, R.V. & Meakins, J.C. (1934). The intrapleural pressure in congestive heart failure and its clinical significance. *Journal of Clinical Investigation*, **13**, 323–345.

Clague, H.W. & Hall, D.R. (1979). Effect of posture on lung volume, airway closure and gas exchange in hemodiaphragmatic paralysis. *Thorax*, **31**, 438–442.

Collins, J.V., Clark, T.J.H., & Brown, D.J. (1975). Airway function in healthy subjects and patients with left heart disease. *Clinical Science and Molecular Medicine*, **49**, 217–228.

Collins, J.V., Cochrane, G.M., David J., Benatar, S.R. & Clark, T.J.H. (1973). Some aspects of pulmonary function after rapid saline infusion in healthy subjects. *Clinical Science*, **45**, 407–410.

Cooper, D.M., Velasquez Rojas, J., Mellins, R.B. , Keun, H.A. & Mansele, A.L. (1984). Respiratory mechanics in adolescents with idiopathic scoliosis. *American Review of Respiratory Disease*, **130**, 16–22.

Cotes, J.E., Dabbs, J.M., Elwood, P.C., Hall, A.M., McDonald, A. & Saunders, A.M. (1972). Iron deficiency anaemia: its effect on transfer factor for the lung and ventilation and card frequency during submaximal exercise. *Clinical Science*, **42**, 325–335.

Critanic, O. & Marino, P.L. (1989). Improved use of arterial blood gas analysis in suspected pulmonary embolism. *Chest*, **95**, 48–51.

D'Alonzo, G.E., Bower, J.S., Rettart, P. & Dantzker, D.R. (1983). The mechanisms of abnormal gas exchange in acute massive pulmonary embolism. *American Review of Respiratory Disease*, 128, 170–172.

D'Alonzo, G.E. & Dantzker, D.R. (1984). Gas exchange alterations following pulmonary thromboembolism. *Clinics in Chest Medicine*, **5**, 411–419.

Davies, H. & Gazetopoulos, N. (1965). Dyspnoea in cyanotic congenital heart disease. *British Heart Journal*, 27, 28–41.

Dawson, A., Rocamora, J.M. & Morgan, J.R. (1976). Regional lung function in chronic pulmonary congestion with and without mitral stenosis. *American Review of Respiratory Disease*, **113**, 51–59.

de Troyer, A. & Borenstein, S. (1980). Acute changes in respiratory mechanics after pyridostigmine injection in patients with myasthenia gravis. *American Review of Respiratory Disease*, **121**, 629–638.

de Troyer, A., Borenstein, S. & Cordier, R. (1980). Analysis of lung volume restriction in patients with respiratory muscle weakness. *Thorax*, **35**, 603–610.

de Troyer, A., Estenne, M. & Yernault, J.C. (1980). Disturbance of respiratory muscle function in patients with mitral valve disease. *American Journal of Medicine*, **169**, 867–873.

de Troyer, A. & Heilporn, A. (1980). Respiratory mechanics in quadriplegia: the respiratory function of the intercostal muscles. *American Review of Respiratory Disease*, **122**, 591–600.

Easton, P.A., Fleetham, J.A., de la Rocha, A. & Anthonisen, N.R. (1983). Respiratory function after paralysis of the right diaphragm. *American Review of Respiratory Disease*, **127**, 125–128.

Edelman, N.H., Lahiri, S., Braudo, L., Cherniack, N.S. & Fishman, A.P. (1970). The blunted ventilatory response to hypoxia in cyanotic congenital heart disease. *New England Journal of Medicine*, **282**, 405–411.

Engel, L.A. & Ritchie, B. (1971). Ventilatory response to inhaled $CO_2$ in hyperthyroidism. *Journal of Applied Physiology*, **30**, 173–177.

Eriksson, L., Wollmer, P., Olsson, C-G. *et al.* (1989). Diagnosis of pulmonary embolism based upon alveolar dead space analysis. *Chest*, **96**, 357–362.

Evans, C.C., Hipkin, L.J. & Murray, G.M. (1977). Pulmonary function in acromegaly. *Thorax*, **32**, 322–327.

Fennerty, A.G., Gunawardene, K.A. & Smith, A.P. (1988). The transfer factor and its subdivisions in patients with pulmonary emboli. *European Respiratory Journal*, **1**, 98–101.

Freedman, S. (1971). Lung volumes and distensibility and maximum respiratory pressures in thyroid disease before and after treatment. *Thorax*, **33**, 785–790.

Gibson, G.J., Edmonds, J.P. & Hughes, G.R.V. (1977). Diaphragm function and lung involvement in systemic lupus erythematosus. *American Journal of Medicine*, **63**, 926–932.

Gibson, G.J., Pride, N.B., Newsom Davies, J. & Loh, L.C. (1977). Pulmonary mechanics in patients with respiratory muscle weakness. *American Reviews of Respiratory Disease*, **115**, 389–395.

Gilmour, D.G., Spiro, S.G., Raphael, M.J. & Freedman, S. (1976). Exercise tests before and after heart valve replacement. *British Journal of Diseases of the Chest*, **70**, 185–194.

Goodman, P. (1984). Pulmonary angiography. *Clinics in Chest Medicine*, 5, 465–478.

Green, M. & Laroche, C.M. (1990). Respiratory muscle weakness. In *Respiratory Medicine*, ed. R.A.L. Brewis, G.J. Gibson, D.M. Geddes, pp. 1373–1387. London: Baillière.

Hales, C.A. & Kazemi, H. (1974). Small airways function in myocardial infarction. *New England Journal of Medicine*, **290**, 761–765.

Hillderal, G., Malmberg, P. & Hemingsson, A. (1990). Asbestos related lesions of the pleura: parietal plaques compared to diffuse thickening studied with chest roentgenography, computed tomography, lung function and gas exchange. *American Journal of Industrial Medicine*, **18**, 627–639.

Horn, M., Ries, A., Neveu, C. & Moser, K. (1983). Restrictive ventilatory pattern in precapillary pulmonary hypertension. *American Review of Respiratory Disease*, **128**, 163–165.

Huisman, M.V., Buller, H.R., ten Cate, J.W. (1989). Unexpectedly high prevalence of silent pulmonary embolism in patients with deep venous thrombosis. *Chest*, **95**, 498–502.

Irwin, R.S., Pratter, M.R., Stivers, D.H. & Braverman, L.E. (1985). Airway reactivity and lung function in triiodothyronine-induced thyrotoxicosis. *Journal of Applied Physiology*, **58**, 1485–1488.

Jones, R.S., Kennedy, J.D., Hoshan, F., Owen, R. & Taylor, J.F. (1981). Mechanical inefficiency of the thoracic cage in scoliosis. *Thorax*, **36**, 456–461.

Kafer, E.R. (1975). Idiopathic scoliosis: mechanical properties of the respiratory system and the ventilatory response to carbon dioxide. *Journal of Clinical Investigation*, **55**, 1153–1163.

Kapitan, K., Buchbinder, M., Wagner, P.D. & Moser, M. (1989). Mechanisms of hypoxaemia in chronic thromboembolic pulmonary hypertension. *American Review of Respiratory Disease*, **139**, 1148–1154.

Kendrick, A.H., O'Reilly, J.F. & Laszlo, G. (1988). Lung function and exercise performance in hyperthyroidism before and after treatment. *Quarterly Journal of Medicine*, **68**, 615–627.

Kilburn, K.H. & Warshaw, R.H. (1991). Abnormal lung function associated with asbestos disease of the pleura, lung and both: a comparative analysis. *Thorax*, **46**, 33–38.

Kreitzer, S.M., Saunders, N.A., Tyler, H.R. & Ingram, R.H. (1978). Respiratory muscle function in amyotrophic lateral scoliosis. *American Review of Respiratory Disease*, **117**, 437–447.

Laine, G.A., Allen, S.J., Williams, J.P., Katz, J., Gabel, J.C. & Drake, R.E. (1986). A new look at pulmonary oedema. *News in Physiological Science*, **1**, 150–153.

Langley, F., Even, P., Duroux, P., Nicolas, R.L. & Cumming, G. (1975). Ventilatory consequences of unilateral pulmonary artery occlusion. *Inserm*, **51**, 209–212.

Lansdorfer, J., Bogui, P., Otayeck, A., Bursaux, E., Pejart, C. & Cabannes, K. (1987). Cardiorespiratory adjustments in chronic sickle cell anaemia. *Bulletin Européen Physiopathologie Respiratoire*, **19**, 339–344.

Ledsome, J.R. & Sharp, J.M. (1981). Pulmonary function in acute cervical cord injury. *American Review of Respiratory Disease*, **124**, 31–44.

Lee H.Y., Stretton, T.B. & Barnes, A.B. (1975). The lungs in renal failure. *Thorax*, **30**, 46–53.

Linderholm, H. & Lindgren, V. (1978). Prediction of spirometric values in patients with scoliosis. *Acta Orthopaedica Scandinavica*, **49**, 469–474.

Litchfield, R.L., Kerber, R.E., Benge, J.W., Bhatnagar, R.K. & Markus, M.L. (1982). Normal exercise capacity in patients with severe left ventricular dysfunction – compensatory mechanisms. *Circulation*, **66**, 129–134.

Littler, W.A., Brown, K. & Roaf, R. (1972). Regional lung function in scoliosis. *Thorax*, **27**, 420–428.

Lopata, M. & Önal, E. (1982). Mass loading, sleep apnoea and the pathogenesis of obesity hypoventilation. *American Review of Respiratory Disease*, **126**, 640–645.

Lurie, P.R. (1953). Postural effects in tetralogy of Fallot. *British Journal of Medicine*, **15**, 292–306.

Manier, G., Castaing, Y. & Guénard, H. (1985). Determinants of hypoxaemia during the acute phase of pulmonary embolism in humans. *American Review of Respiratory Disease*, **132**, 332–338.

Manier, G. & Castaing, Y. (1992). Influence of cardiac output on oxygen exchange in acute pulmonary embolism. *American Review of Respiratory Disease*, **145**, 130–136.

Manier, G., Mora, B., Castaing, Y. & Guénard, H. (1984). Pulmonary oedema after pulmonary embolism. *Bulletin Européen Physiopathologie Respiratoire*, **20**, 55–60.

McDougall, K., Lewis, N.P., Saunders, M.J., Cochlin,

D.L., Davies, M.E., Hutton, R.D., Fox, K.A., Coles, G.A. & Williams J.D. (1990). Long term cardiorespiratory effects of amelioration of renal anaemia by erythropoietin *Lancet*, **335**, 489–493 and 614 (erratum).

McEvoy, R.D., Drew, M.J.R. & Mahar, L.J. (1986). The effect of exercise on ventilation perfusion relationship in patients with mitral stenosis. *Bulletin Européen Physiopathologie Respiratoire*, **22**, 239–246.

Mead, J., Sly, P., Leboeuf, P., Hibbert, M. & Phelan, P.D. (1985). Rib cage mobility in pectus excavatum. *American Review of Respiratory Disease*, **132**, 1223–1228.

Melot, C., Naeije, R., Dechamps, P., Hallemans, R. & Lejeune, P. (1989). Pulmonary and extrapulmonary contributions to hypoxaemia in liver cirrhosis. *American Review of Respiratory Disease*, **139**, 632–640.

Miller, L.R., Greenberg, S.D, & McLarty, J.W. (1985). Lupus lung. *Chest*, **88**, 265–269.

Moore, D.P., Weston, A.R., Hughes, J.M.B., Oakley, C.M. & Cleland, J.G.F. (1992). Effect of increased inspired oxygen concentrations on exercise performance in chronic heart failure. *Lancet*, **339**, 850–853.

Mortolo, J.P., Sant'Ambrogio, G. (1978). Motion of the rib cage and the abdomen in tetraplegic patients. *Clinical Science*, **54**, 25–32.

Mustaf, K.T., Nour, M.M., Shuhaiber, H. & Yousof, A.M. (1984). Pulmonary function before and sequentially after valve replacement surgery with correlation to preoperative haemodynamic data. *American Review of Respiratory Disease*, **130**, 400–406.

Mutoh, T., Lamm, W.J.E., Embree, L.J., Hildebrandt, J. & Albert, R.K. (1992). Volume compression produces abdominal distension, lung compression and chest wall stiffening in pigs. *Journal of Applied Physiology*, **72**, 575–582.

Neu, H.C., Connolly, J.J., Schwertley, F.W. *et al.* (1967). Obstructive respiratory dysfunction in Parkinsonian patients. *American Review of Respiratory Disease*, **95**, 33–47.

Newsom Davis, J., Goldman, M., Loh, L. & Casson, M. (1976). Diaphragm function and hypoventilation. *Quarterly Journal of Medicine*, **45**, 87–100.

Otulana, B.A., Higenbottam, T., Scott, J., Clelland, C., Igboaka, G. & Wallwork, J. (1990). Lung function associated with histologically diagnosed acute lung rejection and pulmonary infection in heart-lung transplant patients. *American Review of Respiratory Disease*, **142**, 329–332.

Patterson, R.W., Nissenson, A.R. & Muller, J. (1981).

Hypoxaemia and pulmonary gas exchange during haemodialysis. *Journal of Applied Physiology*, **50**, 259–264.

Pelletier, C., Lapointe, L. & LeBlanc, P. (1990). Effects of lung resection on pulmonary function and exercise capacity. *Thorax*, **45**, 497–502.

Perks, W.H., Horrocks, P.M., Cooper, R.A., Bradbury, S., Allen, A., Baldock, N., Prowse, K. & Van't Hoff, W. (1980). Sleep apnoea in acromegaly. *British Medical Journal*, **i**, 894–897.

Phillips, M.S., Kinnear, W.J.M., Shaw, D.M. & Shneerson, J.M. (1989). Exercise response in patients treated for pulmonary tuberculosis by thoracoplasty. *Thorax*, **44**, 268–274.

Pison, C., Malo, J-L, Rouleau, J.-L. *et al.* (1989). Bronchial hyperresponsiveness to inhaled methacholine in subjects with chronic left heart failure at a time of exacerbation and after increasing diuretic therapy. *Chest*, **96**, 230–235.

Polak, J.F. & McNeil, B.J. (1984). Pulmonary scintigraphy and the diagnosis of pulmonary embolism: a perspective. *Clinics in Chest Medicine*, **5**, 457–464.

Radwan, L., Strugalska, M. & Koziorowski, A. (1988). Changes in respiratory muscle function after neostigmine in myasthenia gravis. *European Respiratory Journal*, **1**, 119–121.

Ray, C.S., Sue, D.Y., Bray, G., Hansen, J.E. & Wasserman, K. (1983). Effects of obesity on respiratory function. *American Review of Respiratory Disease*, **128**, 501–506.

Rhodes, K.M., Evemy, K., Nariman, S. & Gibson, G.J. (1982). Relation between the severity of mitral valve disease and routine lung function tests in non-smokers. *Thorax*, **37**, 751–755.

Rhodes, K.M., Evemy, K., Lariman, S. & Gibson, G.J. (1985). Effects of mitral valve surgery on static lung function and exercise performance. *Thorax*, **40**, 107–112.

Ringqvist, I. & Ringqvist, T. (1971). Changes in respiratory mechanics in myasthenia gravis with therapy. *Acta Medica Scandinavia*, **190**, 509–518.

Rodriguez-Roisin, R., Agusti, A.G.N. & Roca, J. (1992). The hepatopulmonary syndrome: new name, old complexities. *Thorax*, **47**, 897–902.

Rolla, G., Bucca C, Brussino, L., Bugiani, N., Bergerone, S., Malara, D. & Morea, M. (1992). Bronchial responsiveness, oscillation of peak flow rate and symptoms in patients with mitral stenosis. *European Respiratory Journal*, **5**, 213–218.

Ruff, F., Hughes, J.M.B., Stanley, N., McCarthy, D., Green, R., Aronoff, A., Clayton, L. & Milic-Emili, J. (1971). Regional lung function in patients with hepatic cirrhosis. *Journal of Clinical Investigation*, **50**, 2403–2413.

Saunders, K.B. (1966). Physiological dead space in left ventricular failure. *Clinical Science*, **31**, 145–151.

Schilling, J.A. (1965). Pulmonary resection and sequelae of thoracic surgery. In *Handbook of Physiology*, section 3, vol. 2, ed. W.O. Fenn & H. Rahn, pp. 1531–1552. Bethesda: APS.

Sciurba, F.C., Owens, G.R., Sanders, M.H., Constantino, J.P., Paradis, I.L. & Griffith, B.P. (1991). The effect of obliterative bronchiolitis on breathing pattern during exercise in recipients of heart-lung transplants. *American Review of Respiratory Disease*, **144**, 131–135.

Seidman, J.M. & Mark, E.J. (1992). A 33-year-old woman with cirrhosis and right ventricular failure. *New England Journal of Medicine*, **326**, 1682–1692.

Serisier, D.E., Mastaglia, F.L. & Gibson, G.J. (1982). Respiratory muscle function and ventilatory control. I. In patients with motor neurone disease. II. In patients with myotonic dystrophy. *Quarterly Journal of Medicine*, **51**, 205–226.

Shneerson, J.M. (1978*a*). The cardiorespiratory response to exercise in thoracic scoliosis. *Thorax*, **33**, 457–463.

Shneerson, J.M. (1978*b*). Pulmonary artery pressure in thoracic scoliosis during and after exercise while breathing pure air and oxygen. *Thorax*, **33**, 747–754.

Silberstein, S.L., Barland, P., Grazsel, A.I. & Koerner, S.K. (1980). Pulmonary dysfunction in systemic lupus erythematosus. *Journal of Rheumatology*, **7**, 187–195.

Skatrud, J., Iber, C., Ewart, K. *et al.* (1981). Disordered breathing during sleep in hypothyroidism. *American Review of Respiratory Disease*, **124**, 325–329.

Snashall, P.D. (1980). Pulmonary oedema. *British Journal of Diseases of the Chest*, **74**, 7–22.

Stanley, N.N., Williams, A.J., Dewar, C., Blendis, L.M. & Reid, L. (1977). Hypoxia and hydrothoraces in a case of liver cirrhosis: correlation of physiological, radiographic, scintographic and pathological findings. *Thorax*, **32**, 457–471.

Stanley, N.N. & Woodgate, D.J. (1972). Mottled chest radiograph and gas transfer defect in chronic liver disease. *Thorax*, **27**, 315–323.

Stewart, R.M., Ridyeard, J.B. & Pearson, J.D. (1976). Regional lung function in ankylosing spondylitis. *Thorax*, **31**, 433–437.

Thompson, P.J., Dhillon, D.P., Ledingham, J. & Turner-Warwick, M. (1985). Shrinking lungs, diaphragmatic dysfunction and systemic lupus erythematosus. *American Review of Respiratory Disease*, **132**, 926–928.

Toppell, K.L., Atkinson, R. & Whitcomb, M.E. (1973). Lung growth in acromegaly. *American Review of Respiratory Disease*, **108**, 1254–1258.

von Basch, S. (1887). Uber eine Function des Capillardruckels in der Lungenalveolen. *Wien. Med. Blatt*, **10**, 466.

Warley, A.R.M., Finnegan, O.C., Nicholson, E.M. & Laszlo, G. (1987). Grading of dyspnoea and walking speed in cardiac disorders and chronic airflow obstruction. *British Journal of Diseases of the Chest*, **81**, 349–355.

Weinberger, S.E, Weiss, S.T., Cohen, W.R., Weiss, J.W. & Johnson, T.S. (1980). Pregnancy and the lung. *American Review of Respiratory Disease*, **121**, 559–581.

Williams, N.H., Adler, J.J. & Colp, C. (1969). Pulmonary function studies as an aid in the differential diagnosis of pulmonary hypertension. *American Journal of Medicine*, **47**, 378–383.

Wimalaratna, H.S.K., Farrell, J. & Lee, H.Y. (1990). Measurement of diffusing capacity in pulmonary embolism. *Respiratory Medicine*, **83**, 481–486.

Wood, T.E., McLeod, P., Anthonisen, M.R. & Macklem, P.T. (1971). Mechanics of breathing in mitral stenosis. *American Reviews of Respiratory Disease*, **104**, 52–60.

Wright, P.H., Hansen, A., Kreel, L & Capel, L.H. (1980). Respiratory function changes after asbestos pleurisy. *Thorax*, **35**, 31–36.

Yernault, J-C. & de Troyer, A. (1980). Mechanics of breathing in patients with aortic valve disease. *Bulletin Européen Physiopathologie Respiratoire*, **16**, 491–500.

# 10 Physiological principles underlying the treatment of respiratory failure

Respiratory failure occurs when the lungs are unable to maintain normal arterial blood gas concentrations breathing room air at sea level. It has two components (Roussos, 1985):

1. Lung failure (gas exchange disturbances manifested by hypoxaemia); $CO_2$ retention may also occur.
2. Pump failure (ventilatory failure: elevation of arterial $P_{CO_2}$).

$P_{CO_2}$ rises if there is:

1. Central depression of respiration.
2. A severe disturbance of gas exchange.
3. A severe mechanical ventilatory defect.
4. Respiratory muscle fatigue.

Generally, abnormal blood gases in exercise are not treated as respiratory failure, though the causes and mechanisms of transient hypoxaemia and elevation of arterial $P_{CO_2}$ during exercise are identical.

This chapter discusses the problem of the patient in whom arterial $P_{CO_2}$ is found to be elevated during spontaneous ventilation at rest (Table 10.1). This may develop over many weeks, months or years or it may occur acutely both in normal individuals and in patients whose arterial blood gases are already deranged.

## Arterial blood gases

Radial, brachial or femoral artery puncture are used to sample arterial blood for analysis in blood gas electrodes. A little technical knowledge is necessary to anticipate the possible errors. For accurate analysis, blood should ideally be sampled into self-filling syringes over several respiratory cycles, with buffered heparin (1/1000) used to fill the dead space. To achieve the greatest accuracy the syringes should made of glass and the blood analysed immediately, without cooling. Samples should be cooled only if analysis is likely to delayed by more than 30 minutes; cooling is supposed to reduce the oxygen consumption of the blood cells, but it also delays equilibration in the electrodes. Most analyses are performed on highly complex automated systems, regularly calibrated with gases or liquids of known $P_{CO_2}$ and $P_{O_2}$.

Machines calibrated with gas may show a systematic error in $P_{O_2}$, caused by setting $P_{O_2}$ too high because of blood gas differences within the electrode. Blood equilibrated with gases of known composition in a tonometer is used to determine the characteristics of the analyser. Modern equipment uses liquid standards at 37 °C. If blood is added in a syringe $P_{O_2}$ falls by a factor of ×0.9 for each degree Celsius fall of $P_{O_2}$, so that a febrile patient with a temperature of 39 °C may erroneously be thought to have a low $P_{O_2}$ when the blood is analysed at 37 °C. $P_{CO_2}$ similarly falls by a factor of × 0.95 for each degree Celsius. Certain machines make the necessary correction automatically. A single air bubble rapidly ejected with only one passage through the sample exchanges very little gas, and produces no inaccuracy of importance in clinical evaluation. Very strange results are obtained if the syringe is contaminated with too much heparin or with numerous bubbles of air.

The relationship of pH to $P_{CO_2}$ is fundamental

Table 10.1. *Ventilatory failure*

Respiratory depression by drugs: anaesthetics
Unexplained ('primary') alveolar hypoventilation
Damage to brainstem respiratory centres
  Malignant infiltration
  Cerebrovascular accidents

Damage to spinal respiratory pathways
  Cervical cordotomy
  Myelitis

Paralysis of respiratory muscles
  Poliomyelitis
  Polyneuritis
  Muscular dystrophy

Thoracic cage disorders
  Kyphoscoliosis

Bronchopulmonary diseases, acute
  Central airway obstruction
  Bronchial asthma
  Pneumonia
  Pulmonary oedema:
  (*a*)  cardiogenic
  (*b*)  exudative (ARDS)
  (*c*)  inhalation

Bronchopulmonary disease, chronic
  Chronic airflow obstruction
  Pulmonary fibrosis

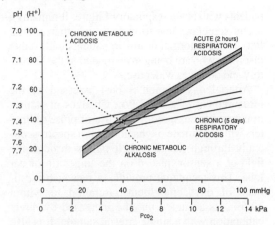

Fig. 10.1. Relationship between pH (and hydrogen ion activity) and $Pco_2$ in arterial blood drawn from patients with various metabolic disorders. An acute rise of $Pco_2$ results in a steep fall of pH and a steep, linear rise of hydrogen ion activity. The fall of pH is less than if whole blood is subjected to the same rise of $Pco_2$ because there are fewer protein ions to buffer the changes in the extracellular fluid than in blood. Renal excretion of bicarbonate results in a degree of metabolic compensation with a fall in the degree of acidity. Metabolic acid–base disturbances cause respiratory compensation via effects on the chemoreceptors (Chapter 14). The limits are rather wide and not shown on the graph. Very severe falls of pH are seen in patients with metabolic acidosis who develop ventilatory failure and who cannot compensate for this by hyperventilation.

to the assessment of acid–base disturbances (Fig. 10.1). It will not be discussed in detail. Elevation of arterial $Pco_2$ in life results in respiratory acidosis. An acute rise of $Pco_2$ results in a change of about 0.1 pH units per 1 mmHg (0.13 kPa) elevation. This takes up to 10 minutes (Laszlo, Clark & Campbell, 1969). If $Pco_2$ remains elevated renal compensation occurs with chloride excretion and bicarbonate retention. This process is complete in about 5 days. Commonly, patients with longstanding ventilatory failure have pH levels above 7.4: this is usually related to potassium depletion resulting from the administration of diuretics which are used to treat the fluid retention accompanying hypoxic cor pulmonale.

### Rebreathing estimates of $Pco_2$

Mixed venous $Pco_2$ can be estimated by equilibrating the alveolar gas with the contents of a small rebreathing bag (1.5 litres) with air enriched with oxygen. The procedure is described in detail in Chapter 14. During normal respiration at rest, arterial $Pco_2$ is close to 40 mmHg (5.5 kPa) and rebreathing oxygenated mixed venous $Pco_2$ is about 46 mmHg (6.3 kPa). The difference is determined mainly by the cardiac output and the metabolic rate (Chapter 3) according to the Fick principle. As respiratory failure worsens, arterial $Pco_2$ rises and the difference widens so that the elevation of arterial $Pco_2$ is amplified when assessed by the rebreathing method. This is therefore a sensitive indicator of changes in the condition of patients with acute respiratory failure. It remains a useful screening test to indicate whether arterial $P_{CO_2}$ is high, normal or low in patients with stable disorders who are being investigated in the laboratory and deserves wider use.

Arterial oxygenation is best assessed by the measurement of arterial $P_{O_2}$. Changes of saturation may be measured by the use of pulse oximeters which estimate oxyhaemoglobin spectroscopically through the skin as it pulses through the field of a sensor, placed on the finger tip or ear lobe. This technique provides a reasonable estimate of oxyhaemoglobin saturation to within ±2.5%. Its accuracy may be increased by direct calibration with a single arterial sample. It is also possible to improve the accuracy of the equipment by measuring $O_2$ saturation after 5 minutes of breathing 100% $O_2$. This results in full saturation except in the presence of a true shunt (Chapter 3) and the difference between the reading and that obtained at 100% can be used to correct the analysis. Oximeters are used to detect changes of oxygen saturation during the polysomnography in the study of respiration during sleep (Chapter 15), general anaesthesia and bronchoscopy and in the intensive monitoring of acutely ill patients with respiratory problems.

## Chronic respiratory failure in patients with hypoxaemic lung diseases

Chronic hypoxaemia leads to pulmonary arteriolar constriction. This in turn results in permanent narrowing of the walls of arterioles, but generally some reversibility remains. Pulmonary arterial pressure is elevated above the normal value (24/6 or less at rest) in chronically hypoxaemic subjects with lung disease.

The clinical manifestations of chronic hypoxaemia are fatigue, enlargement of the pulmonary arteries, loss of consciousness on exertion, right ventricular hypertrophy and peripheral oedema. These may present before the individual becomes aware of any breathlessness associated with the underlying disorder. Examination reveals signs of secondary polycythaemia and of congestive heart failure.

Right ventricular hypertrophy secondary to hypoxaemic lung disease (cor pulmonale) has to be distinguished from the other causes of pulmonary hypertension without hypoxaemia:

1. Thromboembolic disease: this in any case may complicate hypoxic pulmonary hypertension and may be found at post-mortem. Usually, the pulmonary hypertension appears gross in the presence of no desaturation or only modest hypoxaemia.
2. Primary pulmonary hypertension: in this condition, arterial $P_{O_2}$ is rarely less than 70 mmHg (9 kPa).
3. Atrial septal defect with reversed shunt.

### Nocturnal oxygen desaturation in chronic airflow obstruction

Ventilation tends to become irregular and shallow during rapid eye movement sleep. This process normally causes no desaturation. Individuals whose daytime $P_{O_2}$ is close to 60 mmHg (8 kPa) are prone to desaturate at night, because minor changes in ventilation have a profound effect on oxygen saturation as well as $P_{O_2}$ under these circumstances (Chapter 3). This is not synonymous with the sleep apnoea syndrome: patients have normal changes of ventilation but the consequences are different because of alterations in dead space and physiological shunt.

The evidence that it is a factor in pulmonary hypertension is not very strong (Flenley, 1978; Connaughton *et al.*, 1988), but it is associated with decreased longevity in patients with normal daytime oxygen saturation and $P_{O_2}$ greater than 60 mmHg (8 kPa) (Fletcher *et al.*, 1992).

### Long-term oxygen therapy

Long-term inhalation of supplementary oxygen (approximately 30%, or 2 litres per minute via nasal cannulation) reduces pulmonary hypertension, reduces polycythaemia and improves well-being and longevity over a period of time (Weitzenblum *et al.*, 1985). Not less than 15 hours a day is required (Medical Research Council Working Party, 1981) and the results are even better if 24 hours are attempted, at least at the start of treatment (Nocturnal Oxygen Therapy Trial Group, 1980). Lung function may improve and reduce the need for therapy.

This treatment is expensive, requiring the delivery of a large cylinder of oxygen daily or the installation of a concentrator in the patient's home. Oxygen concentrators pump air over crystals which absorb nitrogen and deliver 96% oxygen at 4 litres per minute. Because of the cost, guidelines have been published in the United Kingdom indicating which patients are likely to be helped by long-term oxygen at home. These are based on the results of British trials.

1. $FEV_1$ less than 1.0 litre.
2. Arterial $PO_2$ less than 55 mmHg (7.5 kPa).
3. Rise of $PCO_2$ of no more than 5 mmHg (0.8 kPa) after nocturnal inhalation of oxygen.
4. A documented episode of oedema or heart failure.
5. Assessment in a stable condition, at least 3 weeks after any acute exacerbation.

These guidelines are frequently ignored. They may be excessively restrictive, especially in recommending waiting until heart failure develops (Baudouin et al., 1990). Treatment of nocturnal oxygen desaturation may improve longevity (Fletcher et al., 1992). Nevertheless, as long-term oxygen is expensive and breathing oxygen for 15 hours per day is very restrictive, attempts to improve longevity by earlier prescription of long-term oxygen, supposedly to prevent the development of pulmonary hypertension, may fail through lack of use. Research is needed in this group of patients and among those with fibrosing alveolitis and other causes of hypoxic lung disease. In these, as in patients with terminal malignant disease or heart failure, oxygen therapy may relieve dyspnoea in the short term. There are no trials to show that it improves longevity.

## Acute deterioration of $PO_2$ and $PCO_2$

### Management of acute ventilation failure in chronic airflow obstruction

The principles of treatment of acute exacerbations of chronic bronchitis and emphysema are well known (Campbell, 1965, 1967, 1979). They include:

- Treatment of reversible disease (asthma, infection, pulmonary oedema).
- Controlled oxygen therapy using systems delivering known concentrations (p. 160).
- Respiratory stimulant when appropriate (p. 160).
- Arousal.
- Avoidance of sedation.
- Hydration with 5% dextrose (supplemented with potassium chloride).

### Arterial blood gases in respiratory failure

Untreated patients are generally hypoxaemic, with arterial $PCO_2$ levels between 50 and 75 mmHg (6.5 and 10 kPa). Patients with $PCO_2$ levels higher than this have probably received oxygen as explained in Chapter 3 (McNicol & Campbell, 1965).

Most patients with chronic airflow obstruction who develop acute $CO_2$ retention recover with conservative management; a few will require assisted ventilation.

Progressive hypoventilation or respiratory arrest are caused by:

1. Respiratory muscle weakness.
2. Central depression of ventilation, partly because of reduction of chemoreceptor activity in the presence of the rising $PO_2$.
3. Changes in the acid–base status of the blood due to the acidifying effect of oxyhaemoglobin after injudicious oxygen therapy.
4. Worsening distribution of ventilation and blood flow, because relief of hypoxic vasoconstriction distributes more mixed venous blood to poorly ventilated zones; as a result both $O_2$ and $CO_2$ shunt are increased (Dunn, Nilson & Hubmayr, 1991).

On average, $PCO_2$ rises by only 5 mmHg (0.7 kPa) on changing from air to 24% oxygen and by 7–10 mmHg (1–1.5 kPa) if 28% oxygen is used (Warrell et al., 1970).

Flenley and his colleagues proposed guidelines for treatment (Warren et al., 1980) and evaluated their performance (Jeffrey, Warren & Flenley, 1992).

1. Oxygen therapy by mask to raise $PO_2$ above 50 mmHg (6.6 kPa), but not higher, to avoid progressive hypoventilation.

Table 10.2. *Masks delivering fixed $O_2$ concentrations at high flow rates*

| Mixture (% $O_2$) | Entrainment rates | Minimum $O_2$ flow ($l \cdot min^{-1}$ to deliver 40 $l \cdot min^{-1}$) |
|---|---|---|
| 24 | 20 : 1 | 2 |
| 28 | 10 : 1 | 4 |
| 35 | 5 : 1 | 8 |

2. Infusion of a respiratory stimulant if pH fell below 7.25 ([H⁺] 55 $mmol \cdot l^{-1}$) as a result of therapy.
3. Avoidance of sedation.

Risk factors for death included:

* Acidosis: pH less than 7.25 after oxygen therapy.
* Uraemia.
* Hypotension.

Mortality, at about 12% appeared to be unrelated to $Po_2$ and $Pco_2$ on admission to hospital (Jeffrey *et al.*, 1992; Portier, Defouilloy & Muir, 1992).

These guidelines have to be modified in the presence of gross pulmonary oedema, lobar or segmental pneumonia or pulmonary embolism. These patients are more ill in relation to $Po_2$ than those with infective exacerbations, tend towards hypotension and often are severely breathless.

Progressive hypoventilation, $CO_2$ narcosis and profound hypoxaemia may call for artificial ventilation, which is given if there is a reasonable prospect of recovery.

#### Masks for controlled oxygen therapy

Simple masks delivering fixed concentrations of oxygen work on the Bernouilli principle. A jet of not less than 2·$l.min^{-1}$ of oxygen from a cylinder or wall source entrains air from the room through side holes, like a Bunsen burner. The concentration depends on the design of the side ports, which determines the entrainment ratio. To manufacture 28% oxygen from 21% oxygen and 100% oxygen requires an entrainment ratio of 10 parts air to 1 part oxygen. This creates a draught which blows away the expired $CO_2$, but it is necessary to

blow a sufficiently fast stream to exceed the peak inspiratory flow rate. This is generally about 40 $l·min^{-1}$ (7 $l·s^{-1}$). The entrainment ratios of some available masks, together with their minimum flow rates, are given in Table 10.2. These masks need cylinder pressure to drive them. If it is thought necessary to humidify the oxygen, a special system is needed as the jet will not entrain air if the pressure is too low.

Simple plastic masks and nasal cannulae should not be used in the acute stage of ventilatory failure, because the concentration they deliver is determined by the rate and depth of breathing, such that a patient with very shallow breathing may receive very high concentrations.

#### Treatment with respiratory stimulants

Doxapram and similar agents stimulate respiration by increasing the output of the chemoreceptors, but they also increase the metabolic rate. They therefore have a limited use in patients with transient hypoventilation when no specific antidote exists. They are highly likely to cause convulsions if given to patients with extreme hypoxaemia; therefore this must be corrected with oxygen to a $Po_2$ of at least 45 mmHg (6 kPa). They only work if the patient can be shown to have considerable unused respiratory reserve, demonstrated by the ability to take a markedly deeper breath on command than during spontaneous respiration. Patients breathing maximally cannot improve gas exchange by the use of these agents, which increase oxygen requirement.

### Respiratory muscle fatigue

Respiratory muscle fatigue is an important contributor to respiratory failure in acute illness (Roussos, 1985; Green & Moxham, 1985) (Chapter 2). It occurs for a number of reasons:

#### 1. Failure of blood supply

The human respiratory muscles, including the diaphragm, receive a high proportion of the cardiac output when operating at their maximum. This may be maintained when the circulation to the other tissues becomes inadequate, which results in severe lactic acidosis. This is relieved by resting the respiratory muscles by means of artificial ventilation. Severe cardiogenic shock is itself an indication for artificial ventilation.

If respiration is also impeded by a high abdominal pressure, or by continuous contraction of the diaphragm as in severe bronchial asthma, the diaphragmatic circulation itself is impeded and fatigue is hastened.

### 2. Prolonged excessive respiratory work

Neuromuscular fatigue may be central or peripheral. In fatigued muscle the force generated declines in relation to the firing of the motor nerve. Contraction slows down. Firing rate also decreases and this may be considered either as central fatigue or as adaptation. Normal subjects develop fatigue when pleural pressure exceeds around 30% of the maximum at halfway between FRC and TLC over several respiratory cycles. A rapid shallow breathing pattern avoids this situation for as along as possible. Adopting this breathing strategy increases the ratio of dead space to tidal volume and therefore increases the likelihood of a rise of $PCO_2$. Eventually, a raised $PCO_2$ is tolerated without further stimulating breathing. This reduces the effort of breathing. It is not known whether this adaptation is achieved by acclimatising the respiratory centres to abnormal blood gases or whether it represents a chronic fatigue state. In chronic airflow obstruction, the problem is compounded by the high lung volumes.

Respiratory muscle weakness and fatigue may be recognised at the bedside. One palm is placed on the epigastrium with the thumb and fingers palpating the lower costal margins. The sternomastoid muscle is palpated with the other hand. The weak or failing diaphragm cannot exert a downward pressure on the palm or expand the lower ribs either during spontaneous respiration, during deep breathing or sniffing, or in response to a request to push out the abdominal wall. Alternate use of the sternomastoid and the diaphragm, for three or four breaths in each case, is called 'respiratory alternans'. Finally, diaphragmatic fatigue is characterised by a falling respiratory rate, below 30 per minute. Respiratory rate also falls when the patient improves, but patients with respiratory failure breathe at a rate of 28 per minute or more, until the respiratory

reserve improves and the inspiratory capacity is at least twice the tidal volume. These bedside observations, in conjunction with measurement of VC and the arterial blood gases and pH, identify patients who need to be transferred to the intensive care ward for artificial ventilation.

Movement of the diaphragm is impeded by pain and other nociceptive reflexes after upper abdominal surgery.

## Acute respiratory failure: principles of respiratory intensive care

Respiratory intensive care has advanced in 25 years from the use of simple positive and negative pressure ventilators in medical wards to a highly sophisticated system of applied physiology and pharmacology. Little justice can be done to this subject by a brief summary, but certain basic principles have to be understood if the referring physician is to take a useful part in the work of the intensive care unit; this section attempts to summarise these. Acute emergencies, such as the inhalation of foreign bodies, are not discussed.

Patients are generally admitted to respiratory intensive care units when spontaneous ventilation is inadequate and requires mechanical assistance (Ponte, 1990). Such units generally are able to deal with failure of multiple systems including the circulation and the kidneys. The purpose of intensive care is to maintain a sufficiently normal level of arterial $PO_2$ and $PCO_2$ and to sustain the circulation to the brain and kidneys. The patients generally arrive because of one or more conditions:

1. **Severe diffuse obstruction to peripheral airways**: bronchial asthma, chronic bronchitis.
2. **Excessive lung fluid.** This interferes with gas exchange and makes breathing difficult. The fluid may be inhaled, transuded because of raised pulmonary venous or lymphatic pressure, or exuded because of inflammation.

*Drowning*, in fresh or hypotonic water, causes haemolysis if the water is ingested in sufficient quantities. Salty water draws fluid from the circulation into the lungs. Both reduce the surface areas for gas exchange. Other liquids, such as acid gastric contents, exert their effects by inflaming the airways and causing exudation into the alve-oli. Secondary bacterial infection occurs fre-quently, often with anaerobic agents or with *Staphylococcus aureus*. The use of corticosteroids as inflammatory agents is unproved; similarly, the use of prophylactic antibiotics is questionable, although they are important in the treatment of established infection.

*Acute cardiogenic pulmonary oedema* occurs in left ventricular failure, or in patients with mitral valve obstruction in whom left atrial pressure rises above a critical value under conditions in which blood flow would normally increase. It rarely requires referral to the intensive care unit because it usually responds quickly to vasodila-tors and diuretics: loop diuretics such as frusemide are believed to combine these proper-ties. Patients do not usually develop respiratory failure as a complication of ventricular failure unless they have some underlying disease of the lungs which disadvantages them from the outset; the commonest is chronic airflow obstruction which does not need to be severe to cause this problem.

Exudative lung disease in its extreme form is called *adult respiratory distress syndrome (ARDS)*, and is characterised by the loss of pro-tein-containing fluid into the alveolar walls and spaces because of damage to capillary endo-thelium. A very large number of injurious materials cause such damage. These include infectious agents, inhaled chemicals and circulat-ing toxins. ARDS especially complicates multiple trauma and septicaemia with circulating endo-toxin. Fat embolism is a special case in which circulating products of lipid metabolism probably damage the capillary endothelium as well as tem-porarily obstructing the pulmonary microcircula-tion.

### 3. Respiratory muscle disease

Generally, patients are referred for assisted venti-lation if a muscle disease is potentially reversible or self-limiting, such as polyneuritis, myasthenia gravis, poliomyelitis or tetanus. Patients with progressive chronic conditions are admitted if they have a potentially reversible chest infection which has precipitated respiratory failure. A few susceptible individuals require prolonged ventilation after the use of anaesthetic relaxant agents.

### 4. Chest wall disorders

Bilateral rib fractures, or fractures of the sternum, impair spontaneous ventilation. Quite minor infections precipitate respiratory failure in indi-viduals with scoliosis. Patients with ankylosing spondylitis cannot tolerate interference with the function of the diaphragm, such as occurs during upper abdominal surgery, but generally do not have blood gas disturbances unless some pul-monary disorder is also present.

### 5. Central respiratory depression

Most respiratory depressants, including benzodi-azepines, are well tolerated by those with healthy lungs. Overdoses of antihistamines or barbiturate drugs cause respiratory failure. Individuals vary in their sensitivity to the respiratory depressant effects of opiates, which can be reversed pharma-cologically. Patients with chronic lung disease and impaired blood gases may require ventilation after the injudicious use of uncontrolled oxygen therapy or respiratory depressants.

## Mechanical ventilation of the lungs

When spontaneous ventilation of the lungs is thought to be inadequate, mechanical assistance is provided. In practice, intermittent positive pres-sure ventilation through an endotracheal tube (IPPV) is the only feasible method of instituting adequate ventilation at speed. Advances in tech-nology have rendered this much safer than hith-erto: classical accounts of respiratory failure describe artificial ventilation as something to be avoided if at all possible. Behind this lay the fact that the institution of mechanical ventilation in medical wards carried a 50% mortality. Furthermore, endotracheal tubes were formerly very rigid and their cuffs inflated to a pressure of 20–25 cm $H_2O$ (2.5 kPa) which resulted in stenosed segments of the trachea in at least 25% of patients. Early tracheostomy was the rule, and this was considered mandatory after 5 days of endotracheal intubation. Reluctantly, this time limit crept up to 10 days. The problem was largely solved by the development of cuffs which require inflation to much lower pressures (5 cm $H_2O$, 0.5 kPa) which rarely cause tracheal ulceration. Because of this and numerous other improvements in the management of respiratory failure, artificial ventilation should not be considered as a last resort. This is not to recommend careless management of oxygen therapy on medical wards, but it is not necessary to maintain a state of precarious hypoxaemia for fear of causing hypoventilation.

More arguably, it is not necessary to worry unduly about the ethical problems associated with the artificial ventilation of patients with chronic lung disease. Failure to breathe spontaneously after treatment of the acute exacerbation is a well-known problem when dealing with progressive neuromuscular diseases, but this unfortunate outcome is extremely unusual among patients with chronic airflow obstruction. A chairbound, depressed bronchitic living alone may not be grateful for a new lease of life, but most patients with chronic airflow obstruction have time to acclimatise to their disability and live useful lives giving moral support to their families. A period of assisted ventilation results in normalisation of the arterial $Po_2$ which improves ventricular function and lung function for quite long periods. Patients with chronic airflow obstruction who slip into acute respiratory failure can and should be ventilated, unless there is a record of frequent episodes of hospital admission or unless the patient or the relatives, on the patient's behalf, decline this treatment.

The use of nasal masks to administer intermittent or continuous positive pressure without intubation is being investigated. The technique requires considerable skill and is often not successful (Strumpf *et al.*, 1991).

## Principles of assisted ventilation

Assisted ventilation units depend on the principles of respiratory mechanics and gas exchange that have been described. A few comments follow which place these principles into context. What follows is a physiologist's view of assisted ventilation.

### Setting the ventilator

Traditional inexpensive ventilators allow control of:

1. Rate of inspiration, time of expiration.
2. Tidal volume. Usually a preset tidal volume is delivered by a piston up to the limit of pressure that can be generated within the device. Certain instruments allow maximal inspiratory pressure to be set in these; tidal volume varies according to the dynamic compliance of the lungs and chest wall.

The rules for these ventilators were very simple. Obstructive syndromes were treated with the slowest possible inspiratory and expiratory times. The first ensured a reasonably even distribution of inspired gas, because a rapid inspiration under positive pressure forces the air into the least obstructed airways and overdistends the alveoli distal to these. Slow expiration allows time for the recoil of the lungs to return the thorax to FRC. Patients with stiff or oedematous lungs require shallow breaths under low pressure with incomplete relaxation. If the airways are patent, a short inspiratory time at rapid rate maintains the tidal volume required to achieve the desired minute ventilation.

Modern ventilators using microprocessor technology are able to deliver the inspired air according to carefully regulated flow or pressure patterns. A slow rate of inspiration is best for airflow obstruction. Tidal volume is usually set at around 0.4–0.5 litre in patients with alveolar disorders without airflow obstruction, and 0.5–0.75 litre in patients with airflow obstruction.

When ventilation is instituted, the aim is to achieve a normal pH. Patients who have experienced $CO_2$ retention for some days have elevated levels of plasma bicarbonate, so $Pco_2$ will not need to be reduced as low as 40 mmHg (5.5 kPa).

The pressure required to generate the required tidal volume depends on the compliance of the lungs and chest walls. Ventilation of young subjects with neuromuscular paralysis, but without concomitant lung disease, requires less than 20 cm $H_2O$ (2 kPa); that is, compliance is less than 40 cm $H_2O \cdot l^{-1}$ (4 $kPa \cdot l^{-1}$). The actual pressure is recorded regularly. A rise of dynamic compliance at a known frequency, or simply of the pressure setting, without any worsening of blood gases, is a good indicator of improvement of lung function.

Pressures above 40 cm $H_2O$ (6 kPa), greatly increase the risk of IPPV-induced pneumothorax or pneumomediastinum: above 70 cm $H_2O$ (9 kPa) these are virtually inevitable and, in addition, venous return falls dramatically. Occasionally, pressures of around 70 mmHg (9 kPa) may be required to sustain life in patients with severe bronchoconstriction or acute severe asthma. This can only be delivered by a powerful volume-cycled device fitted with the facility to turn off the safety valve. Very major damage can be done to the alveoli distal to the remaining patent airways when this pressure is transmitted to them. Pneumothoraces induced by IPPV have to be drained. Surgical emphysema is a distressing complication of this and of pneumomediastinum. In this situation, a high $Pco_2$ is preferable to excessive ventilation pressures. Modern instruments can reduce barotrauma by optimising frequency and rise of inspiratory pressure.

The ventilatory requirement may be calculated from the considerations expounded in Chapter 1. Artificial respiration rests all the muscles, so $CO_2$ production and oxygen consumption fall to basal levels, allowing for alterations of body temperature. About 5 litres per minute of *alveolar* ventilation excretes $CO_2$ from well-ventilated and perfused compartments. Wasted ventilation to areas of high ventilation–perfusion ratio (dead space) is usually 50% of tidal volume or greater, and is of course dependent on pattern of breathing.

### Sedation

Sedation is needed initially to maintain artificial ventilation, and abolish spontaneous ventilatory efforts ('fighting the ventilator') (Flick, Bellamy & Simmons, 1989). Intravenous opiates, such as morphine, provide the best sedation in most instances with minimal hypotension. Later, the patient may tolerate being awake and may learn to relax, allowing the ventilator to provide pressure support by augmenting spontaneous breathing.

### Oxygen requirement

Areas of very low ventilation–perfusion ratio account for hypoxaemia which is relieved by sup-

plementary oxygen. Low cardiac output causes mixed venous $Po_2$ to be low and aggravates the effect of 'physiological shunting' of reduced haemoglobin in the lungs, because the shunted blood is highly desaturated. Even in the absence of extrapulmonary shunting, it may be impossible to maintain a normal arterial $O_2$ saturation. This situation tends to arise in pneumonia or severe ARDS in which the chest X-ray shows massive and widespread consolidation.

Oxygen consumption, and thus oxygen requirement, falls dramatically when artificial ventilation is given to breathless patients. This occurs mainly because of the removal of the need to ventilate maximally. The fall of oxygen consumption conversely improves mixed venous oxygenation, with the result that arterial $Po_2$ improves even without any amelioration of the distribution of blood to poorly ventilated areas. Unfortunately, three factors conspire to reduce blood pressure or cardiac output and thus worsen mixed venous $Po_2$.

1. Blood pressure falls if $Pco_2$ is reduced rapidly with a concomitant rise of arterial pH.
2. Blood pressure may fall because of the use of sedatives.
3. Venous return to the heart is impeded by the institution of positive pressure breathing, because the intrathoracic pressure rises from a mean value of below atmospheric to a mean positive pressure, which raises pulmonary arteriolar resistance.

Oxygen in concentrations of greater than 50% is toxic to the alveoli and tends to worsen ARDS, especially in those regions which are well-ventilated and perfused. As well as this direct effect, ventilation with gases low in nitrogen or insoluble gas content with a high $O_2$ concentration is said to result in progressive atelectasis, because of the speed with which alveoli become de-aerated when ventilation is temporarily obstructed. The importance of this has been questioned (Lemaire *et al.*, 1985; Lampron *et al.*, 1985). The prognosis of patients requiring ventilation with 60% oxygen or higher concentrations is very poor. To combat this problem, devices which allow the venous blood to exchange oxygen and $CO_2$ outside the body (extracorporeal membrane oxygenators) are likely to be used more generally. These devices have been introduced into intensive care practice in many parts of the world.

### Sudden worsening of ventilator pressures and arterial oxygenation

One of two easily identified and remediable situations may cause ventilator pressures to rise or arterial $O_2$ saturation to fall:

1. Slippage of the endotracheal tube into the right main bronchus so that it obstructs, or partially obstructs, the left main bronchus. This may be diagnosed clinically or on chest X-ray and is easily remedied by repositioning the tube.
2. Restlessness and arousal of the patient, because of inadequate sedation. The ventilator pressures swing as inspiratory efforts are made out of time with the machine (Flick, Bellamy & Simmons, 1989).

### Positive end-expiratory pressure

Subjects with ARDS have a low FRC and a high closing volume. Usually they are helped by the addition of positive pressure at the end of expiration (PEEP), or traditionally by a valve which prevents expiration when a positive pressure is still present in the alveoli. The effect is to maintain continuity between the alveoli and the conducting airways and to reduce the speed at which the mixed venous blood runs out of oxygen in closed lung units. A pressure of 5–10 cm $H_2O$ (0.5–1 kPa) is usually applied. The benefits of PEEP on gas exchange are offset to some extent by the rise of mean intrathoracic pressure which reduces venous return and eventually lowers mixed venous $Po_2$. Trial and error is generally required to set PEEP at its optimal level.

It follows that PEEP is not always useful in patients with chronic airflow obstruction. They breathe near TLC and many of their airways close before the end of expiration. PEEP, therefore, worsens hyperinflation, but may occasionally be helpful to splint the airways when there is airway closure above FRC.

## Support of the circulation

This aspect of intensive care calls for great skill, experience and pharmacological insight. A few basic physiological principles need to be recalled at the outset.

The problem may roughly be divided into

1. Control of blood pressure.
2. Maintenance of cardiac output.
3. Treatment of arrhythmia.

### High blood pressure

Hypertension may be treated on its merits, remembering that it is usually better to reduce the dose of pressor drugs than to give antidotes.

$CO_2$ retention in acute respiratory acidosis causes hypertension (typically 180/110 mmHg) with peripheral and cerebral vasodilation. This is reversed promptly when artificial ventilation is started. A rapid fall of $Pco_2$ may elevate pH abruptly into the alkalotic range in patients with compensated respiratory acidosis and a high plasma bicarbonate level. Transient hypotension may occur.

### Hypotension: circulatory failure

A low blood pressure is usually associated with a fall of cardiac output, poor tissue perfusion and inadequate flow to all areas. The clinical manifestations of this event depend on the prior condition of the patient and on the circumstances. A sudden fall of blood pressure causes faintness and inability to remain upright, with a loss of the powerful mechanisms maintaining cerebral arterial flow within narrow limits. Tissues with atheromatous impairment of local circulation may infarct, especially the heart, brain and bowel. Mild hypotension causes a transient fall of renal plasma flow, of glomerular filtration and therefore of urine output. Profound hypotension causes reversible tubular necrosis of the kidneys, or, if prolonged, permanent cortical necrosis.

In patients lying in bed, hypotension is caused by combinations of:

1. Severely impaired myocardial function (cardiogenic shock).
2. Loss of circulating red cell or plasma volume either by haemorrhage or by extravasation into the extracellular fluid because of damage to the systemic capillary endothelial tight junctions.
3. Faulty ventilation technique, particularly excessive PEEP or respiratory alkalosis.

These factors interact in subtle ways and cannot be separated. Circulating bacterial endotoxin causes peripheral venodilatation as well as hypotension, as a result of which the circulating blood is pooled in the peripheral vessels and cardiac output falls because of lack of venous return.

The important consequences of hypotension with a low cardiac output are:

1. Oliguria leading to renal failure.
2. Increased extraction of oxygen in tissues, with a fall of mixed venous oxygen concentration and a rise of mixed venous $P_{CO_2}$. This in turn causes arterial hypoxaemia because of the admixture of venous blood at very low $P_{O_2}$ into the arterial circulation. Shunted $CO_2$ is compensated by increased ventilation, but hypoxaemia is not improved by this mechanism, or indeed by oxygen therapy if there is extensive lung damage with a large fraction of the blood coming from unventilated alveoli.

### Acute deterioration of left ventricular function

The falls of cardiac output and of blood pressure that would be expected after acute myocardial infarction are mitigated by baroreceptor and volume receptor reflexes, which provoke the secretion of adrenaline and noradrenaline. These act as inotropic agents and increase the force of contraction as well as the rate of beating of the heart, but they also cause peripheral vasoconstriction. This in turn increases the work of the heart, sometimes to the point of raising blood pressure above normal. The first event is generally cardiogenic pulmonary oedema (alveolar and bronchial transudation of fluid as a result of raised left atrial pressure). Treatment is with vasodilators and diuretics which counteract the adverse effects on the peripheral circulation and reduce the venous return to the heart. Opiates act in a similar way by reducing the sympathetic outflow of the central nervous system: this relieves pulmonary oedema, but at the expense of some systemic hypotension. This in turn may be treated to a limited extent by inotropic agents such as dopamine and dobutamine; these are preferable to noradrenaline, which impairs renal blood flow and reverses therapeutically induced venodilatation. When left ventricular function is so severely impaired that pulmonary oedema is accompanied by a low cardiac output, life support is extremely tenuous. It should be attempted along the same lines. Assisted ventilation may be needed to control hypoxaemia, and should not be delayed until severe $CO_2$ retention is present.

### Haemorrhage, dehydration and shock

Hypotension secondary to haemorrhagic shock or dehydration is readily identified and treated by appropriate transfusion of blood, blood substitute or crystalloids. In certain clinical situations such as burns, cholera or profound haemorrhage, the great deficit and continuing loss of circulating fluid may call for the replacement of very large volumes.

The simplest approach to therapy is to observe or monitor the central venous pressure and to reinfuse blood, protein or crystalloids until blood pressure and urine flow are restored, or until central venous pressure rises above a normal level. This is known as a fluid challenge, and is the standard procedure for determining whether oliguria is secondary to hypovolaemia. Difficulties arise when there is hypoproteinaemia or capillary endothelial damage. The hypovolaemia is exaggerated because the normal Starling forces fail to maintain an adequate plasma volume. As a result tissue oedema develops, in extreme cases even before the volume of the intravascular circulation is restored. The administration of powerful diuretics transiently relieves such oedema, but at the expense of causing further hypovolaemia and secondary hyperaldosteronism.

After fluid challenge, patients with left ventricular failure develop pulmonary oedema when the systemic venous pressure rises above a critical value, above which a further increase in filling pressure does not result in a rise of cardiac output. The situation is readily reversed by diuretics and no major permanent damage is done to the lung by minor degrees of pulmonary fluid transudation. Theoretically, the measurement of pulmonary capillary (arteriolar wedge) pressure can be used to monitor the rate and volume of infusions by indicating the onset of pulmonary venous hypertension. This is not quite as reliable as it sounds, especially when there is chronic lung disease, and the catheters are expensive. In practice, it is usually sufficient to infuse fluid until central venous pressure is just below normal, and to look for the development of pulmonary complications by watching for:

1. An increase in ventilator pressure at a fixed tidal volume.
2. Worsening of arterial oxygenation in spite of improving blood pressure and urine flow.
3. The appearance of plethoric changes or overt oedema on the chest X-ray.

In the supine ventilated patient, cardiogenic oedema, and oedema associated with fluid overload, obscure the main pulmonary artery outlines, in contrast with pneumonia or ARDS.

## ARDS

Non-cardiogenic shock is associated with circulating vascular toxins and cytokines which are also responsible for initiating the inflammatory damage of ARDS. These vasoactive toxins:

1. Damage the endothelial junctions, allowing exudation of protein-rich fluid into the alveolar walls.
2. Impair vascular reactivity. This interferes with the normal hypoxic pulmonary vasoconstrictor mechanism which matches the distribution of pulmonary perfusion to local alveolar ventilation.

The exudation of protein-containing fluid into damaged lungs is enhanced by a raised systemic central venous pressure (Ando *et al.*, 1991). This occurs because pulmonary lymphatic flow is usually increased in this condition, and a rise of venous pressure obstructs its return from the lung. Exudated fluid itself causes severe disturbances of gas exchange. Overload of the pulmonary and systemic circulations must be avoided in ARDS, or in conditions where the latter may develop. Pulmonary exudate is poorly reabsorbed after diuretic and vasodilator therapy.

ARDS is characterised by pulmonary oedema without pulmonary venous hypertension. The Swan-Ganz pulmonary arteriolar catheter may be used to detect whether there is an additional component of left ventricular failure and to titrate the dose of inspired oxygen, inotropic agents and vasodilators to optimise $O_2$ delivery to the tissues:

$$O_2 \text{ delivery} = \text{Cardiac output} \times \text{arterial } O_2 \text{ content} \quad (10.1)$$

The presence of clearly defined pulmonary vessels on the chest X-ray makes cardiogenic oedema unlikely. The distinction is important, because of the differences in treatment.

### Fluid balance

It follows from what has been said that watchful prevention of fluid overload is the most important preventive measure in protecting lung function. When a normal venous pressure and blood pressure have been restored, peripheral and sacral oedema should be sought and treated with diuretics if there is no associated hypovolaemia, provided that these do not impair $O_2$ delivery. The excess of intake over output has to be accumulated 12 hourly and steps taken to check any excess over 1.5 litres, counting insensible loss. In ventilated patients, insensible loss amounts to about 0.5 litre in 24 hours, if oral and rectal estimates of core temperature do not exceed 37 °C, but rises by about 0.75 litre for each degree Celsius rise in temperature.

## Weaning from artificial ventilation

Restoration of spontaneous ventilation requires:

1. Improvement of the conditions for which artificial ventilation was instituted.
2. Restoration of acid–base status compatible with normal ventilation. Chloride ion is needed to enable individuals who have had an elevated $P_{CO_2}$ for long periods to excrete an alkaline urine and restore the plasma bicarbonate towards normal. This is best achieved by infusing generous quantities of potassium chloride.
3. Retraining of the respiratory muscles.

Successful weaning may be predicted under the following conditions:

1. The patient must be conscious when sedative drugs are withdrawn.
2. The chest X-ray should be improving.
3. Arterial $O_2$ saturation should be above 95% on no more than 35% oxygen.
4. Dead space/tidal volume ratio is less than 50%.
5. Thoracic compliance should be better than at the onset of artificial ventilation.

6. On temporarily discontinuing artificial ventilation, the patient should be able to increase the force of diaphragmatic contraction by sniffing. Resting tidal volume should be at least 0.4 litre and inspiratory capacity at least twice the resting tidal volume.

More subtle indices have been constructed based on endurance and respiratory pressures measured on the ventilator (Jabour *et al.*, 1991). Retraining of the respiratory muscles is achieved simply if the ventilator is sophisticated and can supplement tidal volume during spontaneous ventilation by pressure support (see Younes, 1992). If a simple volume or pressure cycled machine is in use, weaning is started by removal of assistance for 5 minutes in each hour and increased as tolerated. Nocturnal assisted ventilation is helpful for several nights while inspiratory capacity returns towards normal.

### Failure to wean

An acute episode of respiratory failure requires about 5 days of intubation except in cases of oxygen or drug-induced respiratory depression, so some patience is needed. In patients with chronic airflow obstruction, failure to re-establish spontaneous ventilation in spite of cardiac and pulmonary improvement often means that there is an associated diaphragmatic paralysis or neuromuscular disease. Other causes include prolonged fatigue and metabolic imbalance causing hypokalaemia.

### Nocturnal assisted ventilation

The benefits of a spell of assisted ventilation generally last for several months or years if a reversible precipitating cause, such as infection or pulmonary oedema, have been identified. Some individuals with severe chronic thoracic cage or neuromuscular diseases may benefit from lifelong nocturnal assisted ventilation. This rests the respiratory muscles and maintains an adequate oxygen saturation without allowing $P_{CO_2}$ to rise. In this way, it may be superior in some instances to long-term nocturnal oxygen supplementation (Kinnear & Shneerson, 1985; Carroll & Branthwaite, 1988; Branthwaite, 1990).

### Conclusion

Patients with chronic respiratory disorders rarely need artificial ventilation in acute exacerbations of chronic airflow obstruction, because they generally respond to suitable oxygen therapy, diuretics, antibiotics and, where appropriate, corticosteroids.

Patients subjected to artificial ventilation rarely remember their admission to the intensive care ward, or indeed, anything other than a sore throat and dysphonia at the end of the procedure. Many patients with chronic lung or neuromuscular disease perform better after recovery than for many months previously. Often, ways are found of maintaining this improvement which include cessation of smoking, the use of inhaled steroids, diuretic therapy, long-term nocturnal oxygen or nocturnal assisted ventilation. The artificial ventilation of patients with chronic respiratory disorders rarely results in severe circulatory problems. Only intravenous and arterial cannulae are required; expensive disposable monitoring devices are not needed, and ventilators with few gadgets are usually adequate for the task. Technology is secondary to experience and an understanding of the basic principles of respiratory physiology.

Artificial ventilation, when needed, is usually successful and should not be regarded as inappropriate (Bovornkitti, Maranetra & Pushpakom, 1989). It should not be withheld unless the physician, the patient and the family are certain that the time has come for compassionate terminal care. Then, it should be remembered that death on a ventilator, while signifying that everything possible was done to preserve life, may not be a fitting end for someone whose life expectancy and quality of life have been compromised for many years.

### References

Ando, F., Arakawa, M., Kambara, K., Miyasaki, H., Segawa, T. & Hirakawa, S. (1990). Lung water and superior vena caval hypertension. *Journal of Applied Physiology*, **68**, 478–483.

Baudouin, S.V., Waterhouse, J.C., Tahlathouri, T., Smith, J.A., Baxter, J. & Howard P. (1990). Long term domiciliary oxygen treatment for chronic respiratory failure reviewed. *Thorax*, **45**, 195–198.

Bovornkitti, S., Maranetra, N. & Pushpakom, R.

(1989). A critical respiratory care unit at Siriraj Hospital. *Internal Medicine*, **5**, 31–34.

Branthwaite, M.A. (1990). Home mechanical ventilation. *European Respiratory Journal*, **3**, 743–745.

Campbell, E.J.M. (1965). Respiratory failure. *British Medical Journal*, **i**, 1451–1460.

Campbell, E.J.M. (1967). The management of acute respiratory failure in chronic bronchitis and emphysema. *American Review of Respiratory Disease*, **96**, 626–639.

Campbell, E.J.M. (1979). Respiratory failure. *Bulletin Européen Physiopathologie Respiratoire*, **15** (Suppl.), 1–12.

Carroll, N. & Branthwaite, M.A. (1988). Control of nocturnal ventilation by nasal intermittent positive pressure ventilation. *Thorax*, **43**, 349–353.

Connaughton, J.J., Catterall, J.R., Elton, R.A., Stradling, J.R. & Douglas, N.J. (1988). Do sleep studies contribute to the management of patients with severe chronic obstructive pulmonary disease? *American Review of Respiratory Disease*, **138**, 341–344.

Dunn, W.F., Nilson, S.B. & Hubmayr, R.D. (1991). Oxygen induced hypercarbia in obstructive pulmonary disease. *American Review of Respiratpry Disease*, **144**, 526–530.

Flenley, D.C. (1978). Clinical hypoxia: causes, consequences and correction. *Lancet*, **i**, 542–546.

Fletcher, E.C., Donner, C.F., Miagren, B., Zielinski, J., Levi-Valensi, P., Braghiroli, A., Rida, Z. & Miller, C.C. (1992). Survival in COPD patients with a daytime $Pao_2 > 60$ mmHg with and without nocturnal oxyhaemoglobin desaturation. *Chest*, **101**, 649–655.

Flick, G.R., Bellamy, P.E. & Simmons, D.H. (1989). Diaphragmatic contraction during assisted mechanical ventilation. *Chest*, **96**, 130–135.

Green, M. & Moxham, J. (1985). The respiratory muscles. *Clinical Science*, **68**, 1–10.

Jabour, E.R., Rabil, D.M., Truinit, J.D. & Rochester, D.F. (1991). Evaluation of a new weaning index based on ventilatory endurance and the efficiency of gas exchange. *American Review of Respiratory Disease*, **144**, 531–537.

Jeffrey, A.A., Warren, P.M. & Flenley, D.C. (1992). Acute hypercapnic respiratory failure in patients with chronic obstructive lung disease: risk factors and use of guidelines for management. *Thorax*, **47**, 34–40.

Kinnear, N.J.M. & Shneerson, J.M. (1985). Assisted ventilation at home: is it worth considering? *British Journal of Diseases of the Chest*, **79**, 313–351.

Lampron, N., Lemaire, F., Teissiere, B., Harf, A., Palot, M., Matamis, D. & Lorino, A.M. (1985). Mechanical ventilation with 100% oxygen does not increase intrapulmonary shunt in patients with severe bacterial pneumonia. *American Review of Respiratory Disease*, **131**, 409–413.

Laszlo, G., Clark, T.J.H. & Campbell, E.J.M. (1969). The immediate buffering of $CO_2$ in man. *Clinical Science*, **37**, 299–309.

Lemaire, F., Matanis, D., Lampron, N., Teissiere, B. & Harf, A. (1985). Intrapulmonary shunt is not increased by 100% oxygen ventilation in acute respiratory failure. *Bulletin Européen Physiopathologie Respiratoire*, **21**, 251–256.

McNicol, M.W. & Campbell, E.J.M. (1965). Severity of respiratory failure: arterial blood gases in untreated patients. *Lancet*, **i**, 336–341.

Medical Research Council Working Party (1981). Report: Long term domiciliary oxygen therapy in chronic hypoxic cor pulmonale complicating chronic bronchitis and emphysema. *Lancet*, **i**, 681–685.

Nocturnal Oxygen Therapy Trial Group (1980). Continuous or nocturnal oxygen therapy in hypoxaemic chronic obstructive lung disease. *Annals of Internal Medicine*, **93**, 391–398.

Ponte, J. (1990). Indications for mechanical ventilation. *Thorax*, **45**, 885–890.

Portier, F., Defouilloy, C. & Muir, J.-F. (1992). Determinants of immediate survival among chronic respiratory insufficiency patients admitted to an intensive care unit for acute respiratory failure. *Chest*, **101**, 204–210.

Roussos, C. (1985). Function and fatigue of respiratory muscles. *Chest*, **88**, 127S–132S.

Strumpf, D.A., Millman, R.P., Carlisle, C.C., Grattan, L.M., Ryan, S.M., Erickson, A.D. & Hill, N.S. (1991). Nocturnal positive pressure ventilation via nasal mask in patients with severe chronic destructive pulmonary disease. *American Review of Respiratory Disease*, **144**, 1234–1239.

Warrell, D.A., Edwards, R.H.T. & Godfrey, S. (1970). Effect of controlled oxygen therapy on arterial blood gases in acute respiratory failure. *British Medical Journal*, **i**, 452–455.

Warren, P.M., Flenley, D.C., Millar, J.S. & Avery, A. (1980). Respiratory failure revisited: acute exacerbations of chronic bronchitis between 1961–68 and 1970–76. *Lancet*, **i**, 467–471.

Weitzenblum, E., Sautejeau, A., Ehrhard, M., Maumosser, M. & Pelletier, A. (1985). Long term oxygen can reverse the progression of pulmonary hypertension in patients with chronic obstructive pulmonary disease. *American Review of Respiratory Disease*, **131**, 493–498.

Younes, M. (1992). Proportional assist ventilation: a new approach to ventilatory support. *American Review of Respiratory Disease*, **145**, 114–120

# 11 Acute breathlessness

Acute breathlessness is a common and taxing situation in emergency practice. This account concentrates on the diagnostic aspects of the problem, with emphasis on the diagnosis of psychogenic hyperventilation.

## Differential diagnosis of acute breathlessness

The differential diagnosis depends firstly on whether there are clinical, radiographic or spirometric abnormalities suggesting bronchopulmonary disease. When the dyspnoea is severe, physiological tests are usually restricted to peak flow and blood gas analysis. Measurement of $FEV_1$ and VC is useful when the patient can cooperate.

The first step is to determine by clinical examination, ECG, chest X-ray, pulmonary function tests and sometimes echocardiography whether there are any signs of damage to the lungs or heart.

1. Wheezing.
2. Crackles.
3. Signs of consolidation.
4. Signs of pneumothorax or tension pneumothorax.
5. Signs of pleural fluid.
6. Normal chest with hyperventilation
   with signs of right heart strain suggesting massive pulmonary embolism;
   with abnormal gas exchange suggesting pulmonary embolism;
   with an acid–base disturbance;
   with no signs other than those attributable to respiratory alkalosis.

The measurement of blood gases, noting the inspired oxygen at the time of sampling, is essential in the management of severely ill, breathless patients. The interpretation of the results is described in Chapter 3. PEF less than 100 $l\cdot min^{-1}$ after bronchodilators or $FEV_1$ less than 1 litre indicate that the patient is at risk from ventilatory failure and requires careful monitoring of $P_{CO_2}$ during oxygen therapy.

### Breathlessness with crackles

Widespread crackles suggest pulmonary oedema or inflammation of the lower respiratory tract. The chest X-ray will often be diagnostic. *Pulmonary oedema* rarely occurs without some evidence of acute or chronic heart disease in the history, or examination or electrocardiogram. Spirometric tests are almost invariably abnormal, typical results showing VC reduced to 30–70% of predicted normal (1.5–2.2 litres) and peak flow around 200 $l\cdot min^{-1}$. $FEV_1$/VC ratio is usually 70% or more and nearly always above 60%. PEF of 100 $l\cdot min^{-1}$ or less indicates concomitant chronic airways disease.

### Breathlessness with wheezing

Widespread wheezing may indicate acute or chronic airflow obstruction. It is usually present when a patient with chronic airflow obstruction develops acute pulmonary oedema or an acute infection of the lower respiratory tract.

Ventilatory tests are not often useful in discriminating different types of wheezing in acute emergencies. PEF less than 180 $l\cdot min^{-1}$ is usually

170

associated with chronic airflow obstruction or acute asthma. Response to bronchodilators is usually lost in severe asthma, and spirometric traces, if obtained at all, usually show $FEV_1/VC$ of greater than 85% because the patient cannot exhale for longer than 2 seconds. When PEF is greater than 150 $l·min^{-1}$ the spirometric trace may be helpful. At this level heart failure causes $FEV_1$ and VC to fall proportionally, $FEV_1/VC$ being normal. $FEV_1/VC$ in asthma often is below 70% and responds to bronchodilators, while chronic bronchitis and emphysema alone is unlikely to cause acute shortness of breath but can be detected because $FEV_1/VC$ is 50% or less.

Localised wheezing may point to obstruction of a large airway by tumour or foreign body. In unilateral disease there may be clinical or radiological signs of reduced ventilation or accompanying vena caval obstruction. In central airway disease, breath sounds may be stridulous. Peak flow may be reduced more than expected for measurement of $FEV_1$ (see Figs. 6.6 and 6.7). Tumours of the airway should be remembered when severe wheezing fails to respond to measures directed against bronchial asthma.

Acute gasping, with or without wheezing, suggests laryngeal or tracheal obstruction. These result in acute respiratory failure and are the commonest causes of collapse in restaurants and during meals.

Severe bronchial asthma and emphysema do not always cause wheezing. Patients with these conditions may present with severe dyspnoea, clinical or radiological evidence of ventilatory failure: peak flow is usually unrecordable; hyperinflation, tachycardia and pulsus paradoxus are usually present.

### Treatment of breathlessness with wheezing

Immediate treatment is based on physiological findings. Treatment strategies are directed against bronchoconstriction, inflammation, infection and pulmonary oedema. Nebulised selective beta-2-adrenergic bronchodilators such as salbutamol are not harmful in heart disease provided that arterial $Po_2$ is kept above 50 mmHg (7 kPa): intravenous aminophylline may be given slowly with the same precautions. These bronchodilators are mildly inotropic and may bring transient relief to patients with heart failure. A single dose of a rapidly acting loop diuretic is added, which may cause an output of more than 2.0 litres greater than intake over a 24-hour period if there is fluid retention. Antibiotics may be given if there is a risk of bacterial infection or evidence that it is present. Except in cases of severe pain opiates are best avoided altogether when there is marked reduction of ventilatory capacity, whatever the cause. $CO_2$ retention may occasionally occur if patients with severe pulmonary oedema are given opiates (Chapter 9). Monitoring of blood gases after the administration of morphine and oxygen usually averts serious consequences, as opiate antagonists are effective, and a short period of artificial ventilation is normally all that is required to overcome the problem if pain relief cannot be achieved in any other way.

Suspected or known bronchial asthma is treated with corticosteroids which cause no harm if given in the short term. Fluid retention may exacerbate the most severe cases of heart failure.

Acutely breathless, wheezing patients are usually treated at presentation with more than one strategy. The mechanism of the dyspnoeic attack may only be elucidated after recovery, when the clinical state of the patient can be assessed in convalescence. The questions to be answered are:

1. Is the patient suffering from chronic airflow obstruction?
2. Is there evidence of bronchial asthma? (see Chapter 7) If there is some evidence of the condition (attacks in childhood, family history, blood eosinophilia when not on oral steroids, characteristic diurnal variation of peak flow during recovery, bronchial hyperreactivity) the patient should remain well when steroids are given by inhalation. Oral steroids, diuretics and antibiotics can then be withdrawn.
3. Are diuretics necessary? Acute cardiogenic pulmonary oedema occurs only when there is a cause for it. Continued diuretic therapy is necessary only if the patient is found to have cardiac insufficiency or hypertension. Diuretics may certainly be withdrawn if there is never any evidence of definite pulmonary oedema, cardiomegaly, cardiac arrhythmia, gallop rhythm, or structural malformation.

Table 11.1. *Causes of hyperventilation*

*Physiological*
Altitude
Anxiety
Speech
Voluntary
Exercise above anaerobic threshold

*Psychological*
Panic
Chronic anxiety

*Pathological: cardiac and pulmonary*

| Acute | Chronic |
|-------|---------|
| Lung inflammation | Moderate airflow obstruction |
| Airflow obstruction | Interstitial lung disease |
| Pulmonary oedema | Heart failure |
| Pulmonary embolism | |

*Metabolic*
  Acidosis
  Hypoxaemia

*Neurogenic*
  Brain stem disease
  Raised intracranial pressure

### Beta-adrenergic antagonists

Beta-adrenergic antagonists cause chronic bronchoconstriction in susceptible individuals even when bronchial asthma had previously been mild or unsuspected. They also impair myocardial function, and have therefore to be withdrawn as part of the treatment of acute breathlessness, except when this is caused by a tachyarrhythmia associated with thyrotoxicosis.

## Hyperventilation presenting as a medical emergency

The causes of hyperventilation are shown in Table 11.1. All the serious causes should be excluded: most are obvious or easily ascertained.

Arterial blood gas analysis identifies patients with abnormal acid–base balance. Measurement of $FEV_1/VC$ and PEF identifies patients with abnormal lung mechanics who have not been diagnosed by means of clinical examination or the chest X-ray.

The relationship between arterial $Pco_2$ and $Po_2$ in hyperventilation has been discussed (Chapter 3). If the lungs are normal, low $Pco_2$ should be accompanied by high arterial $Po_2$ (Chapter 3). When alveolar–arterial $Po_2$ difference is normal, $Po_2$ should be at least 100 mmHg (15 kPa) if $Pco_2$ is 20 mmHg (3 kPa) and if the blood is drawn at the height of hyperventilation. If it is less, the interpretation depends on the respiratory pattern at the time of sampling. During hyperventilation, a low or normal $Po_2$ implies a wide alveolar–arterial $Po_2$ difference. After hyperventilation, R falls so $Po_2$ falls to low levels even if the lungs are normal. Measurement of R during the period of blood sampling distinguishes these two situations, but as the problem usually arises in wards or emergency departments this is rarely feasible. Unexpectedly high levels of $Po_2$ are found if the patient has received oxygen supplements in the previous 30 minutes.

Nevertheless, blood drawn over several respiratory cycles during hyperventilation can be helpful in confirming that the alveolar–arterial $Po_2$ difference is abnormal. This distinction is useful because patients with major embolism with right heart strain and electrocardiographic change who are hyperventilating nearly always have abnormal $Po_2$ levels, and this is often true in cases of presumed minor embolism (Chapter 9).

## Acute hyperventilation attacks of psychogenic origin

### Psychiatric background

Hyperventilation attacks have different backgrounds in different communities. They occur quite frequently in regions where 'conversion hysteria' is a common phenomenon either as a symptom of psychiatric disorder or as a manipulative technique. The patient, usually female, hyperventilates to tetany, with carpopedal spasm and loss of consciousness. The breathing pattern looks as if it is voluntary with deep, forced breaths. Blood gas analysis is usually not necessary or indeed feasible and the vasoconstriction induced by the respiratory alkalosis may make it hard to enter an artery.

Overt conversion hysteria is becoming more rare in Western countries. Some instances are associated with religious ecstasy. Hyperventilation can be induced by excitement during musical concerts and by amphetamine abuse. Generally, psychogenic hyperventilation attacks are more commonly associated with acute anxiety and panic disorder. They may complicate respiratory and cardiac diseases.

Acute hyperventilation often follows attacks of pain in the chest or upper abdomen, perhaps because of the fear of serious consequences. There is often medical concern about the possibility of pulmonary embolism, particularly in young women of child-bearing age. Often, anticoagulants will be prescribed and withdrawn when subsequent investigation reveals that there is no abnormality of pulmonary gas exchange and no defect on the chest X-ray or ventilation–perfusion scan. Hyperventilation occurring after or during an attack of non-anginal chest or upper abdominal pain is often accompanied by a slow or normal pulse rate (personal observation), when subsequent investigation usually proves normal.

Attendance at hospital is most likely in young women and men of about 25–40 years old who are anxious about heart attacks or are suffering from paroxysmal tachycardia which has not been investigated. In the latter there is tachycardia and the breathing is often of the cog-wheel type. A few basal wheezes are sometimes audible, presumably because of simultaneous sympathetic and vagal overactivity. The distinction of these attacks from supraventricular tachycardia or from early heart failure requires clinical examination, electrocardiography and radiology. Pulmonary gas exchange may be normal at rest during short-lived episodes of mild pulmonary oedema.

## Blood gas analysis in hyperventilation with normal lungs

During the period of hyperventilation, $P_{CO_2}$ falls to below 25 mmHg (3.5 kPa) and pH rises correspondingly to around 7.6. $P_{O_2}$ is correspondingly high and should be around 130 mmHg (17 kPa)

while breathing air, or above 200 mmHg (25 kPa) breathing oxygen-enriched gas, if the lungs are normal. When the patient loses consciousness and the attacks cease, respiration ceases for a while because of the loss of $CO_2$ drive. As discussed later, individuals vary in the degree of post-hyperventilation apnoea but there is then a pause of sufficient length to cause reduction of the arterial $P_{O_2}$ usually to about 60 mmHg (8 kPa). $P_{CO_2}$ rises slowly after hyperventilation because the body tissue bicarbonate concentration falls as $CO_2$ is lost from the body and blood $P_{CO_2}$ falls. When hyperventilation ceases, $CO_2$ liberated in the metabolising tissues of the body is retained in part in intracellular and extracellular fluid. Mixed venous $P_{CO_2}$ rises slowly, and the respiratory exchange ratio, R, falls below normal, because oxygen consumption continues normally while $CO_2$ elimination virtually ceases. This fall of $P_{O_2}$ may be sufficiently great to cause convulsions in susceptible individuals, the cerebral hypoxia being aggravated by the fall of cerebral blood flow and hypotension caused by the respiratory alkalosis. The recovery period is generally longer than after voluntary hyperventilation in normal subjects because of continued hyperventilation. Respiration may be irregular or cyclical, according to the degree of hypoxaemia. This produces an uncomfortable awareness of breathing which may be a cause of further involuntary hyperventilation.

## Management of acute hyperventilation

Monosymptomatic hyperventilation attacks in manipulative healthy individuals are best ignored if possible, or watched from a distance. Panic disorder is characterised by multiple symptoms, as described later. Caffeine and bronchodilator overdosage may induce panic, especially when compounded by acute or chronic stress (Lane et al., 1990). Gentle, confident reassurance may be aided by the short-term use of nonselective beta-adrenergic blockade in patients with sinus tachycardia who are not asthmatic.

Rebreathing is often advised: this is misguided. If air is rebreathed, dangerous hypoxaemia may occasionally follow. Oxygen rebreathing is safe but may cause distressing dyspnoea, although it may relieve the dizziness of respiratory alkalosis.

Table 11.2. *Panic attacks (DSM3: American Psychiatric Association 1986, 1987)*

At least four of the following symptoms plus apprehension or fear not attributable to phobic stimulus:

Shortness of breath: having trouble catching the breath
Heart pounding
Chest pain, discomfort, tightness
Dizziness, unsteadiness
Feelings of unreality
Choking or smothering sensations
Tingling in hands or feet
Hot or cold flushes
Sweating
Faintness
Trembling or shaking
Fear of dying
Fear of going crazy
Fear of losing control

Moving about speeds up the reaccumulation of $CO_2$ in the tissues. The attacks are self-limiting.

### Prolonged hyperventilation

Hyperventilation which is less profound and more prolonged presents differently, because there is sufficient time for renal pH adjustments and consequent sodium and potassium loss. The metabolic consequences can be deduced from hyperventilation experiments of various sorts although there is no information derived from such studies in patients so affected. The immediate consequence is that if there has been chronic hyperventilation it can be detected from the relationship between arterial $P_{CO_2}$ and pH. If arterial pH is lower (more acid) than would be expected from the known effect of lowering body $P_{CO_2}$ it will take several hours or days after the cessation of the attack to return to normal, and during this time tiredness, lassitude and shortness of breath are the rule.

### Panic disorder and acute hyperventilation

It is now recognised that hyperventilation attacks form part of the spectrum of panic disorder, as defined rigorously (American Psychiatric Association, 1980) and redefined to include milder cases (American Psychiatric Association,

1987, see Rushford, 1992). This disorder responds to psychological treatment and should be recognised. There is compelling evidence that the respiratory problems are secondary to the behaviour disorder, although subtle genetically determined aspects of ventilatory control such as the rate and depth of breathing during $CO_2$ stimulation (Arkinstall *et al.*, 1974) may affect the clinical findings during anxiety attacks.

There is an overall similarity between symptoms reported during panic attacks provoked by identifiable stress and those which occur spontaneously (Tables 11.2, 11.3). They are the same as those which have been attributed to hyperventilation. Early accounts of this, many of which are graphic and valuable clinical and biochemical portraits, probably reflect the referral bias that is seen in most multi-system disorders (Lum, 1975; Magarian, 1982; Howell, 1990). These accounts emphasise:

1. The complaint of inability to take a satisfying breath.
2. Irregular breathing during spirometry (Christie, 1935: fig. 2.15).
3. Frequent sighing.
4. Exaggerated upper thoracic expansion during inspiration.
5. Reproducibility of symptoms by a period of voluntary hyperventilation (often standardised: for example, 3 minutes at an end-tidal $P_{CO_2}$ of less than 20 mmHg (3 kPa)).
6. Low resting values of arterial $P_{CO_2}$ or end-tidal $P_{CO_2}$ are helpful if they are found to be present but are not essential to the diagnosis.

Recent work has attempted to characterise these patients more rigorously with partial success. Similar psychiatric morbidity is found in many patients with the related condition of chest pain with normal exercise ECG and coronary arteries (Bass & Wade, 1984; Bass & Gardner, 1985; Pearce, Mayou & Klimes, 1990).

In an extensive and fully documented series of investigations, Rushford (1992) has shown that there is no unifying respiratory abnormality which explains the manifestations of panic disorder. Only 9% of her 42 patients had an end-tidal $P_{CO_2}$ of lower than 35 mmHg (5 kPa) at rest, in contrast to 5% of the normal subjects. They were not abnormally sensitive to $CO_2$ inhalation, which

Table 11.3. *Frequency of panic symptoms (from Rushford, 1992)*

| Recalled[a] | % | Diary record[b] | % |
|---|---|---|---|
| Palpitation | 95 | Fear of dying or loss of control | 95 |
| Fear of dying | 90 | Palpitation | 90 |
| Trembling | 85 | Dizzy | 80 |
| Shortness of breath | 80 | Shortness of breath | 75 |
| Chest pain/tightness | 75 | Chest pain/tightness | 75 |
| Sweating | 75 | Shaking | 75 |
| Hot or cold | 70 | Sweating | 75 |
| Dizzy | 70 | Unreality | 70 |
| Choking | 60 | Hot or cold | 50 |
| Tingling | 60 | Choking | 45 |
| Faint | 55 | Tingling | 45 |
| Unreality | 55 | Faint | 30 |

[a] Thirty-three subjects were inverviewed to yield the figures for recalled symptoms, which are similar in frequency to the studies.
[b] Sixteen subjects successfully recorded the symptoms during attacks and these were listed if graded or more than mild. The second list reflects the symptoms of a witnessed attack, for example in an accident room.

did not reproduce symptoms of panic. The characteristic loss of control was not reproduced by voluntary hyperventilation.

Some interesting findings did shed light on the respiratory pattern in panic disorder:

1. Many patients responded to the inhalation of $CO_2$ with a more rapid, shallow breathing pattern though total ventilation was the same as in the control subjects.
2. Some of the patients, though none of the controls, found it difficult to gauge the magnitude of resistances added to the respiratory circuit; normal subjects can do this with accuracy. This is probably related to the increased use of the upper thoracic muscles and the increased activity of these throughout the respiratory cycle, especially the parasternal intercostals.
3. After voluntary hyperventilation, patients with panic disorder showed a slower recovery of $P_{CO_2}$ than that seen in the normal subjects, but the differences were slight and not discriminatory (75% recovery in 3 minutes compared with 85%). Apnoea in inspiration was more prolonged in the normal subjects, while some patients with panic disorder showed irregular

breathing patterns for long periods after voluntary hyperventilation.
4. Patients with panic tended to breathe in more slowly, the duration of inspiration being 70% of that of expiration compared with 60% in the normal subjects. Upper thoracic movement lagged behind the lower thoracic expansion; this did not occur in the normal subjects and confirmed the idea of a clinically recognisable, stress-related breathing pattern.
5. A proportion of the patients failed to complete 3 minutes of voluntary hyperventilation; this appeared to be related to prolonged inactivity as these subjects adopted a sedentary lifestyle to avoid symptoms.

There is evidence that panic attacks are associated with mitral valve prolapse, which has to be re-evaluated in the light of more rigorous definitions. This emphasises the importance of careful counselling when informing patients of the presence of functionless murmurs, and of recognising the coexistence of panic disorder in those presented with a diagnosis of chronic airflow obstruction or bronchial asthma (Karajgi *et al.*, 1990).

It follows that the best interests of patients with clearly recognisable panic disorder are served by a positive psychological diagnosis and rapid exclusion of important disease by examination and simple screening tests. The commonest traps in young subjects are bronchial asthma, thyrotoxicosis and the Wolff-Parkinson-White syndrome. When panic is a presenting feature, this may dominate the clinical course and appropriate psychological help is necessary. Incidental findings are common and have to be treated on their merits. Amongst the most distressing complaints is fear of the next attack.

# References

American Psychiatric Association: Committee on Nomenclature and Statistics. (1980). *Diagnosis and Statistical Manual of Mental Disorders*, 2nd edn. Washington D.C.: American Psychiatric Association.

American Psychiatric Association: Committee on Nomenclature and Statistics. (1987). *Diagnostic and Statistical Manual of Mental Disorders*, 3rd edn, revised. Washington D.C.: American Psychiatric Association.

Arkinstall, W.W., Nirmel, K., Klissouras, V. & Milic-Emili, J. (1974). Genetic differences in the ventilatory response to inhaled $CO_2$. *Journal of Applied Physiology*, **36**, 6–11.

Bass, C. & Gardner, W.N. (1985). Respiratory and psychiatric abnormalities in chronic symptomatic hyperventilation. *British Medical Journal*, **290**, 1387–1390.

Bass, C.& Wade, C. (1984). Chest pain with normal coronary arteries: a comprehensive study of psychiatric and social morbidity. *Psychological Medicine*, **14**, 51–61.

Christie, R.V. (1935). Some types of respiration in the neuroses. *Quarterly Journal of Medicine*, **4**, 427–432.

Howell, J.B.L. (1990). Breathlessness. In *Respiratory Medicine*, ed. R.A.L. Brewis, G.J. Gibson & D.M. Geddes, pp. 221–228. London: Baillière Tindall.

Karajgi, B., Rifkin, A., Poddi, S. & Koth, R. (1990). Prevalence of anxiety disorders in patients with chronic obstructive pulmonary disease. *American Journal of Psychiatry*, **147**, 200–201.

Lane, J.D., Adcock, R.A., Williams, R.B. & Kunn, L.M. (1990). Caffeine effects on cardiovascular and neuroendocrine responses to acute psychosocial stress and their relationship to habitual caffeine consumption. *Psychosomatic Medicine*, **52**, 320–336.

Lum, L.C. (1975). Hyperventilation: the tip and the iceberg. *Journal of Psychosomatic Research*, **19**, 375–383.

Magarian, G.J. (1982). Hyperventilation syndromes: infrequently recognised common expressions of anxiety and stress. *Medicine*, **61**, 219–236.

Pearce, M.J., Mayou, R.A. & Klimes, I. (1990). The management of atypical non-cardiac chest pain. *Quarterly Journal of Medicine*, **76**, 991–996.

Rushford, N. (1992). Panic disorder: a model integrating psychological and respiratory variables. PhD Thesis, University of Melbourne.

# 12 Breathlessness during exertion

Shortness of breath on exertion is the clinical problem most commonly referred to the respiratory laboratory, usually asking:

1. What respiratory and other diseases are present?
2. How severe are they?
3. How disabled is the patient?
4. Is the incapacity all accounted for by the measured abnormalities?

In this chapter we consider ways in which breathlessness can be measured as it affects daily living and as it limits an exercise test. This leads to a progressive approach to the investigation of the symptom of shortness of breath on exercise.

In general, breathlessness is caused by one or more of the following mechanisms (Killian & Campbell, 1983; Leblanc *et al.*, 1986):

1. An increased hindrance to breathing.
2. Decreased neuromuscular power.
3. An increased drive to breathing.

## Declared disability

Walking briskly uphill requires as much ventilation as the majority of occupations. Cardiorespiratory abnormalities sufficient to cause breathlessness are, therefore, readily detected by questions relating to the ability of the patient to walk or hurry under different conditions, especially in the company of other people. Patients will often notice the onset of a disease process because of the effect it has on their ability to perform short bursts of exercise such as climbing stairs. Direct questions about this give less reliable information about the severity of the condition than the subject's observations about steady exercise. It is normal for stair climbing to cause dyspnoea and the severity of this depends as much on the impatience of the subject as on effort tolerance.

The British Medical Research Council's questionnaire assigns the patient to one of five categories or grades (Fletcher *et al.*, 1959; Medical Research Council, 1966). The following adaptation contains an additional grade (I-) found useful in the laboratory where technicians ask the question routinely.

I:    Normal exercise tolerance on hills and stairs.
I-:   Within normal limits but less than accustomed level.
II:   Able to walk at normal speed on the flat, but reduced effort tolerance on hills and stairs.
III:  Able to maintain a steady but reduced speed on level ground.
IV:   Has to stop at intervals even on level ground (distance stated).
V:    Uncomfortable at rest or minimal exertion indoors.

The limiting factor may be angina pectoris or arthritis rather than breathlessness and this has to be noted.

Grade I- is not used in epidemiology but is helpful in preparing reports of lung function tests. Note is taken of the duration and variability of the symptoms and whether the patient's condition at the time of questioning is usual or has deteriorated.

These categories are broad, but have the merit of being easy to assign if some flexibility is

Table 12.1. *Borg's scale of perceived exertion, breathlessness and discomfort*

| 0 | Nothing at all |
|---|---|
| 0.5 | Very, very slight (just noticeable) |
| 1 | Very slight |
| 2 | Slight |
| 3 | Moderate |
| 4 | Somewhat severe |
| 5 | Severe |
| 6 | |
| 7 | Very severe |
| 8 | |
| 9 | Very, very severe (almost maximal) |
| 10 | Maximal |

allowed in the sequence of questioning. It is easiest to begin with the enquiry: 'Are you able to walk at a steady pace on level ground without stopping?' If the answer is yes, then the grade is defined as III or better, and ability to keep up with others can be determined. If the answer is no, then the grade is IV or worse and the stopping distance can be defined.

There is wide experience with this questionnaire, which is simple to apply and which correlates with indices of lung function and self-selected walking speed.

More sensitive questionnaires are being validated. One which scores change of status as well as current disability has been investigated. It is rather long, but likely to be useful for epidemiological work (Mahler *et al.*, 1984).

Another questionnaire assigns categories based on limitation at work and at home and on the amount of effort needed to perform tasks that the patient can only just manage. This produces a more sensitive index which correlates well with lung function indices and with respiratory muscle strength (Stoller, Ferranti & Feinstein, 1986).

## Measurement of perceived exertion

Exercise tests, bronchial challenges and other experiments are often used to induce breathlessness. Various methods have been developed to study this (Adams & Guz, 1991).

10 cm (100 mm) visual analogue
scale marked at 40 mm

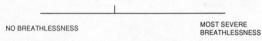

NO BREATHLESSNESS                    MOST SEVERE
                                     BREATHLESSNESS

Fig. 12.1. 100 mm visual analogue scale for breathlessness marked at 40 mm.

### Borg's scale of perceived exertion

The simplest method of measuring this, or any aspect of the severity of effort, is Borg's scale of perceived exertion (Table. 12.1) (Borg, 1978). Categories varying from 'very, very slight' to 'very, very severe' are numbered from 1 to 10. The subject can be asked to grade current or recent muscular effort or dyspnoea by use of the numbers.

The categories were chosen to correspond approximately to a logarithmic scale so that the average subject perceives exercise at 100 watts as twice as hard as 50 watts. This concept follows from the work of Stevens (1975) on the psychophysics of the estimation of the magnitude of sensations. Many sensations are perceived according to the logarithm of their intensity. Stevens employed 'open magnitude scaling' for his experiments. In this technique, subjects were asked to assign any number to an initial sensation such as pain, noise or light and then to assign numbers, greater or smaller, to successive examples of the stimulus at varying severity. Generally, the plot of perceived magnitude against intensity was a power function, the logarithm of the stimulus being proportional to the logarithm of the perceived magnitude. Stevens' elegant technique requires more practice than might at first be supposed, and calls for more sophistication on the part of the subjects than is often available. It is difficult to apply if the stimulus to the sensation being measured cannot be quantified exactly.

### Visual analogue scale

Breathlessness at a given instant can also be scored reproducibly by means of a visual analogue scale (Fig. 12.1) on which the subject marks a straight unbracketed line labelled 'not breathless' at one end, and 'extremely breathless' at the other (Aitken, 1969; Bond & Laver, 1974; Adams *et al.*, 1985). This may be used to measure subjective changes of dyspnoea during exercise tests or under changing conditions. Provided that the last mark is available for inspection, the technique may be used over periods of several days. A similar test may be used to measure other symptoms or to allow a patient to record the overall severity of the disorder. Visual analogue scores asking 'How is your asthma?' move in parallel with peak flow measurements (Higgs *et al.*, 1986). The way in which individuals use the scale is to some extent related to personality and is affected by recent experience, so that symptoms which would normally be considered as severe are scored much lower during recovery from a severe exacerbation. Visual analogue scaling of symptoms is being used increasingly in therapeutic trials.

In experimental work, the Borg scale is slightly more stable but the visual analogue scale is more sensitive to minor changes (Adams & Guz, 1991).

### The language of breathlessness

Patients use or accept different terms to describe their sensations of disordered breathing (Simon *et al.*, 1990). This may become useful clinically, if regional differences are taken into account.

### Definitions of breathlessness

Comroe (1966) called breathlessness (dyspnoea) an unpleasant type of breathing and pointed out that it is not tachypnoea (rapid breathing), hyperpnoea (increased ventilation) or hyperventilation (increased breathing causing a low $PCO_2$) and is partly subjective.

Dyspnoea means 'disordered breathing' and would be a useful phrase if it were restricted to shortness of breath caused by disease or accompanied by discomfort, reserving 'breathlessness' for the physiological condition also experienced by healthy individuals. This distinction has not been achieved and the terms tend to be used interchangeably in this book and elsewhere. Most definitions include the idea of discomfort (Adams & Guz, 1991). For most purposes, breathlessness is simply an awareness of the need to breathe and has three clinical connotations and three forms.

1. It may reduce exercise tolerance and lower the threshold above which exercise is uncomfortable.
2. It may be present at rest.
3. It may develop with change of posture.

Patients may recognise three distinct types of disordered breathing:

1. The need for excessive ventilation.
2. A sensation of undue difficulty when increasing the rate and depth of breathing.
3. Alteration of the pattern of breathing by soreness, pain or associated discomfort.

## Clinical investigation of factors influencing breathlessness induced by exercise

Breathless patients fall into three physiological categories which are discussed separately in the following pages:

1. Airflow obstruction ($FEV_1$/VC ratio reduced below 70%, or below 60% if VC is greater than 120% of predicted normal).
2. Low $FEV_1$, low VC, normal $FEV_1$/VC ratio.
3. Normal $FEV_1$ and VC.

### Airflow obstruction (Chapters 6 and 7)

When $FEV_1$ is reduced, ventilatory limitation to exercise is the rule. $FEV_1$ is closely related to maximum voluntary ventilation in patients with chronic airflow obstruction (Chapter 6). VC correlates better with self-selected walking speed (McGavin *et al.*, 1978). This discrepancy may be explained by the extent to which emphysema, rather than bronchial narrowing, is the cause of the obstruction. Patients with emphysema may have very low $FEV_1$/VC ratios, sometimes less than 40%, without much disability, as long as VC remains normal. Patients without much radiographically demonstrable emphysema presumably have obstructive bronchitis, with or without small areas of centrilobular emphysema. In these patients, $FEV_1$, VC and $FEV_1$/VC deteriorate *pari passu* with disability and all these indices are equally useful as guides to the severity of the obstruction (Chapter 6).

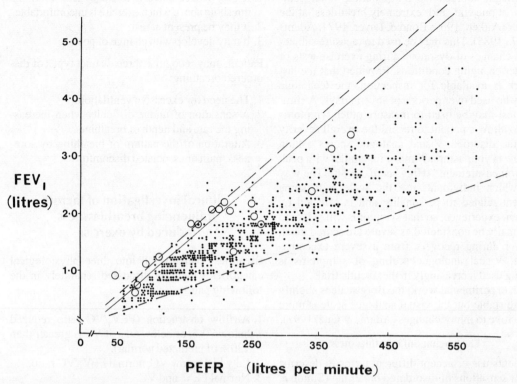

**Fig. 12.2.** Relationship of $FEV_1$ to PEF in a large series of patients with diffuse airflow obstruction (bronchial asthma, chronic bronchitis, pulmonary emphysema), with $FEV_1/VC < 65\%$. The open circles represent individual patients with central airway obstruction. The relationship $FEV_1/PEF = 1/100$ is shown by the continuous line, which is close to the upper 95% confidence limit. Approximately half of the patients with central airway obstruction could have been diagnosed by calculation of $FEV_1/PEF$. There is some overlap with bronchial asthma, perhaps because some asthmatics have a central airway component to their obstruction.

The shape of the spirometric trace should always be examined. This is most simply achieved by looking at the expired volume–time curve from the spirometer, but numerical indices derived from the flow–volume curve are equally satisfactory. A fixed extrapulmonary obstruction, such as that caused by a tumour of the trachea or by laryngeal obstruction, results in a rather constant expired flow rate (Fig. 6.7). The volume–

time curve looks as if it is linear through the origin, in contrast to the curve of severe emphysema in which the linear portion is preceded by a short segment of relatively rapid expiratory flow. It follows (Fig. 12.2) that peak flow is relatively low in relation to $FEV_1$. The ratio of $FEV_1$ (ml) to PEF ($l \cdot min^{-1}$) is rarely more than 10 in patients with diffuse airflow obstruction. Similarly, $FIV_1$ tends to fall below $FEV_1$, whereas in normal subjects these ususally have similar values (Chapter 6). The ratio $MEF_{50}/MIF_{50}$ is reversed if the obstruction is fixed, but not if it is variable; but this test is less specific because it is affected by muscle power and pulmonary compliance. Nevertheless, measurements of forced inspiratory flow rates do help to distinguish extrathoracic from intrathoracic obstruction. Forced expiration compresses the intrathoracic airways, while forced inspiration applies suction to the extrathoracic airway, causing airway closure if the muscles which normally dilate the pharyngeal and laryngeal apertures are weak. Air contrast radiography, laryngoscopy and bronchoscopy are required to confirm the suspicion of central airway obstruction. Audible stridor should lead to the diagnosis, but this sign is often missed or misinterpreted in practice.

Tracheobronchial collapse is illustrated in Fig. 6.4. The commonest cause is severe emphysema. Tracheomalacea occurs without emphysema, but is rather rare.

A difference of greater than 0.5 litre between slow (relaxed) vital capacity and forced vital capacity is characteristic of pulmonary emphysema.

### Variability of airflow obstruction

In the first instance reversibility is assessed by measuring the change of PEF and spirometry after a bronchodilator drug, such as salbutamol (Chapters 6 and 7).

Random variation of the measurements and of physiological increases of bronchial calibre causes difficulty. Salbutamol increases airway conductance and flow rates near FRC in most normal subjects. This is not reflected in the measurement of $FEV_1$ and PEF because full inspiration decreases bronchomotor tone, so the airways are fully patent at the time of the test. It is not certain whether this phenomenon occurs in all patients with chronic bronchitis, and it is absent in patients with asthma, who tend to bronchoconstrict after full inspiration. Small but useful increases of $FEV_1$ are often found after salbutamol, and after inhalations of anticholinergic drugs in patients with no other evidence of bronchial asthma. An improvement in $FEV_1$ of at least 20% and at least 0.4 litres appears to define a group of patients who are hyperreactive and likely to respond to treatment (Chapters 6 and 7). Insisting on this definition will, however, exclude many true asthmatics, especially if they have taken bronchodilator drugs on the day of the test. In patients referred to the laboratory with a clinical diagnosis of bronchial asthma, the mean increase of $FEV_1$ after bronchodilator from a metered dose inhaler is only 10%.

Serial tests must be performed in the same position: VC can fall by up to 25% when the patient lies down from standing. Intermediate results are obtained in the sitting position. The random error of duplicate measurements made

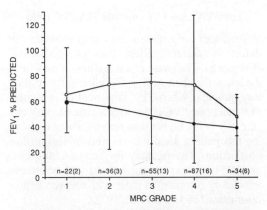

Fig. 12.3. Relationship between MRC dyspnoea grade and $FEV_1$ in patients with chronic airflow obstruction (lower line, filled circles) and patients with a combination of airflow obstruction and ischaemic heart disease (upper line, open circles). The brackets enclose the whole range of measurements made in the patients without heart disease.

seated or standing is 0.1 litre or less when $FEV_1$ is less than 1.0 litre, but may be as high as 0.3 litre above this level.

Improvement of VC, but not of $FEV_1$, after salbutamol is common in patients with chronic bronchitis and emphysema. Increased patency of small peripheral airways is the likely explanation, though there is no evidence to indicate whether this is because of bronchodilatation or because the airways become less collapsible. The clinical importance of this improvement, which may be 1 litre or more if high doses of salbutamol are given, is not known as many patients derive better effort tolerance from the use of bronchodilators, but the improvement is poorly correlated with the magnitude of the bronchodilator response and other mechanisms may be operating.

The relationship between MRC dyspnoea grade and spirometric measurements in patients with chronic airflow obstruction is shown in Fig. 12.3. Often, the reduction of $FEV_1$ is appropriate to the degree of declared disability. Further detailed respiratory tests are then likely to contribute little to the assessment of dyspnoea, and are used when necessary to determine the presence of respiratory failure, the severity of emphysema and the degree of variability.

## Low FEV$_1$, low FVC, normal FEV$_1$/VC ratio

When associated with low static lung volumes, this defect is correctly described as 'restrictive' (Chapter 8). The cause of the restriction may lie in the lungs, the chest wall or abdomen or the respiratory muscles. When TLC is normal or increased, the reduction of VC is due to premature airway closure, RV being higher than normal. Patients showing this pattern usually have predominant airflow obstruction. The relationship between dyspnoea and VC is similar among patients with restrictive ventilatory disorders to those with chronic airflow obstruction (McGavin et al., 1978).

Measurements of TLC distinguish restriction from obstruction, but clinical examination, or an assessment of the lung volume derived from the inspiratory chest X-ray, may be equally useful. PEF tends to be normal in the fibrotic lung diseases but low if there is reduced inspiration, respiratory muscle weakness, or associated airway obstruction.

Respiratory muscle weakness is likely to be the cause of an unexplained fall of VC if there are no clinical or radiographic signs of lung disease or deformity of the thoracic cage. Isolated paralysis of one or both hemi-diaphragms is not rare and may be detected by measuring VC in the lying and standing position (Chapter 2). TLco/V$_A$ is usually normal, unless there is concomitant lung disease, when the danger of respiratory failure increases substantially.

## Normal FEV$_1$ and VC

Dyspnoeic patients with normal spirometry and PEF require further investigation to diagnose the cause of their disability. Clinical examination, chest X-ray and resting ECG have to be reviewed as discussed below. The majority of such patients have exercise-induced asthma, alveolitis or diffuse pulmonary fibrosis, undiagnosed heart disease, pulmonary thromboembolism, neurological diseases or metabolic causes of dyspnoea. Some have 'functional' or psychogenic hyperventilation, the proportion depending on the source of referral (de Paso et al., 1991). Most of these diagnoses can be made clinically or by appropriate lung function tests. Haemoglobin, thyroid function, radionuclide ventilation–perfusion scanning and echocardiography or cardiac catheterisation may be needed in some instances.

*Exercise-induced asthma.* Minimal abnormalities of the FEV curve in a non-smoker without chronic bronchitis may draw attention to this diagnosis. Exercise-induced asthma is by far the commonest cause of habitual exertional dyspnoea in young, apparently healthy, individuals. The diagnosis may be confirmed by a suitable exercise test, or by measuring the response of the airways to a bronchoconstrictor challenge (Chapter 7). PEF is a good indicator of variable airflow obstruction. A child may be asked simply to run as fast as possible around the house for 6 minutes. PEF should be measured before, and 5–10 minutes after exercise, remembering the delayed onset of bronchoconstriction. The characteristic wheezing is usually brought on, and may be terminated by inhalation of a standard dose of bronchodilator. Obviously, recent use of a bronchodilator may invalidate the test. There should not have been breathless attacks on the day of the test, because an attack of bronchoconstriction usually resolves spontaneously after 20 minutes rest and will be followed by a variable refractory period of 2–4 hours.

*Defective pulmonary gas exchange.* This may be detected in most instances by careful measurements of TLco, which is reduced in patients with fibrosing alveolitis and interstitial lung disease, and in the few patients with early pulmonary emphysema careful attention to the technique is essential if weight is to be placed on minor abnormalities. Nevertheless, if the test is technically satisfactory and haemoglobin is normal, a value of less than 1.6 RSD below the predicted normal (about 90%) in a non-smoker and 1.9 RSD (80%) in a smoker, raises a strong possibility of some disease at the level of the alveoli. Conversely, alveolar–arterial Po$_2$ difference is usually normal in exercise if spirometric tests are normal and TLco greater than 70% of the appropriate reference value (Mohsenifar et al., 1992).

Some patients with radiographically distinct granulomatous pulmonary disease, notably sarcoidosis and coal-workers' pneumoconiosis, complain of mild or moderate dyspnoea but spirometric tests, lung volumes and TLco are in the normal range. Appropriate exercise tests in the majority of these patients show a combination of abnormalities of dead space and $Po_2$ which are sufficient to account for the abnormal ventilatory requirement (Chapter 8).

Persistent pulmonary thromboembolism (Chapter 9) is often accompanied by signs and electrocardiographic changes of right ventricular hypertrophy and pulmonary hypertension. It causes a characteristic disturbance: increased $V_D/V_T$ is accompanied by a low $Pco_2$ during exercise. Ventilation–perfusion scanning demonstrates the abnormality. TLco is not invariably reduced. When the emboli are small and distributed diffusely the condition is very similar to primary pulmonary hypertension. Ventilation–perfusion scans may fail to show any regional disturbances. TLco is usually, but not always, low and it is hazardous for patients with primary or severe thromboembolic pulmonary hypertension to perform exercise tests, as unaccustomed exercise appears to cause occasional deaths within the following 48 hours.

*Unsuspected heart disease, without physical signs.* Patients with congenital heart failure or pulmonary oedema often complain frequently of persistent coughing, with or without expectoration and shortness of breath, attributed at first to bronchitis. These patients usually have a restrictive ventilatory defect with a high $TLco/V_A$ with mild airflow obstruction. Occasionally this is borderline. Review of the chest X-ray reveals the diagnosis. A patient with unexplained dyspnoea of effort who has normal lung volumes and TLco should be re-examined for congenital or valvular heart disease. If examination and ECG are unhelpful, the next step is to perform an ultrasound examination of the heart which may reveal aortic stenosis, obstructive cardiomyopathy or impairment of left ventricular emptying. The murmur of aortic outflow obstruction is usually audible, but 'silent' aortic stenosis occasionally complicates mild chronic airflow obstruction, and is suspected when there is undue disability in relation to the ventilatory impairment. Echocardiography is technically difficult when hyperinflation causes herniation of the lungs into the mediastinum, but this problem can sometimes be overcome.

Surprisingly, more than three quarters of patients with breathlessness due to valvular or ischaemic heart disease have some impairment of VC (Warley *et al.*, 1987), perhaps because of previous heart failure or the effect of raised left atrial pressure on the lung. Patients with ischaemic heart disease who are limited by angina pectoris, usually have normal resting lung function tests.

Coronary artery disease, or outflow obstruction sufficient to cause significant impairment of activity, usually cause changes in the resting ECG. Sometimes, combinations of quite mild pulmonary and cardiac disease cause disabling breathlessness, which is difficult to evaluate when diffuse coronary artery disease causes deterioration of cardiac function without overt angina. Coronary artery disease may often be diagnosed by means of a progressive treadmill exercise test with monitoring of 12 ECG leads, employing the usual criteria of abnormality (1 mm plane depression sustained for at least 80 milliseconds beyond the J point: see Chapter 13). If this is normal, the diagnosis can only be made by left ventricular function tests, such as measurement of systolic arterial pressure or left atrial (pulmonary wedge) pressure during exercise. So-called non-invasive tests of cardiac function are accurate in severe cases only. Of particular interest to respiratory physiologists has been the possibility that respiratory measurements may point to the diagnosis of cardiac insufficiency. So far, nothing reliable to distinguish mild or moderate heart disease from 'unfitness' has emerged. There are a few indicators which may be helpful, in addition to the obvious development of severe angina, if exercise tests are undertaken. This is discussed further in Chapter 13.

Right-to-left shunting is a common problem in patients with known septal defects. Patients with pulmonary hypertension may have unexpectedly severe hypoxaemia secondary to shunting through intrapulmonary arteriovenous anastomoses such as those seen in liver disease or in hereditary telangiectasia or through a patent foramen ovale. Dyspnoea has been described in patients with normal lungs, a result of shunting through a patent foramen ovale, with complete relief following open heart surgery (Pitcher *et al.*, 1986), though this is commoner when there is existing lung or liver disease. The diagnosis is suspected if arterial $P_{O_2}$ or arterial $O_2$ saturation falls during exercise and fails to rise as expected while the patient breathes 100% oxygen.

*Metabolic and neurological causes of effort dyspnoea.* Thyrotoxicosis, hypothyroidism, anaemia, uraemia, uncontrolled diabetes and neurological disorders may cause disorders of breathing. Acute febrile illnesses of all types result in effort intolerance, which may require a surprisingly long convalescence. The mechanisms are not fully understood, but are linked with the question of training.

*'Functional hyperventilation'.* Functional or inappropriate hyperventilation is diagnosed when a patient with normal lung function overbreathes such that arterial $P_{CO_2}$ is below 35 mmHg (5 kPa).

This diagnosis cannot be made if there are abnormalities of $P_{O_2}$ or pH which would be expected to cause hyperventilation. A minor degree of hyperventilation is usually found during attacks of asthma or acute pulmonary oedema, and in patients with moderate airflow obstruction. Arterial $P_{O_2}$ is not abnormally high in this situation. What is inappropriate hyperventilation in patients with damaged lungs has never really been defined, although the problem is well described (King & Cotes, 1989; Burns & Howell, 1969).

Patients with psychogenic hyperventilation have high levels of arterial $P_{O_2}$ and of arterial $O_2$ saturation. The diagnosis is confirmed by exclusion of the conditions discussed above, but there are certain features which are characteristic of the condition and it can often be made as a clinical diagnosis. A defensive or hypochondriacal history alone is not diagnostic, because many patients with exercise-induced asthma and chronic neurological disorders present with effort intolerance and have sometimes been called 'neurotic' for many years (Chapter 11).

## Physiological features and clinical aspects of psychogenic exercise hyperventilation

Psychogenic hyperventilation may be classified for the purposes of respiratory investigation under three headings:

1. Acute attacks of shortness of breath. This is discussed in Chapter 11.
2. A variety of symptoms associated with chronic anxiety which will not be discussed further. Many patients present with more than 12 different symptoms referable to different systems, and have evidently somatised their problems over a number of years.
3. Shortness of breath on exertion, sometimes associated with non-anginal chest pains. The latter tend to occur at the end of exercise or after it, and tend to last for several hours.

The diagnosis of hyperventilation as a cause of effort intolerance may be difficult to demonstrate, because the patients often tolerate investigation rather poorly. Usually, the subject is comfortable at rest but complains that mild exercise provokes respiratory discomfort, coughing and hyperventilation.

Investigation has to proceed in stages, to accustom the patient to the laboratory apparatus. Spirometry, single-breath TL$_{CO}$ and lung volumes are measured. The respiratory pattern during quiet breathing is most useful. An irregular rate of breathing with deep breaths and frequent sighing is characteristic of the disorder, and may be detected readily if closed circuit spirometry is employed to measure lung volumes, or by some device which measures the movement of the chest wall (Fig. 2.15). Rebreathing $P_{CO_2}$ may be low, and the test may cause marked hyperpnoea.

Severe hyperventilators find difficulty in performing exercise tests in the laboratory because they tend to become dizzy. The essential measurements are ventilation, expired and arterial $P_{CO_2}$ and $P_{O_2}$ and heart rate during some form of steady-state exercise, straight leg raising while lying on a couch being better than nothing if cycle or treadmill ergometry is likely to cause problems. Exercise usually stops well before the expected limit. Those with normal pulmonary function will have low $P_{CO_2}$ in the arterial blood and in the expired gas, with normal measurements of dead space and alveolar–arterial $P_{O_2}$ difference. The pulse rate is usually normal for the exercise load. Oximetry may show a high $O_2$ saturation.

The pattern of breathing during exercise is rather variable. It may be rapid and shallow in spite of encouragement to breathe as slowly as possible. This makes measurements of dead space very unreliable.

The presence of abnormal dead space or alveolar–arterial $P_{O_2}$ difference indicates that some other disease is present. Occasionally, patients suspected of having functional hyperventilation are found to have a normal arterial $P_{CO_2}$ on exercise, the excessive ventilation being caused entirely by an increased dead space. This may occur in patients with ischaemic heart disease or aortic outflow problems who may also have effort syncope, but this is rare in the presence of an apparently normal ECG unless lung disease is present.

The sensitivity and reliability of these investigations is not really known.

When the condition follows an episode, such as acute respiratory infection or pulmonary embolism, which has required a period of treatment, the patient usually assumes that the condition still requires the same therapy. Firm reassurance is required. Serial tests may be used therapeutically to reassure the patient that the lesion is resolving, and thus help to prevent this problem from developing.

Hyperventilation associated with psychological problems is often rather resistant to formal psychotherapy. Death of the patient's father, husband, close relative or friend may precede the symptoms, often by several months. A mistake easily made is to assume that the patient requires reassurance about heart disease, when in fact it is lung cancer or tuberculosis that is suspected to be the cause of the symptom. It is most important to find out what patients think might be the problem, rather than asking directly what they are worried about, as the latter approach often provokes a firm denial of any anxiety. All this information is more easily obtained at the first interview than later.

There is no evidence that tricyclic antidepressants are of any value, and the benefit of benzodiazepines taken occasionally has never been proved.

The physiological basis of functional exercise hyperventilation is not known: theoretically, there may be a disturbance of cortical control or some abnormality of receptors in the lungs or of the chemoreceptors mediated by the autonomic nervous system.

The prognosis is best in patients with bronchial hyperreactivity whose symptoms follow an acute infection. The majority of patients with longstanding functional hyperventilation settle down to a restricted, but acceptable life, avoiding physical exercise in the same way as patients with valvular heart disease. In contrast to the well-studied problem of panic attacks (Chapter 11), a detailed discussion about management of exercise-related functional hyperventilation is not possible, because there is no well-substantiated published work.

## Mechanical limitation to breathing: theoretical considerations

The relationship between ventilatory capacity and ventilatory requirement was discussed in Chapter 1. A more detailed approach takes into account the power of the respiratory muscles and the respiratory effort needed to increase ventilation (Killian & Campbell, 1983; Killian & Jones, 1984, 1988; Leblanc et al., 1986).

1. The ventilatory requirement to the alveoli ($\dot{V}_A$) is determined by requirement for $O_2$ uptake and $CO_2$ output and any additional drive to due to hyperventilation caused by hypoxia or metabolic acidosis. To this is added dead space ventilation ($V_D$).
2. This is achieved by generating tension in inspiratory muscles to create a driving pressure ($P_{insp}$). The frequency of breathing (f), inspiratory duration ($t_i$) and tidal volume ($V_T$) are selected subconsciously to minimise effort, though a rapid shallow breathing pattern results in increased dead space ventilation.

Generating inspiratory pressure ($P_{insp}$) achieves inspiratory flow ($\dot{V}_I$), tidal volume ($V_T$) and acceleration ($V_T/t_i^2$). To do this it has to overcome airway resistance

$$R = \frac{P_{insp}}{V_I} \qquad (12.1)$$

but because $V_I = V_T$/inspiratory time ($t_i$)

$$R = \frac{P_{insp}}{V_T t_i} \qquad (12.2)$$

The elastance E (or recoil) of the lungs ($E = P/V_T$) must also be overcome, as well as the inertia which opposes the acceleration of airflow in the initiation of inspiration $P.t_i^2/V_T$. Inertial forces are numerically of less importance. Ignoring these

$$P_{insp} = [ (V_T/t_i \times R) + (V_T \times E) ] \qquad (12.3)$$

The maximal flow–volume loop represents the reserve that is available for breathing. The inspiratory limb is limited by the mechanical factors outlined (muscle power, elasticity and resistance). Expiration is usually accompanied by only sufficient muscular effort to 'brake' or slow down the flow of air and poses a mechanical problem when it is severely slowed down by airflow obstruction. Then it becomes an important determinant of respiratory frequency because the time available for inspiration is reduced.

Expiratory flow limitation impinges on breathing in patients with severe airflow obstruction. Patients with this problem often breathe at high lung volumes because there is insufficient time to return to FRC. This places the inspiratory muscles at a mechanical disadvantage and increases the elastic work of inspiration (Chapter 6).

The magnitude of perceived exertion therefore depends on the expiratory reserve and on how closely inspiration approximates to the maximum breathing capacity. This is determined by the maximum respiratory pressure and the mechanical limitations to inspiration listed. Continued exercise employing a peak inspiratory pressure at more than half the patient's maximal effort results in disabling dyspnoea and in respiratory muscle fatigue. This may occur because of weakness, mechanical difficulty or a combination of the two. In Fig. 12.4 these concepts are shown diagrammatically. The normal subject, exercising vigorously, employs only a fraction of the available muscle power (horizontal axis, left). The patient with airflow obstruction cannot exercise because of severe breathlessness. The reason is that the respiratory muscles are operating at their limit; the relationship between breathlessness and muscular effort, as a fraction of maximal, remains

normal but the ventilation achieved is much lower than normal (Table 6.3).

A crude estimate of the reserve of power available during exercise may be obtained indirectly from the measurement of maximum inspiratory pressure and the maximal inspiratory flow volume loop (Killian & Jones, 1984).

The insights based on such calculations are important, and contribute to our understanding of groups of patients with disordered breathing, as well as occasionally explaining the nature of effort limitation.

## Assessment of disability: the capacity to meet the demand of work, recreation and everyday life

The assessment of disability in occupational medicine remains controversial and is generally bound by simple rules designed more for convenience than for accuracy. In general, there is poor agreement between those who assess impairment according to the history, to clinical examination or to functional impairment. It is helpful to define four aspects to the overall reduction in the capacity to meet the demands of everyday life and occupation (Jones, 1988):

1. *Lung damage*: identified by clinical signs and imaging techniques.
2. *Impairment*: reduction in organ function.
3. *Disability*: reduction in exercise capacity because of impairment.
4. *Handicap*: the difficulty experienced in following an accepted way of life or occupation.

Very severe lung impairment leads to predictable levels of disability and handicap. When damage and impairment are mild, there is room for other factors such as body build, personality, motivation and unfitness to affect formal exercise tests and the degree of adaptation (Cotes, Zejda & King, 1988; King & Cotes, 1989). These factors confound the formal attempt to evaluate disability purely in terms of impairment (De Coster, 1983; American Thoracic Society, 1986). Nevertheless, care is needed in interpreting the meaning of replies to questions on attitudes to health. Morgan *et al.* (1983) showed that self-assessment as 'deli-

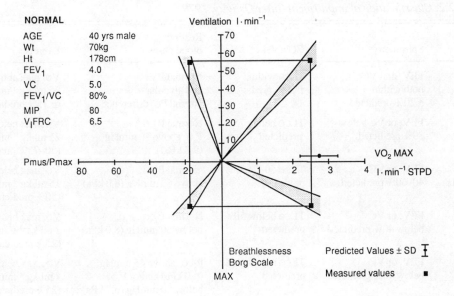

NORMAL

| AGE | 40 yrs male |
|---|---|
| Wt | 70kg |
| Ht | 178cm |
| FEV$_1$ | 4.0 |
| VC | 5.0 |
| FEV$_1$/VC | 80% |
| MIP | 80 |
| V$_I$FRC | 6.5 |

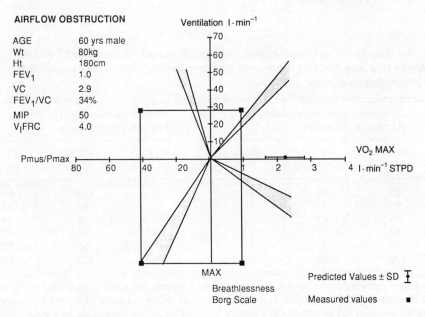

AIRFLOW OBSTRUCTION

| AGE | 60 yrs male |
|---|---|
| Wt | 80kg |
| Ht | 180cm |
| FEV$_1$ | 1.0 |
| VC | 2.9 |
| FEV$_1$/VC | 34% |
| MIP | 50 |
| V$_I$FRC | 4.0 |

Fig. 12.4. Sensation of breathlessness and ventilatory capacity in normal subjects and patients with chronic airflow obstruction. The normal relationships are shown by the fanning lines. The relationship between dyspnoea and muscular effort (Pmus/Pmax: the proportion of the maximal pressure employed during inspiration) is the same in the patient as in the normal subject. This imposes a less than optimal performance in all other respects. For explanation, see text (adapted from Killian & Jones, 1984).

Table 12.2. *Classification of impairment (after Ostiguy, 1979)*

| Class | Spirometry[a] | CO uptake[a] | Resting blood gases | Exercise |
|---|---|---|---|---|
| Class I (none) | $FEV_1$ and VC both within ± 20% predicted | TLco within ± 20% predicted | Normal $P_aCO_2$ and alveolar – arterial $Po_2$ difference | $Vo_2$ max above 25 ml·kg$^{-1}$·min$^{-1}$ or 75% predicted) |
| Class II (mild) | $FEV_1$ or VC below 80% predicted | TLco below 75% predicted | Normal $P_aCO_2$ $P_aO_2$ above 70 mmHg (9.3 kPa) | $Vo_2$ max below 25 ml·kg$^{-1}$·min$^{-1}$ (50–75% predicted) |
| Class III (moderate) | $FEV_1$ or VC 40–60% predicted | TLco 50–75% predicted | Normal $P_aCO_2$, $P_aO_2$ above 60 mmHg (8.0 kPa) | $Vo_2$ max below 15 ml·kg$^{-1}$·min$^{-1}$ (50% predicted) |
| Class IV (severe) | $FEV_1$ or VC below 40% predicted | TLco below 50% predicted | Normal $P_aCO_2$, $P_aO_2$ below 60 mmHg (8.0 kPa) | $Vo_2$ max below 7 ml·kg$^{-1}$·min$^{-1}$ (25% predicted) |
| Class V (very severe) | $FEV_1$ or VC below 40% predicted | TLco below 50% predicted | $P_aCO_2$ above 45 mmHg (6.0 kPa) and/or $P_aO_2$ below 50 mmHg (6.7 kPa) | $Vo_2$ max below 7 ml·kg$^{-1}$·min$^{-1}$ (25% predicted) |

[a] Predicted values on basis of age, sex and size: spirometric defect may be obstructive (low FEV/VC) or non-obstructive (low VC with normal or high FEV/VC).

Table 12.3. *Relationship of spirometric tests and single breath TLco to MRC disability grade in patients referred to a lung function laboratory with irreversible airflow obstruction, interstitial lung diseases or occupational exposure*

| MRC grade | 224 patients with chronic airflow obstruction (not asthma) | | | 196 non-obstructed patients with interstitial lung diseases | | |
|---|---|---|---|---|---|---|
| | $FEV_1$ (% predicted) | VC (% predicted) | TLco (% predicted) | $FEV_1$ (% predicted) | VC % (% predicted) | TLco (% predicted) |
| I | 60 | 94 | 57 | 100 | 104 | 66 |
| II | 55 | 91 | 45 | 86 | 93 | 58 |
| III | 48 | 83 | 43 | 75 | 78 | 49 |
| IV | 42 | 77 | 40 | 74 | 77 | 47 |
| V | 39 | 71 | 36 | 67 | 68 | 30 |
| Lab. normal | 120 | 120 | 100 | 120 | 120 | 100 |

Concomitant known cardiac disorders and asthma are excluded. Normal values are from Cotes (1979), but healthy smoking and non-smoking subjects studied in this laboratory had higher values for $FEV_1$ and VC (author's data). The results given are mean values; individual variation was wide, 1 SD for each grade was about 17%. There is some selection bias in the results for interstitial lung disease in grade I, because asymptomatic subjects with normal spirometry and TLco would be less likely to be assigned to the group of interstitial lung diseases than those with impaired TLco.

Table 12.4. *Oxygen cost of various occupations in l ·min⁻¹*

|  | Highest sustained O$_2$ intake | Highest burst of O$_2$ intake |
|---|---|---|
| *Walking at 2 mph (3 km ·h⁻¹)* |  | 0.5 |
| Telephonist | 0.6 | 0.6 |
| Secretary | 0.7 | 0.7 |
| Consultant physician | 0.75 | 0.75 |
| *Walking at 3 mph (3 km ·h⁻¹)* |  | 0.75 |
| Housework | 1.0 | 1.2 |
| Postman | 1.0 | 1.3 |
| *Walking at 4 mph (6.5 km ·h⁻¹)* |  | 1.2 |
| Farm work | 1.5 | 2.0 |
| *Walking at 5 mph (8 km ·h⁻¹)* |  | 1.7 |
| Mining/construction work | 1.9 | 2.2 |
| *Walking at 6 mph (9.5 km ·h⁻¹)* |  | 2.2 |
| Stevedore | 2.0 |  |

cate' influenced the walking speed of patients with moderate chronic airflow obstruction, but this may merely mean that the subjects had suffered previously from asthma, which we have found to be a major determinant of walking speed in these patients.

A well-recognised classification of impairment in the occupational lung diseases is given in Table 12.2 (Ostiguy, 1979, modified by Jones, 1988). Our data suggest that in an unselected population referred to a lung function laboratory, reduction of VC to below 80% of published predicted values (60% of our laboratory normal subjects) results in a major degree of disability (Table 12.3). Reduction to class II may be sufficient to impair working capacity in a number of heavy occupations (Table 12.4). This is a broad class which contains a number of healthy subjects and the majority of those discovered while at work to have abnormal clinical findings or an abnormal chest radiograph. For these subjects, an exercise test is needed to determine maximal oxygen consumption (Cotes *et al.*, 1988) as the prediction of disability from resting lung function tests is very poor.

## References

Adams, L., Chronos, N., Lane, R. & Guz, A. (1985). The measurement of breathlessness induced in normal subjects: validity of two scaling techniques. *Clinical Science*, **69**, 7–16.

Adams, L. & Guz, A. (1991). Dyspnea on exertion. In *Exercise*, ed. B.J. Whipp & K. Wasserman, pp. 449–494. New York: Marcel Dekker.

Aitken, R.C.B. (1969). Measurement of feelings using usual analogue scales. *Proceedings of the Royal Society of Medicine*, **62**, 989–993.

American Thoracic Society (1986). Evaluation of impairment/disability secondary to respiratory disorders. *American Review of Respiratory Disease*, **133**, 1205–1209.

Bond, A. & Laver, M. (1974). The use of analogue scales in rating subjective feeling. *British Journal of Medical Psychology*, **47**, 211–218.

Borg, G. (1978). Subjective effort and physical activities. *Scandinavian Journal of Rehabilitation Medicine*, **6**, 108–113.

Burns, B.H. & Howell, J.B.L. (1969). Disproportionately severe breathlessness in chronic bronchitis. *Quarterly Journal of Medicine*, **238**, 277–294.

Comroe, J.H. (1966). Some theories of the mechanisms of dyspnoea. In *Breathlessness*, ed. J.B.L. Howell &

E.J.M. Campbell, pp. 1–7. Oxford: Blackwell Scientific Publications.

Cotes, J.E. (1979). Lung function (4th edn). Oxford: Blackwell Scientific Publications.

Cotes, J.E., Zejda, J. & King, B. (1988). Lung function impairment as a guide to exercise limitation in work-related lung disorders. *American Review of Respiratory Disease*, **137**, 1089–1093.

De Coster, A. (1983). Respiratory impairment and disablement. *Bulletin Européen Physiopathologie Respiratoire*, **19**, 1P-3P.

de Paso, W.J., Winterbauer, R.H., Lusk, J.A., Dreis, D.F. & Springmeyer (1991). Chronic dyspnoea unexplained by history, chest examination, chest roentgenogram and spirometry. *Chest*, **100**, 1293–1299.

Elliott, M.W., Adams, L., Cockroft, A., Macrae, K.D., Murphy, K. & Guz, A. (1990). The language of breathlessness. *American Review of Respiratory Disease*, **144**, 826–832.

Fletcher, C.M., Elmes, P.C., Fairbairn, A.S. & Wood, C.H. (1959). The significance of respiration symptoms and the diagnosis of chronic bronchitis in a working population. *British Medical Journal*, **ii**, 257–266.

Higgs, C.M.B., Richardson, R.B., Lea, D.A., Lewis, G.T.R. & Laszlo, G. (1986). Influence of knowledge of peak flow on self-assessment of asthma: studies with a coded peak flow meter. *Thorax*, **41**, 671–675.

Jones, N.L. (1988). Occupational health. In *Clinical Exercise Testing*, pp. 111–122. Philadelphia: Saunders.

Killian, K.J. & Campbell, E.J.M. (1983). Dyspnoea and exercise. *Annual Review of Physiology*, **45**, 465–479.

Killian, K.J. & Jones, N.L. (1984). The use of exercise testing and other methods in the investigation of dyspnea. *Clinics in Chest Medicine*, **5**, 99–108.

Killian, K.J. & Jones, N.L. (1988). Respiratory muscles and dyspnea. *Clinics in Chest Medicine*, **9**, 237–248.

King, B. & Cotes, J.E. (1989). Relation of lung function and exercise capacity to mood and attitudes to health. *Thorax*, **44**, 402–409.

Leblanc, P., Baize, D.M., Summers, E., Jones, N.L. & Killian, K.J. (1986). Breathlessness and exercise in patients with cardiorespiratory disease. *American Review of Respiratory Disease*, **133**, 21–25.

Mahler, D.A., Weinberg, D.H., Wells, C.K. & Feinstein, A.R. (1984). The measurement of dyspnoea. *Chest*, **85**, 751–758.

McGavin, C.R. Artvinli, M., Naoe, H., McHardy, G.J.R. (1978). Dyspnoea, disability and distance walked: comparison of estimates of exercise performance in respiratory disease. *British Medical Journal*, **ii**, 241–243.

Medical Research Council (1966). *Questionnaire on Respiratory Symptoms*. London: Medical Research Council.

Mohsenifar, Z., Collier, J., Belman, M.J. & Koerner, S.K. (1992). Isolated reduction in single-breath diffusing capacity in the evaluation of exertional dyspnea. *Chest*, **101**, 965–969.

Morgan, A.D., Peck, D.F., Buchanan, D.R. & McHardy, G.J.R. (1983). Effect of attitudes and beliefs on exercise tolerance in chronic bronchitis. *British Medical Journal*, **286**, 171–173.

Ostiguy, G. (1979). Summary of task force report on occupational respiratory disease (pneumoconiosis). *Canadian Medical Association Journal*, **121**, 414–421.

Pitcher D., Fletcher, P., Laszlo, G., Keen, G., Rees, J.R. (1986). Onset of right-to-left shunting through a foramen ovale in a 70-year-old woman: successful surgical treatment. *European Heart Journal*, **7**, 541–544.

Simon, P.M., Schwartzstein, R.M., Weiss, J.W., Fencl, V., Teghtsoonian, M. & Weinberger, S.E. (1990). Distinguishable types of dyspnea in patients with shortness of breath. *American Review of Respiratory Disease*, **142**, 1009–1014.

Stevens, S.S. (1975). Sensation and measurement. In *Psychophysics*, ed. G. Stevens, pp. 37–62. New York: John Wiley.

Stoller, J.K., Ferranti, R. & Feinstein, A.R. (1986). Further specification and evaluation of a new clinical index for dyspnea. *American Review of Respiratory Disease*, **134**, 1129–1134.

Warley, A.R.H., Finnegan, O.C., Nicholson, E.M. & Laszlo, G. (1987). Grading of dyspnoea and walking speed in cardiac disorders and chronic airflow obstruction. *British Journal of Diseases of the Chest*, **81**, 349–355.

# 13 Exercise testing

Measuring respiratory, metabolic and cardio-vascular responses to exercise helps to explain why effort tolerance may be limited. Different procedures have been devised to impose a variety of physiological stresses, because no single test answers all the questions that arise.

## Protocols for exercise testing

The choices to be made are:

1. Position: upright or supine
2. Muscle groups: large or small; cycling, walking or arm exercise.
3. Choice of equipment: cycle, treadmill, step, couch, free.
4. Duration and intensity: maximal or submaximal; fixed or incremental work; quasi-steady or non-steady state.
5. Respiratory and cardiac variables to be measured.

### Position

Patients generally find upright exercise easier, but the supine position may be unavoidable if the test forms part of a complex procedure such as cardiac catheterisation. Patients who are quickly exhausted or who suffer from effort syncope cannot easily be investigated in the upright position. Simple measurements may be made after a period of exercise in the semirecumbent position while the patient raises and lowers the legs in turn in time to a metronome.

### Muscle groups

Leg exercise in the upright position is most likely to allow the subject to achieve the permitted maximum oxygen uptake, and is therefore used to investigate cardiorespiratory limitation. The results of leg exercise tests are easy to interpret because the relationship between oxygen requirement and work performed, that is, work efficiency, varies very little from one individual to another. Exercise using smaller muscles is normally limited by pain endurance: there is relatively more anaerobic metabolism.

Isometric exercise causes systolic and diastolic hypertension. There is a relatively greater increase in cardiac work than in isotonic exercise, which causes systolic pressure to rise in normal subjects with little or no fall of diastolic pressure.

### Choice of equipment

To determine maximal performance in athletes it is necessary to make assessments doing the type of exercise for which they have trained.

For clinical purposes, respiratory variables and intravascular pressures are most easily recorded during ergometry on a stationary cycle or treadmill. These also allow the same workload to be administered on different occasions.

There is little to choose between cycles and treadmills for making respiratory measurements. Those accustomed to cycling find it easier to breathe through a mouthpiece while pedalling than when they are walking on a treadmill. It is easier to obtain a stable ECG trace and blood pressure recording on a bicycle than on other types of apparatus, though expensive modern ECG machines designed for treadmill exercise have overcome this problem.

Bicycle ergometers can be adapted for supine exercise, for example during cardiac catheterisation. Walking is the universal form of exercise, while subjects unaccustomed to cycling may be limited by muscle fatigue rather than by the circulation or by pulmonary gas exchange. Treadmill tests should, in theory, provide a better assessment of mobility than cycle ergometers, but the advantage is reduced by the slight difficulty of measuring breathing during exercise. Angina pectoris is more satisfactorily identified on a treadmill than on a bicycle, because some patients with ischaemic heart disease do not develop angina on a bicycle but develop muscle fatigue or become breathless. In cases where exercise is limited by breathing rather than cardiac pain, maximal tests are more easily performed on a bicycle because the subject can stop without having to switch the machine off.

Step tests were supposed to overcome these difficulties. The main value of the costly equipment now used is that procedures can be standardised.

Free running is a satisfactory way of inducing asthma in susceptible children (Chapter 7). Treadmills are better than bicycles for this purposes if room air is breathed, but exercise-induced asthma can reproducibly be provoked on a bicycle if dry air is inhaled.

The elderly and nervous and those with multiple disabilities find this sort of equipment forbidding. Walking tests may help to assess disability, while straight leg raising on a couch is a satisfactory method of inducing exercise stress if measurements requiring a mouthpiece are needed in subjects who are likely to faint if asked to perform upright exercise.

## Maximal or submaximal test

### Tests of maximal exertion

Tests of maximal exertion may be the only way of demonstrating the mechanism of exercise limitation in certain individuals. ECG changes rarely occur before the onset of angina pectoris, so maximal tests are necessary to investigate this condition. Several protocols have been studied extensively:

1. Incremental treadmill test with ECG monitoring, gradient and speed being increased every 3 minutes (the Bruce test), or every minute (Balke protocol) (Bruce & McDonough, 1969; Balke & Ware, 1959).
2. Patients who are disabled by chronic circulatory or respiratory disorders may be investigated on a treadmill at a fixed speed, measuring endurance time.
3. Cycle ergometry with incremental workloads increasing every minute (Jones stages 1 and 2, p. 194) (Jones, 1988).

Serial exercise tests may be valuable in demonstrating improvement in exercise tolerance, for example after certain therapeutic procedures. If the condition of the lungs improves it may be possible to demonstrate improvement in the performance of a submaximal test, examining measured variables such as heart rate and ventilation in relation to exercise load. Very often, however, the question of whether a patient's effort tolerance has improved can be determined only by using discomfort as the end point of the investigation. Patients with angina or claudication should be asked to stop when they would normally do so. Patients limited by dyspnoea or fatigue can be encouraged to continue until further exercise is impossible.

### Safety

Exercise tests are terminated by the operator:

1. If the patient becomes dizzy, apprehensive, confused or looks ashen, clammy or cyanosed.
2. For cardiological reasons:
   If there is chest pain which might be ischaemic.
   Electrocardiographic changes of ischaemia.
   Dysrhythmia.
   If ventricular ectopic beats occur in runs of more than one during exercise, or more than six per minute.
   Heart block.
   If systolic blood pressure fails to rise by 20 mmHg, subsequently falls as exercise progresses, or rises above 280 mmHg.
   In all cases where the heart rate reaches a predicted maximum of (210 - age). This figure is an average at which diastolic time is too short for complete ventricular filling and cardiac output cannot rise further. Sometimes, for exam-

ple after myocardial infarction, a lower maximum is set.

3. If there is intolerable dyspnoea. It is generally safe to allow patients to choose the level at which they stop for this reason.

4. If pain develops in one or both legs.

Maximal exercise testing is safe if certain precautions are observed:

1. The test must be cancelled if an acute intercurrent illness has developed or if the patient is febrile, because of the high incidence of myocarditis in common virus infections.

2. Resuscitation equipment must be available. ECG monitoring is essential in cardiological practice and advisable for all patients over the age of 40. Two trained operators, one experienced in cardiopulmonary resuscitation, should be present. In the case of respiratory limitation, the second need only be available on immediate call.

3. Exercise tests are unsafe in cases of severe pulmonary hypertension and aortic outflow obstruction.

4. Heart failure, systemic hypertension, unstable angina pectoris and unstable cardiac rhythms should be controlled before exercise tests are undertaken.

### Submaximal tests

Submaximal tests are of value in assessing the physiology of the lungs and heart. There are fairly well-defined normal limits for the relationship between ventilation, heart rate, $CO_2$ production and oxygen consumption and for indices of pulmonary gas exchange such as dead space and alveolar–arterial $Po_2$ difference. Abnormalities of these relationships may be detected at workloads considerably below maximum in patients with lung diseases.

Most subjects can sustain 50% of their maximum heart rate for long periods. Submaximal tests are stopped when the patient reaches about 85% of predicted maximum heart rate or for the other reasons listed above.

Self-selected speed tests have recently become popular, formalising the old practice of watching the patient exercise in a measured corridor. These tests are useful but changes have to be interpreted carefully because improvement may take two

forms: either the patient may walk faster, or the same ground may be covered with less respiratory discomfort (Woodcock, *et al.* 1981). Interpretation therefore depends on subjective as well as objective measurements. For serial measurements, improvement may best be shown by endurance testing at a fixed speed, determined by trial and established by rehearsal. End points have to be defined, the most useful being the time which elapses before the onset of a sensation of fatigue.

### Single load tests

Single load tests are occasionally used. It is possible to choose a load which is suitably easy or difficult for the patient to sustain by prior performance of a Stage 1 test, during which the slope of the heart rate/work curve is about 80% of the steady state value in most subjects. It is more difficult to predict the work that will produce a given stress by taking a history. Walking on level ground uses about 1 litre of oxygen per minute, while walking at 2.5 mph (4 km/h) up a slight incline requires about 2 litres per minute.

### Fixed load tests

Fixed load tests which are standard for all patients are occasionally valuable because the normal range of a measured variable is much narrower in mild exercise (usually 150–300 kilopond metres per minute, 25–50 watts) than at rest. Cardiac output, pulmonary arterial pressure and CO uptake are reproducible in moderate exercise. Physiological studies of the circulation and respiratory system, for example to study the effect of drugs, may require repeated exercise at intervals.

### Repeatability

As work rate increases the effect of anxiety and inexperience becomes relatively less important. Several studies have shown the importance of eliminating the effect of unfamiliarity with the procedure and surroundings. Twelve-minute walking distance increases by a factor of about 5% at the second attempt, the test being reproducible thereafter (McGavin, Gupta & McHardy, 1976). During cycle ergometry hyperventilation and tachycardia are also reduced at low workloads during the second trial. In normal subjects,

Table 13.1. *Prediction of maximum exercise variables (formulae from Jones, 1988)*

| | | |
|---|---|---|
| Max. work (watts) | Male | $= 298 \times ht^{2.77} \times age^{-0.52}$ |
| | Female | $= 208 \times ht^{2.59} \times age^{-0.46}$ |
| Max. cardiac frequency | | $= 210 - 0.65\, age \pm 10$ |
| Max. $O_2$ uptake | Male | $= (0.83 \times height^{2.7}) \times$ $(1 - 0.007\, age)$ |
| | Female | $= (0.62 \times height^{2.7}) \times$ $(1 - 0.007\, age)$ |
| Max. voluntary ventilation | | $= 129 + 25\,(FEV_1 - 4)$ $l \cdot min^{-1}$ (normal) |
| | | $= 20 + (20 \times FEV_1)$ $l \cdot min^{-1}$ ($FEV_1 < 1.5$) |
| Max. ventilation ($l \cdot min^{-1}$) | | $= (31 \times FEV_1) - 30$ |
| Max. tidal volume (litres) | | $= (VC \times 2/3) - 0.65$ |
| Max. diastolic blood pressure | | $=$ baseline $+ 15$ mmHg |

Height in metres, $FEV_1$ in litres, BTPS work (power output) in watts. Conversion from watts to kilopond–metres per minute: $\times 6.1$.

Table 13.2. *Relationship of physiological variables to work intensity (formulae from Jones, 1988)*

| | |
|---|---|
| $O_2$ uptake ($ml \cdot min^{-1}$) | $= 3.5 \times weight + (11 \times work)$ |
| Ventilation up to 50% of power output ($l \cdot min^{-1}$) | $= 8 + work/3$ $= 5 + (22 \times O_2$ uptake, $l \cdot min^{-1})$ |
| Anaerobic threshold ($O_2$ uptake, | $= 55\%$ of maximal $O_2$ uptake $l \cdot min^{-1}$ $= 2.4 \times height$ (or metres) $- (0.007\, age) - 2.4$ |
| Cardiac output ($l \cdot min^{-1}$) Upright Supine | $= 4 + 0.006 \times O_2$ uptake $\pm 2$ ($l \cdot min^{-1}$) $= 6 + 0.006 \times O_2$ uptake $\pm 2$ ($l \cdot min^{-1}$) |
| Systolic blood pressure (mmHg) | $= 120 + (0.06 \times work)\,[2 + (0.1 \times age)]$ |

one rehearsal is sufficient and subsequent tests are reproducible but if serial physiological or pharmacological studies are to yield valid results, participants have to practice the techniques until successive tests show abolition of the rehearsal effect. This phenomenon is different from training, which can be shown to improve circulatory variables and maximise oxygen uptake gradually over several days, with effects on muscle metabolism and probably on the distribution of blood to exercising muscle through the microcirculation. Inactivity has dramatic effects in the opposite direction (Jones, 1988).

## One-minute incremental work rate test (Jones Stage 1): measurements and interpretation

The one-minute incremental work rate test, the best studied form of exercise test, consists of asking the patient to cycle seated on a stationary ergometer on which the work rate can be increased in a stepwise manner. Increments should ideally be judged to provide at least 4–8 workloads for study. A normal male subject, able to achieve

150–200 watts, will be studied most efficiently by using 25 watt increments. Very unfit or deconditioned patients or those with low values of predicted maximal oxygen uptake should start at 12.5 watts with 12.5 watt increments.

Most of the information is gained from measurements of heart rate, ECG, ventilation, expired gas concentrations, oxygen uptake and $CO_2$ output. Measurements of oxygen saturation may easily be included. Arterial blood gases, pH and lactic acid, if needed, are best obtained during a submaximal test in which each workload, which may be single or part of a series, is sustained for 3–4 minutes in order to achieve a steady state.

## Relationship between workload and measured variables

The relationship between physical work and cardiorespiratory variables has been studied extensively. The best available formulae are given in Tables 13.1 and 13.2 (data from Jones, 1988).

### Maximal heart rate

Above a certain heart rate, the ventricles cannot fill fully in diastole. The output of the heart is therefore not increased by any rise of rate above

Table 13.3. *Cardiac variables in exercise*

| | $O_2$ uptake ($l \cdot min^{-1}$) | Cardiac frequency beats·$min^{-1}$ | Stroke volume (ml) | Cardiac output ($l \cdot min^{-1}$) | Arteriovenous $O_2$ content difference ($l \cdot min^{-1}$) | Mixed venous $O_2$ saturation (%) |
|---|---|---|---|---|---|---|
| *Normal subject* | | | | | | |
| Gentle exercise | 1.0 | 100 | 100 | 10 | 100 | 45 |
| Maximal exercise | 2.5 | 180 | 110 | 20 | 100 | 45 |
| *Athlete* | | | | | | |
| Gentle exercise | 1.0 | 80 | 125 | 10 | 100 | 45 |
| $O_2$ consumption 2.5 $l \cdot min^{-1}$ | 2.5 | 130 | 140 | 18.2 | 137 | 26 |
| Maximal | 4.6 | 190 | 140 | 26.6 | 175 | 20 |

The relationship between cardiac output and $O_2$ consumption is similar for athletes and normal subjects. The difference lies in the higher values of stroke volume and maximum stroke volume (140 ml in this example) among athletes. In addition, training improves tissue $O_2$ extraction, permitting much lower levels of venous $O_2$ saturation.

the value, which, for subjects of average fitness, equals [210 - 0.65 (age in years)] (Spiro, 1977). Maximal tests should be terminated if the rate reaches this value. Variations of this rule may be advised, especially in untrained subjects. Convenient submaximal tests may be carried out at 80% of this figure, or an added margin of safety introduced for older patients by employing the formula [210 - (age in years)]. Some elderly subjects and a few with ischaemic heart disease lose the capacity to increase their heart rate ('chronotropic incompetence'), which may be an important factor in limiting exercise tolerance.

### Maximal oxygen consumption

In normal people, oxygen delivery to the tissues is limited by the circulation. As discussed in Chapter 3, the oxygen dissociation curve is quite flat at the level of alveolar $Po_2$ usually seen in health. Minor variations of ventilation have very little effect on oxygen uptake. A healthy young man with an $FEV_1$ of 5 litres would extract 6 litres of oxygen per minute from room air with an alveolar $Po_2$ of 110 mmHg (14 kPa) if there were enough pulmonary blood flow to carry this away and enough muscle to metabolise it. The maximal oxygen intake in sedentary young men is between 2.5 and 3 litres per minute. This imposes a greater

load on ventilation because of anaerobic metabolism, discussed below, which increases the amount of $CO_2$ that has to be excreted. Nevertheless, in health there is still a substantial gap between maximal breathing capacity and maximum exercise ventilation, which has been called the breathing reserve (Wasserman *et al.*, 1986). This gap is closed in athletes by training of the circulation. It is also reduced in patients with conditions such as chronic asthma in whom the ventilatory capacity is more severely impaired than is the pulmonary circulation.

The diffusing capacity of the lung for oxygen, calculated from CO measurements, permits an oxygen uptake of around 5.0 $l \cdot min^{-1}$ in a healthy man. The limiting factors in the circulation are:

1. Stroke volume, which determines cardiac output at maximal heart rates.
2. Tissue extraction of oxygen. The capacity for tissue enzymes to function at low $Po_2$ determines the venous $Po_2$ of exercising muscle. Training may improve tissue extraction of oxygen to some extent.
3. Distribution of blood flow preferentially to exercising tissue. The ability of the peripheral circulation to divert the blood to where it is needed may also be influenced by training.

Whether capillaries are generated *de novo* by regular exercise is uncertain.

In the quasi-steady state, there is a linear increase in cardiac output in proportion to workload. In the supine position, this is brought about mainly by increase in rate; in the upright position, stroke volume increases during light exercise, and thereafter remains constant. Moderately severe exercise, for example 150 watts or cycling up a gradient of 1/10, may call for a ninefold increase of oxygen consumption from about 250 ml/min at rest to 2250 ml/min (2.25 l/min). This is achieved by approximately a threefold increase of tissue extraction and a threefold increase of cardiac output. Typical figures are given in a worked example to illustrate the order of magnitude of the changes (Table 13.3).

Healthy trained athletes exercise at a lower heart rate and blood pressure and higher stroke volume than sedentary individuals. The relationship between cardiac output and work is fairly constant, however; mechanisms which result in reduced tissue $Po_2$ operate when the limit is reached. This also applies to patients with reduced cardiopulmonary function in whom arteriovenous blood gas pressure differences may be very wide. Heart rate and stroke output can increase without any increase in cardiac volume at the end of diastole because of the inotropic effect of the sympathetic response to exercise and reduction of vagal tone.

The oxygen-pulse ($O_2$ consumption divided by heart rate) is a moderately useful index of physical fitness, but the normal range is wide. There is a correlation between maximum oxygen uptake and heart rate at 1.5 l·min$^{-1}$ oxygen consumption, but it is not very close and does not take into account the problems posed by respiratory limitation. For these reasons, it is difficult to predict maximal work rate and oxygen uptake from submaximal tests.

## Ventilation and carbon dioxide output

The relationship between $CO_2$ production, excretion and ventilation has been considered in some detail in Chapter 1. Blood gases should remain normal during mild or moderate exercise, to maintain adequate oxygen without wasteful over-breathing, which causes respiratory alkalosis without a useful increase of oxygen uptake. To maintain a constant and normal value of alveolar and therefore of arterial $Pco_2$, ventilation must be appropriate to the metabolic production of $CO_2$. Alveolar ventilation is defined as the ventilation required to excrete the $CO_2$ produced by metabolism at the patient's arterial $Pco_2$, assuming uniformly distributed ventilation and perfusion (Chapter 1). The actual ventilatory requirement will exceed this figure because of the volume of unperfused but ventilated air passage. There is no oxygen uptake in the trachea and bronchi, and only a little $CO_2$ excretion (because a measurable amount occurs from the bronchial capillaries). This adds approximately 150–180 ml per breath to the alveolar ventilation, the 'anatomical dead space'. In addition, the non-uniform distribution of pulmonary blood flow adds a further 30–60 ml in the upright subject at rest (the 'alveolar dead space or wasted ventilation'). This diminishes in the supine position, and virtually disappears in exercise in subjects with normal lungs. The anatomical dead space does increase with tidal volume because as the lungs get larger, so do the airways. The ratio dead space/tidal volume falls with increasing exercise: tidal volume increases by a greater factor than dead space.

### Pulmonary carbon dioxide exchange

The difference between arterial and mixed expired $Pco_2$ is a measure of the total dead space, anatomical and alveolar.

$$\frac{\text{Dead space}}{\text{Tidal volume}} = \qquad (13.1)$$

$$\frac{\text{Arterial - expired } Pco_2}{\text{Arterial } Pco_2 - \text{inspired } Pco_2}$$

or

$$V_D/V_T = \frac{}{P_aco_2 - P_Eco_2 / P_aco_2 - P_Ico_2} \qquad (13.2)$$

$V_D$ may now be calculated by multiplying by tidal volume and subtracting the dead space of the valve box employed. Dead space varies from about 150 ml at rest to about 300 ml at high tidal volumes in exercise. Mixed expired $P_{CO_2}$ may also be corrected by the same calculation for the dilution effect of the valve box. This is important in narrowing the normal range by correcting for the quite substantial contribution of the valve box (60–100 ml) to the dilution of alveolar gas in subjects who adopt a shallow pattern of breathing.

It follows, therefore, that an increased ventilation with respect to $CO_2$ output, with low expired $P_{CO_2}$, may result from:

1. Disturbed pulmonary gas exchange.
2. Low arterial $P_{CO_2}$ (alveolar hyperventilation):
   Stimulated by lactic acidosis.
   Stimulated by hypoxaemia.
   'Functional', which may be due to stimulation of ventilation associated with lung disease to a greater extent than would be expected from hypoxaemia or acidosis or caused by anxiety. Inappropriate or functional hyperventilation is defined as a fall of arterial $P_{CO_2}$ to below 36 mmHg (5 kPa) without any identifiable chemoreceptor stimulus being present. $P_{CO_2}$ may be low for several reasons.

It is unusual for arterial $P_{CO_2}$ to be abnormally high in exercise, except in the presence of severe ventilatory impairment. Therefore, a totally normal corrected expired $P_{CO_2}$, or a normal relationship of ventilation to $CO_2$ production, virtually excludes either of the above abnormalities unless there is a severe disturbance of lung mechanics.

To distinguish between alveolar hyperventilation and disturbed gas exchange, it is necessary to measure arterial $P_{CO_2}$ or to estimate it in some way. When arterial cannulation is justified on clinical grounds this provides the most accurate information. Capillary samples are readily obtained and may be used for this purpose. Earlobe capillary sampling provides a specimen for microanalysis of arterial $P_{CO_2}$ which is nearly as good as arterial sampling for the purposes of this analysis, but it is difficult to be sure of avoiding cross-infection hazards. Transcutaneous $P_{CO_2}$ electrodes are available: these respond slowly to changes of arterial $P_{O_2}$ but give a guide to changes. With care, the earlobe sampling provides reasonably accurate estimates of $P_{O_2}$ as well, except when peripheral perfusion is reduced, but arterial sampling or earlobe oximetry is a more reliable way of detecting arterial desaturation during exercise. Desaturation occurs rapidly after the onset of exercise and may be detected during the course of a 1-minute incremental test.

The mechanisms which cause $P_{CO_2}$ to fall in functional hyperventilation are not known and are the subject of considerable speculation, being loosely categorised as 'reflex' or 'psychogenic' according to whether some disease process known to be associated with breathlessness has been identified or not. Irritant reflexes from the bronchi, larynx and upper airway are associated with hyperventilation, which may be an early feature of bronchial asthma or bronchial hyperreactivity. Pulmonary 'congestion', increased central blood volume and a rise of left atrial pressure appear to cause hyperventilation without hypoxaemia in some instances: this has been ascribed to stimulation of juxta-alveolar or 'J' receptors which have been demonstrated in animal experiments. The mechanism of the alveolar hyperventilation found to be a common feature of thromboembolic pulmonary hypertension is quite unknown. In a few patients, no disease can be found and the condition is regarded as cortical. The neurophysiology of this is not known. A few patients thought on clinical grounds to have psychogenic exercise hyperventilation have mild asthma or respiratory muscle weakness.

Anaemia causes hyperventilation, because of poor oxygen delivery to the tissues, including the peripheral chemoreceptors. Chronic anaemia does not have very much effect on effort tolerance until the haemoglobin level falls to about 50% of normal (Chapter 9).

## Anaerobic metabolism

When tissue $P_{O_2}$ is low, aerobic energy sources are supplemented by anaerobic glycolysis with additional production of lactic acid. This is a relatively inefficient way of generating ATP, but it does impose a respiratory stress because the lactic acid produced is excreted into the blood and buffered by bicarbonate ion, with the production of considerable volumes of carbon dioxide. There is a very trivial increase of blood lactate during relatively low levels of exercise, but the level

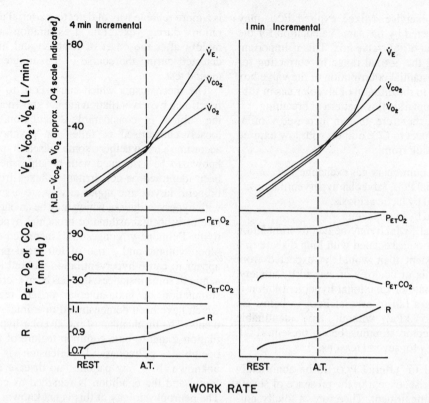

**WORK RATE**

Fig. 13.1. Identification of the anaerobic threshold (A.T.) during incremental and steady state exercise (diagrammatic). The linear relationship between work rate and oxygen uptake is constant regardless of whether a steady state is reached (4-minute test) or whether the increments are applied rapidly (1-minute test). In each case the anaerobic threshold is identified by an upturn in the relationship between ventilation, $CO_2$ output or R to work rate. During the short test, ventilation rises exponentially, because the initial upturn caused by the increase of $CO_2$ output is followed by further hyperventilation as the $H^+$ receptors in the brain begin to sense the increased acidity of the blood. At this point, end-tidal $Pco_2$ ($P_{ET}co_2$) begins to fall. During 4-minute incremental tests, measurements are usually made in the last minute when a steady state has generally been reached. During these few minutes there is time for the brain to sense these changes of acidity, so $Pco_2$ falls steadily, reflecting the ventilatory stimulus. Similarly, the increase of ventilation with increasing workload reflects both the acid stimulus and the increase of R caused by the evolution of $CO_2$ from plasma bicarbonate. See text. (From Wasserman & Whipp, 1975, with permission.)

begins to rise sharply, above 4 $mmol·l^{-1}$, at about 50% of maximum oxygen uptake. The work rate at which this occurs is known as the anaerobic threshold (Fig. 13.1). Below the anaerobic threshold, the respiratory exchange ratio during steady state exercise reflects events in the tissues. R rises progressively from 0.8, the average post-prandial resting value, to around 0.9, assuming that the subject is in a steady state and that sufficient time has been allowed for the tissue $Pco_2$ to rise to the new venous level. This process is slower than the fall of venous $Po_2$ because the buffering capacity of tissues for $CO_2$ exceeds the small storage capacity for oxygen in exercising muscle. When lactic acid production increases, $CO_2$ is liberated from bicarbonate in blood and R rises above 0.9, usually reaching 1.6 at maximum exercise levels (Fig. 13.1; Cooper *et al.*, 1992).

Anaerobic threshold is defined as the oxygen consumption at which the rate of rise of blood lactate accelerates. For the reasons given, this coincides with an accelerated rise of R, ventilation and

$CO_2$ output during progressive exercise. This inflection is most easily recognised during non-steady state incremental exercise (Wasserman & Whipp, 1975; Wasserman, 1984) as will be explained. It cannot always be identified with ease and there is some observer error. Breath-by-breath computer analysis of expired gases and ventilation gives the best results. The inflection is sometimes known as Owles' point, because its relationship to anaerobic metabolism is not fully accepted (Owles, 1930).

Lactic acidosis stimulates alveolar hyperventilation in steady state exercise, with a fall of arterial $P_{CO_2}$, expired $P_{CO_2}$ and end-tidal $P_{CO_2}$. Hyperventilation itself causes a transient increase of R, with an increase of $CO_2$ output without a concomitant increase of $O_2$ consumption (Chapter 3).

It takes about 2 minutes to increase carbon dioxide output, oxygen consumption, cardiac output and ventilation after a step change of work rate; rather less in the exceptionally fit.

These changes are more complicated during tests in which a steady state is not reached before the workload is increased. During such tests $CO_2$ tissue buffers react continuously with $CO_2$ produced by metabolism. The appearance of a metabolic acidosis does not immediately stimulate ventilation. The initial rise of R is attributable almost entirely to the appearance of lactic acid and the evolution of extra $CO_2$ from the blood. After 1 or 2 minutes at the same workload, with increasing lactic acidosis, R rises further because of ventilatory stimulation by $H^+$ receptors. When this occurs, end-tidal $P_{CO_2}$ gradually falls to between 27 and 35 mmHg (3.5 and 4.5 kPa) almost until maximal exercise is reached. Expired $P_{O_2}$ rises because of the increased ventilatory equivalent for oxygen. For these reasons, an increasing slope of ventilation/oxygen uptake during incremental exercise indicates anaerobic metabolism. The slope of ventilation/$CO_2$ output remains constant until the circulating lactic acid stimulates compensatory hyperventilation and $P_{CO_2}$ falls. During incremental exercise, a fall of alveolar, arterial or expired $P_{CO_2}$ at the same time as a rise of R implies a respiratory disorder. The anaerobic threshold occurs at the same level of oxygen consumption regardless of the duration of each workload (normally about 55% of maximal oxygen consumption).

The anaerobic threshold is an indicator of the ability of the circulation to deliver oxygen to exercising muscle. It is lower when the bulk of exercising muscle is small. It is abnormally low in disorders of the peripheral and central circulation and in many types of extreme unfitness, often occurring after illness or bed rest. A specific disorder of effort intolerance has been described, known as vasoregulatory asthenia, which is a form of chronic fatigue syndrome characterised by a low anaerobic threshold and thought to be due to poor control of the peripheral circulation (Holmgren & Strom, 1959). Severe cardiac disease may be distinguished from respiratory dysfunction by the presence of a low anaerobic threshold, but the test is not sufficiently sensitive to distinguish between unfit normal subjects and those with early myocardial insufficiency.

The lactic acidosis of exercise does not necessarily reflect anaerobiasis of exercising muscle alone. Lactate is utilised by some types of muscle fibres and by the liver: the serum level reflects the balance between breakdown and production (Jones, 1988).

Lactic acid production is not the only cause of increasing ventilatory stimulation during exercise, which occurs in MacArdle's syndrome, a muscle phosphorylase deficiency condition in which lactate is not produced in exercising muscle. Rises of body temperature may play a role.

## Arterial oxygenation

Under normal conditions of ventilation and gas exchange, arterial oxygen saturation rises slightly or remains constant. Ideally, arterial $P_{O_2}$ should be measured over several breaths from an indwelling cannula during exercise. As cannulation carries some risk of arterial occlusion, inferior techniques are often used to determine exercise $P_{O_2}$. Arterial sampling, employing a simple needle 'stab', is not always easy during intensive exercise: a sample drawn within 15 seconds of stopping work may be adequate unless subtle analyses of gas exchange are to be performed, as this technique will detect important hypoxaemia ($P_{O_2}$ less than 60 mmHg, 8 kPa).

Measurements of oxygen saturation by earlobe pulse oximetry are accurate to within 2% at around or near normal saturation. They are useful for identifying major falls of $O_2$ saturation such as those seen in severe chronic lung disease, notably emphysema and fibrosing alveolitis. Errors arise if there is intensive vasoconstriction of the earlobe, as occurs in very heavy exercise in normal subjects (this also affects capillary samples).

Nevertheless, many patients with these and other lung diseases show changes of saturation which are unimpressive or within the range of error of oximeters. For rigorous assessment of pulmonary oxygen exchange, it is necessary to measure alveolar–arterial $Po_2$ difference because:

1. Hypoxaemia potentiates breathlessness at a given ventilation, and in some subjects this might occur at levels higher than 60 mmHg (8 kPa).
2. $Pco_2$ is usually low, which tends to restore $Po_2$ to normal.

Many subjects with a mild impairment of $FEV_1$ and VC appear at first sight to be inappropriately limited, but calculation of dead space and alveolar–arterial $Po_2$ difference demonstrates the presence of an increased ventilatory requirement and chemoreceptor drive, which may be sufficient to account for the symptoms.

## Tidal volume, ventilation and pattern of breathing

In general, a slow breathing pattern is the most efficient. Tidal volume normally increases to approximately 55% of VC as ventilation increases (Jones & Rebuck, 1979). Thereafter, further ventilation is achieved by increasing the rate of breathing. Children and patients with small lungs breathe more rapidly, often at rates of up to 60 breaths per minute. Those with airflow obstruction cannot easily increase their rate of expiration; a slow respiratory rate requires the least effort and exercise is limited by tidal volume in patients with severe airflow obstruction. This probably accounts for the good correlation between VC and effort tolerance measured by 12-minute walking distance and by respiratory questionnaires.

Tidal volume normally increases steadily with ventilation but in a curvilinear fashion, so that two thirds of the maximal tidal volume is used at 50% of maximum exercise ventilation. It may be necessary to encourage inexperienced subjects to adopt the slowest possible rate as this may be influenced by pedalling speed or their stride rate. An irregular or changing pattern of breathing is a feature of inappropriate hyperventilation. An abrupt change, accompanied by the sudden development of respiratory discomfort, may indicate the onset of myocardial decompensation or respiratory embarrassment.

### Symptoms

Most laboratories use the Borg scale of perceived exertion (Chapter 12). Usually subjects perceive no dyspnoea or physical effort until exercising at about 25% of maximum. Normally, breathing at the end of cycle exercise is graded at 6–8, and leg effort 7–9 out of a maximum of 10. On a treadmill, the relationship between leg effort and breathing are even more closely coupled. The relationship between perceived exertion and power output are linear between the threshold and maximum ventilation.

### Submaximal indices of exercise performance

Maximal exercise tests of short duration such as the 1-minute incremental work rate test are tolerable and safe. Maximal oxygen uptake cannot be predicted from submaximal indices, and to determine this it is necessary to perform maximal tests; nor indeed is it possible to predict the nature of exercise limitation in every individual from submaximal tests. Abnormal groups may, however, be separated from the normal by studying the relationship between ventilation heart rate and oxygen consumption at 1500 ml·min$^{-1}$ (67 mmol·min$^{-1}$), which is equivalent to a work rate of 1500 kpm·min$^{-1}$ (100 watts). Abnormal responses at this workload reliably indicate disease (Spiro, 1977). The physiological information which may be obtained from an incremental exercise test is summarised in Table 13.4.

Table 13.4. *Interpretation of abnormalities of cardiorespiratory performance during an incremental exercise test*

| Measurement | Fault | Finding |
|---|---|---|
| Relationship between power output and $O_2$ consumption | Ergometer needs calibrating | Systematic difference |
| | Obesity | Increased $VO_2$ at all loads |
| | Circulatory failure (peripheral central or pulmonary) | Low $VO_2$ at maximal work |
| Cardiac frequency and $O_2$ consumption | Cardiac or pulmonary circulatory impairment | Maximal cardiac frequency at low work load |
| | Non-cardiac limitation | Low maximal $O_2$ uptake, normal cardiac frequency |
| Ventilation at maximal exercise compared with predicted maximal ventilation | Ventilatory limitation | Greater than 70% |
| Submaximal ventilation compared with predicted in relation to $O_2$ uptake | Circulatory and pulmonary gas exchange impairment | Increased ventilation is a feature of most disorders of the circulation or of pulmonary gas exchange, except when there is alveolar hypoventilation. Normal ventilation may be found throughout symptom-limited exercise with chronotropic incompetence, angina, painful breathing or impaired mobility, chest wall or neuromuscular disease, poor motivation or malingering |
| Anaerobic threshold (when identifiable) | Unfitness Deconditioning Cardiac disease | Anaerobic threshold below 50% of predicted maximal $O_2$ uptake |
| ECG | Ischaemia Hyperventilation | ST changes, T wave inversion Unstable ST-T segments |
| | Dysrhythmia | Ischaemic change worsens in exercise. Normal resting brady-cardia. Primary heart block and ventricular extrasystoles disap-pear after onset of exercise |
| Symptoms at end of exercise test | Obesity Angina Peripheral vascular disease Respiratory impairment Unfitness | Symptom limitation |
| | Cardiac limitation | Breathlessness, fatigue or test terminated by the operator |
| | Pulmonary vascular disease | Breathlessness |

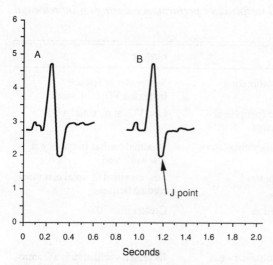

Fig. 13.2. QRS complexes from a 12-lead ECG taken during exercise. A, 'J' depression: not ischaemic. B, plane depression 4.3 mm: probably ischaemic.

## Exercise testing in the evaluation of ischaemic heart disease

The reader is referred to specialist accounts of this topic for full details. It has been known for many years that most patients with typical angina of effort due to ischaemic heart disease develop depression of the ST-T segment of some leads on the electrocardiogram of 2 mm or more with a horizontal or downsloping segment persisting for at least 0.08 second after the 'J' point (Fig. 13.2). The changes occur with the onset of pain sufficient to stop the exercise and persist for up to 15 minutes. Other abnormal patterns include ST-T elevation and U waves. Less rigorous criteria, such as upsloping ST depression lasting 0.08 second or ST depression of between 0.5 or 1 and 2 mm, produce more false positive and fewer false negative results (Diamond & Forrester, 1979).

The end point is generally taken as pain with positive ECG changes, or the achievement of a set proportion of the maximum heart rate (adhering to the safety rules described earlier). Studies employing limited leads give fewer positive results.

Precordial ECG mapping techniques are being developed, but have not yet found a place in routine practice. ST segment changes may be corrected for heart rate, if this is submaximal, and for R wave amplitude (Hollenberg *et al.*, 1985; Sheffield, 1985).

The Bruce protocol is shown in Table 13.5*a*. This progressive treadmill test is a useful measure of effort tolerance when this is limited by the development of angina pectoris. Twelve-lead ECG recordings are made before, immediately after, and 5, 10 and 15 minutes after the test regardless of how it is terminated (p. 192). The test is positive if the criteria for abnormality are met. Some laboratories employ the Balke test, which is less likely to be limited by fatigue as the work rate is increased more rapidly (Table 13.5*b*).

Other indices are derived during the test, which yield an estimate of exercise endurance and maximal power output: these correlate with myocardial function. Failure of systolic pressure to rise with each increment indicates impending myocardial failure, as does failure of the blood pressure to fall to 80% of its peak value within 3 minutes of stopping (Nelson & Deedwania, 1989).

Using coronary arteriography to assess myocardial perfusion, false positive exercise ECG results are common (Table 13.6). False positive results occur, most commonly, among young women with atypical chest pain and hyperventilation and in patients taking digoxin. This instability of the ST segments may be demonstrated by electrocardiography after voluntary hyperventilation, which is helpful when the test is being performed in patients of this type.

Patients complaining of 'chest tightness' may give a description of their symptoms which, rarely, may be difficult to distinguish from airway obstruction however carefully the history is taken. About 30% of asthmatics experience pain, not anginal, when their asthma is severe (Chapter 7). The Bruce test may also be used to provoke exercise-induced asthma in which peak flow, initially normal, typically falls 5–10 minutes after the end of exercise by more than 10% of the initial value. In 50 of our patients with classical angina PEF fell by 10% during the period of severe pain immediately after the exercise test, but had returned to baseline in all instances after 5 minutes of rest.

Patients with anxiety and depression rarely complete maximal exercise tests. Those with very

Table 13.5. *Treadmill tests: modified Bruce and Balke protocols (after Jones, 1988)*

| | Speed (mph) | (km·h⁻¹) | Grade (%) | Approximate power, 80 kg male (watts) | Time (min) |
|---|---|---|---|---|---|
| *(a) Modified Bruce protocol* | | | | | |
| Stage 0 | 1.0 | 1.6 | 5 | | 3 |
| Stage 1 | 1.7 | 2.7 | 10 | 60 | 3 |
| Stage 2 | 2.5 | 4.0 | 12 | 110 | 3 |
| Stage 3 | 3.4 | 5.4 | 14 | 200 | 3 |
| Stage 4 | 4.2 | 6.7 | 16 | >200 | 3 |
| *(b) Modified Balke protocol* | | | | | |
| Step 1 | 1 | 1.6 | 0 | | 1 (2) |
| Step 2 | 2 | 3.2 | 0 | | 1 (2) |
| Step 3 | 2 | 3.2 | 2.5 | 50 | 1 (2) |
| Step 4 | 2 | 3.2 | 5.0 | | 1 (2) |
| Step 5 | 2 | 3.2 | 7.5 | | 1 (2) |
| Step 6 | 2 | 3.2 | 10.0 | 100 | 1 (2) |
| Step 7 | 2 | 3.2 | 12.5 | | 1 (2) |
| Step 8 | 2 | 3.2 | 15.0 | | 1 (2) |
| Step 9 | 2 | 3.2 | 17.5 | 150 | 1 (2) |
| Step 10 | 2 | 3.2 | 20.0 | | 1 (2) |

Table 13.6. *Estimated probability of detecting coronary disease at angiography predicted by 12-lead exercise ECG*

| Depression (mm) | Asymptomatic (%) M | F | Non-anginal pain (%) M | F | Atypical angina (%) M | F | Typical angina (%) M | F |
|---|---|---|---|---|---|---|---|---|
| 0.5 | 3 | 1 | 10 | 3 | 35 | 10 | 75 | 35 |
| 1.0 | 10 | 3 | 20 | 5 | 55 | 35 | 88 | 65 |
| 2.0 | 57 | 20 | 72 | 40 | 90 | 76 | 99 | 96 |
| 2.5 | 83 | 60 | 93 | 85 | 97 | 96 | 99 | 98 |

M, male; F, female; aged 45 years. Note the high incidence of 'false positive' tests among women. For a more detailed analysis see Jones (1988).

high scores in questionnaires designed to detect these conditions are hardly worth subjecting to an exercise test, especially if the symptom is chest pain (Channer *et al.*, 1985).

The recent revival of interest in the exercise ECG is most useful in the group in which the procedure has the greatest discriminating power: patients in whom ischaemic heart disease is prob-able or certain. The test can be used to predict the severity of the changes and to place individual patients in functional categories for the planning of their treatment and the monitoring of therapeutic trials of medical and surgical treatments. There has been a tendency to use tests of this type to exclude asymptomatic individuals at risk of ischaemic heart disease from certain occupations, such as that of airline pilot. For this purpose, radionuclide imaging with thallium-201 may have a higher sensitivity and specificity than ECG monitoring – over 80% and perhaps as high as 90% (Diamond *et al.*, 1980; O'Hara *et al.*, 1985). Magnetic resonance imaging may soon provide a new gold standard.

## Tests to demonstrate exercise-induced asthma

This topic is covered more fully in Chapter 7.

Children who wheeze regularly during play readily exercise sufficiently to induce asthma without risk. They may be asked to run round the building or backwards and forwards along some route that does not provide any traffic hazard for 6 minutes. After a rest of 5 minutes PEF falls by more than 20%.

Adults are most likely to develop exercise-induced asthma under test conditions if supervised. A treadmill test set to provoke a rise of heart rate of 80% maximal for the last 2 minutes of a 6-minute run will provoke exercise-induced asthma in 90% of those who suffer from it in ordinary life. Patients over 40 years old or those at risk of ischaemic heart disease are most safely exercised using a Bruce protocol with ECG monitoring. This will provoke exercise-induced asthma if 80% of maximal heart rate is achieved and even more reliably if dry air is breathed during exercise from a reservoir.

The typical rise of PEF after 6 minutes of running, followed by a fall between 5 and 20 minutes after the end of exercise, is described in Chapter 7.

## Walking tests

The idea of walking the patient up and down a passage and observing what happens without making any measurements is time-honoured. The distance walked when hurrying with encouragement along a flat indoor passage in exactly 12 minutes appears to correlate well with respiratory and cardiac disability. In the test described by McGavin *et al.* (1976), stops are allowed and the total distance measured. The most common complaint which interferes with the assessment is arthritis of the hip, which results in a slower walking than the most severe chronic respiratory disease. Twelve minutes was chosen because it was thought that patients able to perform short bursts of exercise at a fair speed, would be sure to have to compensate by slowing down between 6 and 12 minutes. For the assessment of respiratory disorders, 6 minutes is as good as 12, but shorter tests are probably not (Butland *et al.*, 1982; Guyatt *et al.*, 1985).

The patient is instructed to hurry to some imaginary destination, at such a speed as to arrive as soon as possible but not exhausted. The distance walked, or average speed, is calculated over 12 minutes, including stops for rest which are allowed. A rehearsal effect is noted, the second and subsequent test showing an improvement of 5% in distance walked. A single walk gives a useful measurement, but the rehearsal effect must be overcome if the test is to be used serially.

Walking speed is not limited by respiratory factors, or indeed by dyspnoea in normal individuals, but by stride length and mobility. The correlation between perceived dyspnoea and walking speed is strongest among those with a perceived disability of MRC Grade III or worse.

Self-selected speed tests are not very useful for assessing the benefit of therapeutic measures, because there are two possible patterns of improvement. The patient may select the same speed with less discomfort, or may walk faster, as discussed earlier (Woodcock *et al.*, 1981). The best way of assessing objective improvement in walking of patients with severe limitation is by measurement of the time to exhaustion on a treadmill set at a fixed speed and incline. This is another instance where a maximal test gives more information than a submaximal procedure, in this case by ensuring that the end point of the experiment is similar. Patients with severe respiratory disorders regularly exercise to exhaustion without any important rise in heart rate, because of the ventilatory limitation. These may, in general, be asked to undergo such tests without serious hazard. Where cardiovascular function is suspect, the usual precautions are necessary.

PEF may sometimes fall after a 12-minute walking test, or after a maximal treadmill test.

Table 13.7. *Diagnostic implications of exercise testing (after Wasserman et al., 1986)*

|  | Specific abnormality | Gas exchange | Circulation |
|---|---|---|---|
| Obesity | Increased $O_2$ cost of physical work (lifting weight) | $V_D/V_T$ normal; alveolar–arterial PA–a$O_2$ falls on exercise | Normal if calculated from height |
| Peripheral vascular disease | Leg pain | Low $O_2$ uptake at maximum work | Low anaerobic threshold |
| Pulmonary vascular disease |  | Imparied $O_2$ uptake at maximum work; high $V_D/V_T$; high submaximal $V_E$; high alveolar–arterial $Po_2$ | Low anaerobic threshold; high pulse rate/$\dot{V}o_2$ (low $O_2$ pulse) |
| Anaemia; CoHb; low $P_{50}$ |  | Low maximum $\dot{V}o_2$ normal dead space and alveolar $Po_2$ difference | Low anaerobic threshold; high pulse rate/$\dot{V}o_2$ (low $O_2$ pulse) |
| Airflow obstruction | Abnormal expiratory flow pattern | Low maximal $\dot{V}o_2$ high $V_D/V_T$; wide alveolar–arterial $Po_2$ difference; higher than expected $Pco_2$ low breathing reserve | Submaximal heart rate |
| Restrictive lung disease |  | Low maximal $\dot{V}o_2$; high breathing frequency (> 50); high $V_D/V_T$; increasing alveolar–arterial $Po_2$ difference; low breathing reserve |  |
| Chest wall defects |  | Low maximal $\dot{V}o_2$; high breathing frequency; low breathing reserve; normal alveolar–arterial $Pco_2$ and $Po_2$ difference | Submaximal heart rate |
| Bronchial asthma | Fall of PEF 5–10 min after exercise | Often normal | Often normal |
| Metabolic acidosis | Low $HCO_3^-$ and pH | Steep relationship of ventilation to $CO_2$ output; normal alveolar–arterial $Po_2$ difference; normal $V_D/V_T$ |  |
| Ischaemic heart disease | Chest pain; ECG changes; arrhythmias | Fall of PEF for 30 s after exercise only: often normal | Failure of BP to rise with incremental exercise |
| Ventricular and heart disease |  | Low maximum $O_2$ uptake; high ventilation/$O_2$ uptake relationship | Steep heart rate/$O_2$ uptake relationship; low anaerobic threshold |

This is a useful way of detecting variable airflow obstruction and may explain why some patients appear to complain of disproportionate effort intolerance.

## Simple tests

Patients who are severely disabled by respiratory disease may be unable to perform exercise tests in the upright position. Leg raising in time to a metronome, in the supine position, is a useful substitute. Exercise has to be terminated for the same reason as when walking or cycling. Earlobe pulse oximetry or arterial blood gas analysis can be performed, with measurements of heart rate. A respiratory circuit may be added to obtain an estimate of oxygen uptake and R. These procedures may be used to measure exercise-induced hypoxaemia or hyperventilation and the integrity of pulmonary gas exchange, and are helpful in the clinical evaluation of patients with severe fibrosing alveolitis.

## Clinical usefulness of exercise testing

Numerous important physiological and clinical insights have been obtained from the study of cardiopulmonary variables during exercise in groups of patients with various disorders. Contemporary accounts agree that it is logical to measure exercise tolerance in patients complaining of effort limitation. The physiological view is exemplified by Jones (1988). This philosophy is, roughly, that physicians can use the results of exercise testing in the same way as they do the $FEV_1$, the blood pressure, the blood sugar or the electrocardiogram: as an extension of the clinical examination. Sometimes the information is essential and leads to a diagnosis, such as myocardial ischaemia or asthma. In other cases the physiological responses are used to measure disability, to separate the relative importance of a number of abnormalities, to reinforce advice about the limitations imposed by disease or to monitor changes in the condition of the patient. Most importantly, an exercise test may demonstrate that an individual, perhaps someone with objective abnormalities on clinical examination, is functionally normal. This approach makes use of relatively simple variables.

The diagnostic approach is put forward by Wasserman *et al.* (1986). The implication is that with extra investment of equipment and effort, all the important respiratory variables can be measured, including blood gases, pH, lactate, $V_D/V_T$ and alveolar–arterial $Po_2$ difference. Armed with this information, plus heart rate and 'oxygen pulse', diagnostically useful patterns of abnormality emerge which can then lead on to further investigation of the appropriate system (Table 13.7). Their case reports repay detailed study, but it has to be remembered that the specificity of these highly sensitive procedures has not been established (Table 13.7).

In the last 20 years, cardiological imaging techniques have improved and now allow radiologists and clinicians to assess the severity of valvular and myocardial diseases without turning to invasive procedures. It is not surprising, therefore, that most cardiologists have abandoned exercise testing except for the treadmill ECG, since this is no longer the simplest screening test to decide whether cardiac catheterisation is needed. Nevertheless, the study of the physiological response to exercise in the laboratory is of great, if sometimes indirect, value to patients being investigated for shortness of breath on exertion and to their physicians.

## References

Balke, B. & Ware, R.W. (1959). An experimental study of physical fitness of Air Force personnel. *US Armed Forces Medical Journal*, **10**, 675–688.

Bevegard, S., Holmgren, A. & Jonsson, B. (1960). The effect of body position on the circulation at rest and during exercise with special reference to the influence of the stroke volume. *Acta Physiologica Scandinavica*, **49**, 279–298.

Bruce, R.A. & McDonough, J.R. (1969). Stress testing in screening for cardiovascular disease. *Bulletin of the New York Academy of Medicine*, second series, **45**, 1288–1305.

Butland, R.J.A., Pang, J.A., Gross, E.R., Woodcock, A.A. & Geddes, D.M. (1982). Two, six and twelve minute walks compared. *British Medical Journal*, **284**, 1607–1608.

Channer, K.S., Papouchado, M., James, M.A. & Rees, J.R. (1985). Anxiety and depression in patients with chest pain referred for exercise testing. *Lancet*, **ii**, 820–823.

Cooper, C.B., Beaver, W.L., Cooper, D.L. & Wasserman, K. (1992). Factors affecting the components of the alveolar $CO_2$ output–$O_2$ uptake relationship during incremental exercise in man. *Experimental Physiology*, **77**, 51–64.

Diamond, G.A. & Forrester, J.S. (1979). Analysis of probability as an aid in the clinical diagnosis of coronary artery disease. *New England Journal of Medicine*, **300**, 1350–1358.

Diamond, C.A., Forrester, J.S. & Hirsch, M. (1980). Application of conditional probability analysis to the clinical diagnosis of coronary artery disease. *Journal of Clinical Investigation*, **65**, 1210–1221.

Guyatt, G.H., Sullivan, M.J., Thompson, P.J., Fallen, E.L., Pugsley, S.O., Taylor, D.W. & Berman, L.B. (1985). The 6-minute walk: a new measure of exercise capacity in patients with chronic heart failure. *Canadian Medical Association Journal*, **132**, 919–923.

Hollenberg, M., Zoltick, J.M. & Go, M. (1985). Comparison of a quantitative treadmill exercise score with standard electrocardiographic criteria in screening asymptomatic young men for coronary artery disease. *New England Journal of Medicine*, **313**, 600–606.

Holmgren, A. & Strom, G. (1959). Blood lactate concentration in relation to absolute and relative work load in normal men and in mitral stenosis, atrial septal defect and vasoregulatory asthenia. *Acta Medica Scandinavica*, **163**, 185–193.

Jones, N.L. (1988). *Clinical Uses of Exercise Testing*, 3rd edn. Philadelphia: Saunders.

Jones, N.L. & Rebuck, A.S. (1979). Tidal volume during exercise in patients with diffuse fibrosing alveolitis. *Bulletin Européen Physiopathologie Respiratoire*, **15**, 321–327.

Kearon, M.C., Summers, E., Jones, W.L., Campbell, E.J.M. & Killian, K.J. (1991). Effort and dyspnoea during work of varying intensity and duration. *European Respiratory Journal*, **4**, 917–925.

McGavin, C.R., Gupta, S.P. & McHardy, G.J.R. (1976). Twelve minute walking test for the assessment of disability in chronic bronchitis. *British Medical Journal*, **ii**, 241–243.

Meakins, J.M. (1934). Dyspnoea. *Journal of the American Medical Association*, 183, 1442–1445.

Nelson, J.R. & Deedwania, K. (1989). New exercise parameter for the identification of severe coronary artery disease. *Chest*, **95**, 895–898.

O'Hara, M., Lahiri, A. & Whittington, J.R. (1985). Detection of high risk coronary artery disease by thallium imaging. *British Heart Journal*, **53**, 616–623.

Owles, W.H. (1930). Alterations in the lactic acid content of the blood as a result of light exercise and associated changes in the $CO_2$ combining power of the blood and in the alveolar $CO_2$ pressure. *Journal of Physiology*, **69**, 214–237.

Powers, S.K., Lawler, J., Dempsey, J.A., Dodd, S. & Landry, G. (1989). Effects of incomplete pulmonary gas exchange on $Vo_2$ max. *Journal of Applied Physiology*, **66**, 2491–2495.

Sheffield, L.T. (1985). Another perfect treadmill test (editorial). *New England Journal of Medicine*, **313**, 633–635.

Spiro, S.G. (1977). Exercise testing in clinical medicine (review). *British Journal of Diseases of the Chest*, **71**, 145–172.

Wade, O.L. & Bishop, J.M. (1962). *Cardiac Output and Regional Blood Flow*. Oxford: Blackwell Scientific Publications.

Wasserman, K. (1984). The anaerobic threshold measurement to evaluate exercise performance. *American Review of Respiratory Disease*, **129** (suppl.), S35–S40.

Wasserman, K., Hansen, J.E., Sue, D.Y. & Whipp, B.J. (1986). *Principles of Exercise Testing and Interpretation*. Philadelphia: Lea & Febiger.

Wasserman, K. & Whipp, B.J. (1975). Exercise physiology in health and disease. *American Review of Respiratory Disease*, **112**, 219–249.

Woodcock, A.A., Gross, E.R., Gellert, A., Shah, S., Johnson, M. & Geddes, D.M. (1981). Effects of daily dihydrocodeine, alcohol and caffeine on breathlessness and exercise tolerance in patients with chronic obstructive lung disease and normal blood gases. *New England Journal of Medicine*, **305**, 1611–1616.

# 14 Experimental techniques for the study of respiratory control and pulmonary gas exchange

## Metabolic control of breathing

Breathing is a complex rhythmic motor act with extensive involvement of cranial, cervical, thoracic and upper lumbar motoneuron pools. Rather than dealing with it as a set of simple reflex mechanisms, it should be considered as behaviour which changes quantitatively and qualitatively, according to the prevailing needs of the body (after von Euler, 1986; see also Plum, 1970). These have to be superimposed on the mechanism which produces the cyclical breathing pattern which continues during non-REM sleep. The localisation of this control is probably in the brain stem.

A detailed account of the sensory pathways which contribute to the process of integration is beyond the scope of this book (for lucid essays applicable to human physiology see Cherniack & Widdicombe, 1986). Various types of behavioural breathing, for example speaking, singing, diving or playing dead, occur in different species. Many reflexes which are well described in animals, such as the Hering-Breuer reflex, are poorly developed in man. Information arises in health and disease from:

1. The chemoreceptors.
2. Upper airway receptors.
3. Irritant receptors in the airways and lungs.
4. Stretch receptors in the lungs.
5. Spatial information from the chest wall, which may be responsible for the voluntary and involuntary control of tidal volume.
6. Pain receptors in the pleura and chest wall.
7. Voluntary cortical mechanisms which may override all other inputs.

Patients with transplanted, denervated lungs employ a normal breathing pattern in exercise and in response to other stimuli (Chapter 9). Pulmonary reflexes are probably, therefore, unimportant in the control of breathing under normal circumstances.

The sensors of metabolic control are the chemoreceptors, peripheral and central.

1. The carotid bodies are the only known peripheral chemoreceptors in man. Their contribution to inspiratory power output varies according to arterial $P_{CO_2}$, $H^+$ ion concentration and arterial $P_{O_2}$. They have a rich blood supply controlled by the sympathetic nervous system which can modify chemoreceptor sensitivity.

2. The central chemoreceptors are in the floor of the medulla. These respond to changes of $H^+$ ion concentration in the brain. They are not far from the fourth ventricle and their activity responds fairly closely to changes of $H^+$ in the cerebrospinal fluid. Over short periods of time, the acid–base state of the brain near the chemoreceptor varies with changes of $P_{CO_2}$, because $CO_2$ can cross the blood–brain barrier while ions cannot. Cerebral hypoxia may also act locally by causing an increase of lactic acid generated by anaerobic metabolism in the brain tissue. Changes of the non-respiratory acid–base state of the blood result in slow alterations of brain and cerebrospinal fluid pH, and therefore ventilation, requiring about 24 hours for ventilation to reach a steady state (Read & Leigh, 1967).

Countless experiments have been performed in various species to study the properties of the chemoreceptors, administering different mixtures of $O_2$ and $CO_2$ to breathe, with measurements of

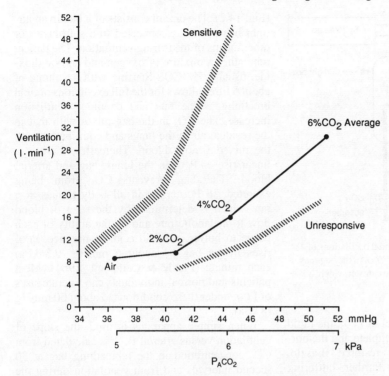

Fig. 14.1. The effects of breathing different mixtures of $CO_2$ in 21% $O_2$. The plot is often linear in individuals, but not when groups are studied. Interventions which depress or stimulate breathing, such as the administration of drugs, may affect the slope and position of the line.

ventilation. When ventilation is impeded by thoracic disease, measuring the electrical activity in the efferent nerves yields a better estimate of the drive from the central nervous system to the respiratory muscles. Different parts of the system may be blocked, ablated or stimulated.

From such experiments it is known that the peripheral chemoreceptors are almost without activity when $Po_2$ is 200 mmHg (27 kPa) or greater. There is a sharp increase of activity when $Po_2$ falls below 60 mmHg (8 kPa) which is lost if the carotid bodies are ablated. In contrast, only 15% of the sensitivity to rises of $Pco_2$ is lost if the peripheral chemoreceptors are ablated or when high concentrations of oxygen are breathed. The remaining 85% is under the control of central receptors. Sensitivity to $CO_2$ is increased in the presence of hypoxaemia. The rate of change of $Pco_2$ may be important. The output of the peripheral chemoreceptors affects ventilation mainly during the first half of inspiration. Profound hypoxaemia and hypercapnia cause central respiratory depression.

Experiments in conscious man have led to similar conclusions, with the cooperation of patients who have had their carotid bodies removed (a treatment, never really fashionable, for bronchial asthma) (Honda *et al.*, 1979).

## Clinical methods of assessment of chemoreceptor sensitivity in man

These tests shed light on the pathophysiology of breathing, but are rarely used in the investigation of individual patients.

### Ventilatory response to carbon dioxide inhalation

The purpose is to obtain an estimate of the slope of increases of ventilation in response to rises of arterial $Pco_2$.

The traditional technique consists of the administration of hyperoxic mixtures of 2 or 3%, 4 or 5% and 6 or 7% $CO_2$ for 10–15 minutes, with measurements of ventilation at the end of this time (Fig. 14.1) (Lloyd, Jukes & Cunningham, 1958). At the end of 10 minutes of experimental

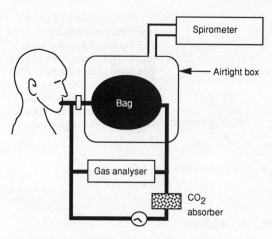

Fig. 14.2. Device for recording the tidal oscillations of $P_{CO_2}$ during rebreathing. The rise of $P_{CO_2}$ in the bag may be modified by means of a soda-lime canister which absorbs $CO_2$.

hypercapnia at a constant level of $P_{CO_2}$, the rapid phase of $CO_2$ absorption is complete and the normal veno-arterial difference restored (Laszlo, Clark & Campbell, 1969). Further buffering mechanisms within the cells result in a gradual rise of extracellular and intracellular bicarbonate with a gradual fall of ventilation, but this change takes place slowly over several hours. Breathing 7% $CO_2$ for several minutes is uncomfortable because

1. $P_{CO_2}$ rises to 55 mmHg (7.3 kPa).
2. At this $P_{CO_2}$, ventilation may be 40–60 l.min$^{-1}$.
3. The ventilatory stimulus persists for some time after returning to normal atmosphere, because it takes some minutes to wash the $CO_2$ out of the chemosensitive area of the brain. The consequence is rebound hyperventilation with a period of time when $P_{CO_2}$ is lower than normal and this may cause tetany.
4. The sequence of acid–base changes during these procedures causes headaches which may sometimes be severe. This sometimes occurs during hypercapnia which causes cerebral vasodilation; in the majority it occurs after the experiment.

*Rebreathing tests of $CO_2$ responsiveness* are much more acceptable and are now standard

(Fig. 14.2). The circuit consists of a bag in an airtight box which is connected to a spirometer or other means of measuring ventilation. The patient rebreathes a mixture of oxygen and carbon dioxide, usually 7% $CO_2$. Starting with a volume of about 5 litres allows for the full excursions of tidal breathing as the rate and depth of ventilation increase. The $CO_2$ in the bag mixes with that in the residual air in the lungs and equilibrates with the mixed venous blood. Thereafter, there is a linear rise of $P_{CO_2}$ in the lungs, bag and arterial blood. The bag prevents $CO_2$ from being excreted, so $P_{CO_2}$ rises in all body tissues at a rate which is determined by the ratio of blood flow to metabolic rate and by the ability of each tissue to buffer carbonic acid. In practice, $P_{CO_2}$ rises in the bag by about 6 mmHg (0.8 kPa) each minute (Fowle & Campbell, 1964). Most patients and normal individuals can tolerate rises of $P_{CO_2}$ under these conditions to about 60 mmHg (8 kPa).

When simple apparatus is used, the slope of ventilation versus arterial $P_{CO_2}$ is calculated from $CO_2$ concentration in the rebreathing bag at 30 second intervals and from ventilation during the preceding 15 seconds (Read, 1967). With facilities for on-line computation it is easy to calculate these variables breath by breath, so it is important, when considering the relationship of arterial $P_{CO_2}$ to ventilation, to look at the starting conditions, the size of the rebreathing bag and the temporal relationship of the measurements. Inspiratory time and the control of rate and depth of breathing may also be calculated. All these variations make little difference to the slope of ventilation on $P_{CO_2}$ ($\dot{V}/P_{CO_2}$).

Interestingly, this slope is similar to that obtained during the 10-minute experiment except when the metabolic acid–base state is deranged (Linton *et al.,* 1973). The intercept of the line is different (Fig. 14.3). The explanation lies in the rapid diffusion of $CO_2$ into the superficial parts of the brain. As $P_{CO_2}$ rises, H$^+$ concentration changes immediately in the chemoreceptors in proportion to the amount of $CO_2$ present. Conversion of $CO_2$ to carbonic acid and buffering is a slow process, so a rise of $P_{CO_2}$ in the cerebrospinal fluid causes little change of bicarbonate ion concentration for several hours. If $P_{CO_2}$ is elevated by rebreathing

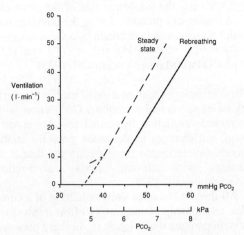

Fig. 14.3. Ventilatory response to CO$_2$: average value (Linton *et al.*, 1973). The slope is similar to the steady state response, but the intercept is greater, reflecting the fact that the measured PCO$_2$ is closer to cerebro-spinal fluid or tissue PCO$_2$.

and then held constant for 10 minutes, ventilation continues to increase. This is because the normal difference between tissue and arterial PCO$_2$ is restored. In other words, PCO$_2$ in the neighbourhood of the chemoreceptors continues to rise, although arterial PCO$_2$ is held constant.

There is a wide range of ventilatory responses to inhaled carbon dioxide (Fig. 14.1). Numerically, they span from 0.5 to 10 litres per minute per mmHg (3.75 to 75 litres per minute per kPa). Those with anxious personality traits tend to have steep slopes. There is evidence that the response is genetically determined. There are normal individuals whose slope is very flat. The degree of sympathetic adrenergic output determines the sensitivity of the peripheral chemoreceptor, probably by altering the relationship of blood flow to metabolism in the carotid body. Under resting conditions, the measurement is reproducible from day to day in most individuals, but there are some who give widely disparate results.

The response of individuals who are regularly exposed to high concentrations of CO$_2$ is flattened, just as breath-holding time may be lengthened by training. This training may be useful. Divers become quite tolerant of hypoxia and elevated arterial PCO$_2$ and this improves their perfor-

mance. It is often surmised that if individuals who have become accustomed to elevated arterial PCO$_2$ develop chronic lung disease, they tend to tolerate hypoxaemia and present with the manifestations of pulmonary hypertension, but there are no epidemiological studies which confirm this notion, and it is not the case in an animal model (Javaheri, Lucey & Snider, 1985).

Most people never experience abnormal elevations of arterial PCO$_2$. That CO$_2$ 'casts its umbrella' over the ventilatory control mechanism (Haldane & Priestley, 1935) seems certain, but the mechanisms which ensure that ventilation normally increases before the development of elevated arterial CO$_2$ whenever metabolic rate increases are not identified. Thus, at the start of physical exercise, most individuals are conditioned to an appropriate increase of ventilation or, in mild exercise, to a mild degree of alveolar hyperventilation. The response may be learned or it may be the result of some more subtle stimulus. Hypothetical explanations include the possibility that the chemoreceptors recognise an increase in the size of the oscillations of blood gas pressures in the arterial blood, that the lung senses CO$_2$ flow or mixed venous PCO$_2$ or that a respiratory stimulant circulates during exercise. There is evidence for and against all these ideas (Wasserman, Whipp & Casaburi, 1986). It appears that loss of spinal cord afferent pathways does not affect the ventilatory adaptation to exercise during electrical stimulation of the legs, so the maintenance of normal levels of PCO$_2$ during exercise cannot be due solely to limb reflexes.

### Pattern of breathing

Changes of respiration in response to experimental stimuli such as CO$_2$ inhalation can be analysed more elegantly by examining the so-called duty cycle of ventilation. This is described by two indices, derived from ventilation and frequency of breathing. This approach is more subtle than the classical technique of measuring ventilation, but is similarly limited in usefulness by the fact that comparisons between experiments can be made only if the mechanical properties of the lung are similar in each case.

$V_T/t_I$ is the mean inspiratory flow rate or 'drive' to the inspiratory muscles. $t_I/t_{TOT}$ is inspiratory time divided by the total time for one breath. This gives an indication of the timing of the controller, and is sometimes known as the 'duty cycle', the period when the inspiratory muscles are working. The product of these two is ventilation, $V_T \times t_{TOT}$. In disorders in which $V_T/t_I$ cannot increase normally, such as respiratory muscle weakness or lung disease, there is a disproportionate decrease of $t_I/t_{TOT}$ which predisposes to respiratory muscle fatigue.

### Measuring the output of the chemoreceptors

These measurements of the ventilatory response to a respiratory stimulus give an accurate picture of the sensitivity of the respiratory control mechanism when the lungs are healthy. Theoretically, this response can be reduced by:

1. Lack of sensitivity.
2. Lack of neural output.
3. Lack of neural pathways or respiratory muscle power.
4. Disordered mechanics of breathing.

Patients with chronic lung diseases have a reduced ventilatory response to $CO_2$ (Flenley & Millar, 1967; Clark, 1968). So, however, do normal individuals breathing through narrow tubes which act as external resistances, and it is clear that the ventilation achieved may depend as much on the work of breathing as on the ventilatory drive. Attempts to assess the work of breathing are informative but cumbersome (Milic-Emili & Tyler, 1963). The neural output, or central drive, to respiration is most commonly assessed by examining the effort recorded at the onset of inspiration during sudden occlusion of the airway. This effort increases as $P_{CO_2}$ rises.

More recent studies have examined the inspiratory effort recorded during sudden occlusion of the airway, as this increases progressively with increasing $CO_2$ pressures. Electromyography has shown that there is a delay of 200 milliseconds before there is any alteration of the pattern of inspiratory effort after airway occlusion. Two techniques have given information:

1. $P_{0.1}$: the pressure generated 0.1 seconds after total occlusion of the airway applied during rebreathing (Whitelaw, Derenne & Milic-Emili, 1975).

2. dP/dt max: the maximum rate of development of inspiratory pressure during the transient initial occlusion of each breath by a valve selected for having a threshold resistance of 10 cm $H_2O$ (0.15 kPa) (Matthews & Howell, 1975).

These techniques may be applied readily to a variety of experimental situations. Correlation with increased ventilation in normal subjects is very good, but changes in occlusion pressure at the mouth underestimate those within the thorax in patients with chronic airway obstruction (Marazzini et al., 1978).

All these techniques show reduction of a complex relationship of inspiratory effort to alveolar $P_{CO_2}$ in patients with high $P_{CO_2}$. In these patients, shortening of $T_I$ and reduction of tidal volume indicate that they have adapted to their condition by breathing in the most economical way, in spite of the deleterious effect on pulmonary gas exchange (Pardy et al., 1982).

The use of these tests to measure respiratory drive depends on normal inspiratory muscle power (Gribbin, Gardiner & Heinz, 1983). In chronic airflow obstruction, increasing FRC reduces the efficiency of the respiratory muscles during the test and limits the value of measuring $P_{0.1}$. The diaphragmatic or intercostal electromyogram may be used to measure the neural drive to the respiratory muscles (Lourenço, 1976). These procedures are not easy, but they provide a different insight into the relationship between central nervous stimulation and power output of the respiratory system. Fatigue of the breathing mechanism may develop during prolonged respiratory effort, when ventilation is increased.

### Chemoreceptor sensitivity to hypoxia

Because arterial hypoxaemia stimulates hyperventilation, the effects of breathing hypoxic gas mixtures are those of hypoxia combined with respiratory alkalosis. Classical experiments have shown that reduction of $P_{O_2}$ increases sensitivity to $CO_2$ (Fig. 14.4) (Lloyd et al., 1958). A number of tests were developed to measure, over a few seconds, the transient ventilatory response to hypoxia or hypoxaemia. Seven breaths of oxygen or three of nitrogen given at rest or during exercise produce a transient fall or rise of ventilation

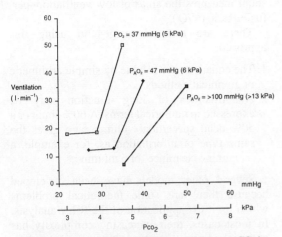

Fig. 14.4. Brisk steady state ventilatory response to $CO_2$ in the presence of alveolar hypoxia. Conversely, the response is flattened above 100 mmHg (13 kPa) partly because hyperoxia switches off the carotid chemoreceptor.

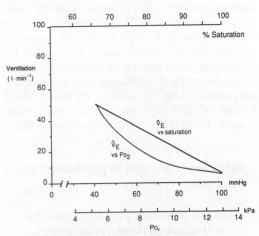

Fig. 14.5. Ventilatory response to hypoxia while rebreathing at constant $P_{CO_2}$ using a circuit similar to Fig. 15.2. As $P_{O_2}$ falls progressively, there is a hyperbolic increase in ventilation. If arterial $P_{O_2}$ is measured in mmHg, the relationship takes the form

$$\dot{V}_E - \dot{V}_E0 = A/(P_AO_2 - 32)$$

where $\dot{V}_E0$ is the asymptote of the flat portion of the curve at high values of $P_{O_2}$. A = 34.4 in the example given: an average value. The relationship of $\dot{V}_E$ to $O_2$ saturation is approximately linear, probably because of the shape of the dissociation curve rather than because the chemoreceptor senses a function of $O_2$ saturation.

which is seen over the subsequent six or seven breaths. These probably assess activity of peripheral chemoreceptors and may be useful, but they are not independent of $P_{CO_2}$.

To examine the effects of hypoxaemia on ventilation separately from those of changes of $P_{CO_2}$, ventilation may be measured while $P_{O_2}$ falls gradually as the subject rebreathes air from a bag fitted with a means of keeping end-tidal $P_{CO_2}$ constant (Fig. 14.5) (Weil, Byrne Quinn & Sodal, 1970; Rebuck & Campbell, 1974). Ventilation increases progressively as $P_{O_2}$ falls. The slope is not linear, as ventilation increases proportionally to $1/P_{O_2}$. The assessment of $O_2$ sensitivity employs the relationship

$$\dot{V}_E = \dot{V}_E0 + A/(P_AO_2 - 32) \qquad (14.1)$$

At about 60 mmHg (8 kPa), ventilation starts to rise sharply. Although $P_{CO_2}$ remains constant during this procedure, the fall of oxygen saturation in the arterial blood causes some rise of pH by the Bohr shift, which has an undetermined effect on ventilation. The procedure is suitable for studying healthy subjects, because the $P_{O_2}$ in the rebreathing bag mirrors closely that in the arterial blood.

When pulmonary gas exchange is abnormal, arterial $P_{O_2}$ may be much lower than that measured in the rebreathed gas. An earlobe oximeter

may be used to monitor the falling arterial oxygen saturation. The relationship of ventilation to arterial $O_2$ saturation ($S_aO_2$) is linear, which makes interpretation easy (Rebuck & Campbell, 1974). This useful test could possibly be hazardous and as the information gained is often of theoretical rather than practical interest, it is performed only occasionally in patients with severe chronic lung disease. Valuable information may be expected from studies of altitude dwellers, subjects acclimatised to unusual environments, in clinical pharmacology and in the investigation of patients with healthy lungs suffering from disorders of ventilatory control.

As in the case of $CO_2$, the ventilatory response to hypoxaemia is affected by racial, familial and environmental factors. Altitude dwellers become desensitised to hypoxaemia regardless of genetic factors (Weil, 1986). There are individuals who tolerate extremes of hypoxia without much increase in ventilation. Those who have this trait cannot survive at the highest altitudes, where the maintenance of tolerable levels of alveolar $Po_2$ depends on a well-developed ventilatory response to hypoxaemia and individuals who lack this cannot exercise at the $Po_2$ found at the top of Mount Everest (West, Lahiri, Maret *et al.*, 1983; West, Hackett, Maret *et al.*, 1983, see also West, 1985).

## Advanced concepts in pulmonary gas exchange

### The use of models to characterise the ventilation–perfusion relationships within the lung

The theory of pulmonary gas exchange is usually explained by treating the lung as a single unit in which tidal ventilation, gaseous diffusion and blood flow may be varied (Fig. 1.1). In reality, the lung contains several million alveoli, all ventilated and perfused at different rates and having different diffusing capacities. Classical descriptions of pulmonary gas exchange therefore employ models, or mathematical representations, of the lung in which simplifying assumptions are made.

The most commonly used is the three-compartment model developed by Richard L. Riley and his colleagues in the 1940s from concepts laid down earlier (Chapter 3). The excitement of this period of research into respiratory physiology has been captured in the accounts by Riley (1980) and Otis & Rahn (1980). To reiterate, the three compartments are:

1. A gas-exchanging compartment.
2. An unventilated, perfused compartment (physiological shunt).
3. A ventilated, unperfused compartment (alveolar dead space).

For any given value of inspired $Po_2$, all possible combinations of arterial $Pco_2$, arterial $Po_2$ and R may be characterised in terms of alveolar ventilation, dead space and physiological shunt. As a first approximation, dead space measures the areas of high ventilation–perfusion ratio, while

shunt measures the areas of low ventilation–perfusion ratio ($\dot{V}/\dot{Q}$).

There are two advantages in using this approach.

1. The equations are soluble by simple arithmetic or graphical methods.
2. Abnormalities of lung function may be expressed in numerical terms. A 60% shunt or a 50% dead space/tidal volume ratio gives the same type of information as, for example, a 'creatinine clearance' of 5 ml·min$^{-1}$.

Several other models have been developed because there are some theoretical problems which limit the application of the Riley analysis. In most cases, their increasing complexity has outweighed any advantage, but some have contributed to our understanding of pulmonary gas exchange and deserve detailed examination.

The main theoretical problems with Riley's three-compartment model are caused by the alinearity of the $O_2$ dissociation curve.

Firstly, the Riley model cannot increase its oxygen saturation by more than about 5% when 'given' oxygen to breathe. If the model is given $O_2$ to breathe, that is, $F_1O_2$ is increased, the extra $O_2$ is available only to the well-ventilated compartment which cannot increase its $O_2$ uptake by more than that required to increase the $O_2$ saturation from 95% to 99.5%. Units with low, but not zero, $\dot{V}/\dot{Q}$ ratios do increase $O_2$ uptake considerably. Therefore, a cyanosed patient with chronic lung disease and a '30% shunt' may have an $O_2$ saturation of nearly 100% when breathing $O_2$. By representing all the areas of low ventilation–perfusion ratio as having zero $\dot{V}/\dot{Q}$, the model will increase its oxygen uptake very little since there will be no additional oxygenation of the non-ventilated blood.

This problem was understood from the beginning. The technique originally described included the administration of 100% oxygen and measurement of the alveolar–arterial $Po_2$ difference, when

$$\text{Alveolar } Po_2 = P_1O_2 - \text{arterial } Pco_2 \quad (14.2)$$

because all the nitrogen has been exhaled from the lung. Under these circumstances, an alveolar–arterial difference for $Po_2$ of 20 mmHg (2.9 kPa) represents 1% shunt when mixed venous oxygen saturation is 75%. This figure is arrived at from the solubility of $O_2$ in plasma at 37 °C (0.03 ml·l$^{-1}$·mmHg$^{-1}$ or 0.01 mmol·l$^{-1}$· kPa). There is enough oxygen dissolved in the plasma of 1000 ml of blood to increase the saturation of 10 ml of blood from 75% to 100%.

Measured in this way, the anatomical shunt of normal individuals is about 5% of the total blood flow. The technique can be used to demonstrate the failure of blood shunted through a septal defect from right to left to saturate after oxygen breathing. The measurement does not quantify accurately the disturbance in chronic lung disease, because the administration of pure oxygen to patients results in resorption atelectasis of lung units of very low ventilation–perfusion ratio.

A more subtle and less well studied problem was spelt out by Farhi in 1966. Riley's model is insensitive to areas of slightly reduced ventilation–perfusion ratio because it expresses these areas as if they were 'true' shunt. The alveolar–arterial $P_{O_2}$ difference is an excellent way of detecting areas of extremely low ventilation–perfusion ratio: quite small mixtures of blood containing reduced haemoglobin have a dramatic effect on the $P_{O_2}$ of the blood from the well-ventilated regions where the $O_2$ dissociation curve is relatively flat and the slope therefore small (Fig. 3.1). The converse is that in a lung where the main abnormality consists of an increase in the number of units having only a slightly low ventilation–perfusion ratio, the apparent shunt is calculated to be trivial. To take into account slightly low as well as very low $\dot{V}/\dot{Q}$ abnormalities, a test gas with a linear dissociation curve is required.

This argument may be extended to show that under normal conditions $O_2$ is at least as good as $CO_2$ for calculating 'dead space' because it has a flat and almost linear dissociation curve in the range between alveolar and expired gas pressure. $CO_2$ with its linear curve is theoretically better for averaging shunts than is $O_2$, but the high blood capacity for $CO_2$ makes it unsuitable for studies on resting subjects because a 20% shunt is required to alter arterial $P_{CO_2}$ by 2 mmHg (0.25 kPa). This sort of accuracy can not reliably be achieved. $N_2$ would theoretically have been more suitable, but the measurement of arterial $P_{N_2}$ is not easy.

In summary, therefore, the three-compartment model is deficient in two ways:

1. Inaccurate reflection of the effects of changes of inspired $P_{O_2}$.
2. Insensitivity to abnormalities of the distribution of ventilation and perfusion involving the presence of slightly under-ventilated or over-ventilated areas.

Alternative models of alveolar gas exchange have been developed for a number of purposes:

1. Teaching.
2. Exploration of the effects of physiological stresses on arterial blood gas pressures.
3. Characterisation of the lung; that is, a lung function test 'result' which provides an index on the non-uniformity of the distribution of ventilation and perfusion.

## Models for teaching and exploration

### Two-compartment models

Gas exchange can be analysed as if it took place in two compartments, one of higher and one of lower $\dot{V}/\dot{Q}$ ratio (Fig. 14.6). Neither compartment is supposed to represent ideal alveolar gas and the difference between the two reflects the width of scatter of $\dot{V}/\dot{Q}$ ratios. Any set of gas exchange data (arterial $P_{CO_2}$, arterial $P_{O_2}$ and $CO_2$ output and oxygen consumption) can be solved in these terms, as in the case of a three-compartment model. This analysis does not yield a value which is instantly recognisable as an index of non-uniformity. It does, however, merit some attention. An example of how to manipulate this model follows.

The starting points are the total ventilation and perfusion, the fractional ventilation and perfusion to each compartment, the inspired gas concentrations and the mixed venous content and partial pressures. The effect of a sudden perturbation of the total ventilation or perfusion may be calculated assuming a constant mixed venous point. The resultant change is first seen as a change of R, arterial $P_{CO_2}$ and arterial $P_{O_2}$. Physiologically, the respiratory controller will re-set $P_{O_2}$ and $P_{CO_2}$ by altering total ventilation, so that eventually a new mixed venous point is reached and a new steady state achieved.

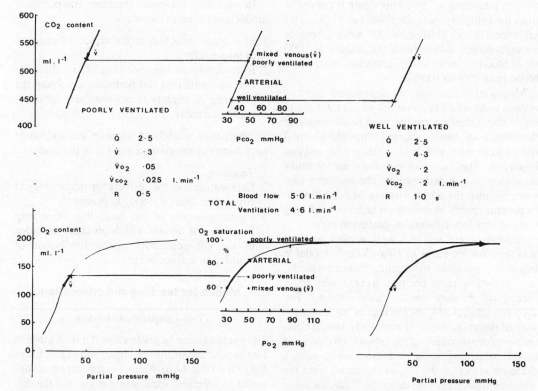

Fig. 14.6. Two-compartment model illustrating the effects of uneven distribution of ventilation and blood flow on pulmonary gas exchange. In this example, the total blood flow ($5\ l\cdot min^{-1}$) is divided equally between a well-ventilated compartment (right: ventilation $4.3\ l\cdot min^{-1}$) and a poorly ventilated compartment (left: ventilation $0.3\ l\cdot min^{-1}$). At the outset, mixed venous $O_2$ saturation is assumed to be 60%, mixed venous $P_{CO_2}$ to be 50 mmHg (6.8 kPa), oxygen uptake to be 250 ml·min⁻¹ and $CO_2$ output to be 225 ml· min⁻¹. These are reasonable values yielding RQ = 0.9. Solving the gas exchange equations for pulmonary blood flow and alveolar ventilation (Chapter 3), the right-hand compartment performs most of the gas exchange. $\dot{V}/\dot{Q}$ is high; $P_{CO_2}$ is low [30 mmHg (4.0 kPa)]; $P_{O_2}$ is high [125 mmHg (16.8 kPa)]; the respiratory exchange ratio R is high. This blood mixes with the poorly ventilated blood from the left-hand compartment where $\dot{V}/\dot{Q}$ and therefore R are low. The example chosen makes it easy to see how the content of the mixed arterial blood leaving the lung can be predicted from the contents of the two hypothetical compartments. $P_{CO_2}$ and $P_{O_2}$ follow from the dissociation curves. This patient has an arterial saturation of 82% and an arterial $P_{CO_2}$ of 40 mmHg. Note: (1) According to the Riley analysis this patient would have an alveolar ventilation of $4\ l\cdot min^{-1}$, calculated

from $CO_2$ output and arterial $P_{CO_2}$. The two-compartment analysis yields a more realistic solution in which total ventilation to the alveoli is greater than it would be in an ideal lung. (2) $P_{CO_2}$ is normal because of 'hyperventilation' in the well-ventilated compartment; $P_{O_2}$ is low because the well-ventilated compartment can take up no more oxygen. (Adapted from Riley & Permutt, 1965. This repays study.)

The example given in Fig. 14.6 illustrates how uneven distribution of ventilation and pulmonary blood flow result in inefficiency of gas exchange. In a uniform system

$$\frac{\dot{V}_A \cdot P_{CO_2}}{P_b - P_{H_2O}} = \dot{V}_{CO_2}$$

(14.3)

In the example, $\dot{V}_A = 4\ l\cdot min^{-1}$, $P_{CO_2}/P_{BAR}-P_{H_2O} = 6\%$, $P_{CO_2} = 42$ mmHg (5.8 kPa) and $\dot{V}_{CO_2} = 240$ ml·min⁻¹.

In the two-compartment model, the low $\dot{V}/\dot{Q}$ alveolus with end capillary $P_{CO_2}$ greater than 40 mmHg (5.5 kPa) is compensated by a high $\dot{V}/\dot{Q}$

alveolus where the blood leaves at a lower $P_{CO_2}$. The example has been chosen to yield a normal $P_{CO_2}$ of 40 mmHg (5.5 kPa); to achieve this, the inefficient lung must be ventilated at 4.6 l·min$^{-1}$ and $P_{O_2}$ is slightly low. In the Riley analysis, the effective, or alveolar, ventilation would be 4.0 l·min$^{-1}$ and the additional ventilation required would be called 'dead space'.

Over the years, more complicated models have been built to explore, theoretically, the behaviour of the imperfect lung in various simulated situations. Five, nine and ten compartments have been set up, to simulate gravitational and other types of inequality. It can be shown that diffusing capacity, as well as ventilation, must be distributed evenly for efficient gas exchange. The reason is intuitively obvious: low D as well as low $\dot{V}$ causes low regional $P_{O_2}$.

### Fifty-compartment model for exploration of the relative importance of diffusion limitation and ventilation–perfusion inequality in pulmonary gas exchange

Wagner and West (1972) used a 50-compartment model to explore the factors limiting gas exchange, assuming a log-normal distribution of $\dot{V}/\dot{Q}$ ratios. This is a convenient way of describing a variety of distributions mathematically by their log standard deviation. Using this model, they re-stated the theoretical importance of diffusion limitation. In discussions of diffusion limitation, most physiology books contained the statement that, under certain circumstances, alveolar–capillary equilibrium for $P_{O_2}$ might not be achieved but that $CO_2$ equilibrated much faster because $CO_2$ is 20 times as soluble as $O_2$ in tissue, and therefore diffuses 20 times as rapidly. Wagner and West pointed out that $CO_2$ equilibration is barely achieved when $CO_2$ output is high. The explanation lies in the very large capacity of the blood to absorb $CO_2$: 4 ml·l$^{-1}$·mmHg$^{-1}$ (300 ml·l$^{-1}$·kPa$^{-1}$), in contrast to 0.3 ml·l$^{-1}$·mmHg$^{-1}$ for $O_2$.

Alveolar–capillary equilibrium is achieved quickly when the gas is poorly soluble in the blood or plasma (so that only small volumes need to be transferred), and when the diffusing capacity through alveolar tissue is fast. In Chapter 5 it was explained how the very high affinity of haemoglobin for CO made the latter a suitable gas

for testing diffusion; $CO_2$ also has a high affinity for blood. Because $CO_2$ is about 20 times as soluble in blood and alveolar partial pressures than is oxygen, it needs to be 20 times as diffusible in tissue to achieve the same percentage equilibrium. Serious disturbances of diffusing capacity, therefore, would be predicted to impede the uptake of $CO_2$ as much as $O_2$ when transfer is expressed in ml·min$^{-1}$. The magnitude of the alveolar–end-capillary partial pressure difference is, however, less for $CO_2$ than for $O_2$, because the capacity of the blood to combine with $CO_2$ is greater.

### Characterisation of the maldistribution of ventilation and perfusion employing gases of different solubilities and a 50-compartment model

Up to now, gas exchange has been considered only in so far as it affects $O_2$ consumption and $CO_2$ output employing measurements in the steady state. However, the dynamics of $CO_2$ and oxygen transport are very complex because of the alinearity of their dissociation curves. The calculations are simpler in studies of foreign gases which dissolve in blood but do not combine chemically with it. These so-called physiologically inert gases obey Henry's law:

$$\frac{P_{gas} \cdot \alpha}{P_{BAR}} = C_{gas} \qquad (14.5)$$

which states that for an ideal gas, the relationship between partial pressure and the amount of gas carried in the blood ($C_{gas}$) is linear. The uptake of inert gases is not limited by diffusion because they are fully soluble in blood and therefore only small volumes need to be transferred.

There are now a number of studies by Wagner and several colleagues in which the distribution of ventilation–perfusion ratios was computed for a 50-compartment lung from the exchange of six gases of different solubilities in vivo. The experiment is essentially simple but has to be carried out with extreme care. Six inert gases are dissolved in saline and infused at a constant rate into a central vein. The output of the gases and their arterial content is measured under steady state conditions by gas chromatography (Wagner, Saltzmann & West, 1974; Wagner, Naumann & Laruso, 1974).

The basic principle is the different rate of excretion of gases according to the blood–gas partition coefficient or solubility. Intuitively, one may see that an almost insoluble gas will be excreted into any alveolar air with which it comes into contact, even if the alveolus is very poorly ventilated. The passage of such a gas into the arterial blood implies the presence of complete shunt or absence of contact of the venous blood with any air at all. At the other end of the scale, the transfer of quite large quantities of highly soluble gas can be effected with little change in the mixed venous partial pressure. As a result, there is little difference between the mixed venous pressure and that in the gas expired from the alveoli (mixed expired/mixed venous partial pressure ratio approaching 1.0). The presence of any difference in the expired and mixed venous pressures of a highly soluble gas must be accountable for by totally unperfused alveoli (dead space). Computer analysis makes it possible to identify distributions of ventilation and perfusion with respect to ventilation–perfusion ratio in a 50-compartment lung from information about the retention and excretion of six gases.

The equations regarding inert gas exchange are very simple and follow from the basic rules of pulmonary gas exchange (Farhi, 1967):

$$\dot{Q} = \frac{\dot{V}_{gas}}{(Pv - a_{gas})S} \quad \text{(Fick equation)} \quad (14.6)$$

and

$$\dot{V} = \frac{\dot{V}_{gas} \cdot P_b}{P_{gas}} \left( \begin{array}{c} \text{Alveolar ventilation} \\ \text{equation} \end{array} \right)$$

$$(14.7)$$

where

$P_{gas}$ = partial pressure in end-capillary blood
$P_b$ = barometric pressure ignoring water vapour
$P_{H_2O}$ = water vapour pressure
$S$ = solubility in litres per litre per pressure unit at 37 °C
$\dot{Q}$ = blood flow in $l \cdot min^{-1}$
$\dot{V}$ = ventilation in $l \cdot min^{-1}$
$Pv\text{-}a$ = venous–arterial pressure difference when a steady state is present, so that tissue gas concentrations are constant

then

$$\dot{V}_A/\dot{Q} = Pv\text{-}a_{gas} \cdot S/Pa_{gas} \cdot P_b \quad (14.8)$$

As $\dot{V}$ is in BPTS units, and gas exchange and solubility are in STPD units, we define S', the blood gas partition coefficient, as S divided by the BTPS to STPD factor for 37 °C and multiplied by barometric pressure (863). In the following, Pc is the pulmonary capillary pressure of the gas under consideration and (S × 863) is called S'.

The retention of an inert gas is the fraction retained in the arterial blood after passage through the lungs. The mixed venous gas flow is (Pv· $\dot{Q}$ · S) and the flow out of the lungs is (Pc · $\dot{Q}$ . S).

Then

$$Pc \cdot \dot{Q} \cdot S / Pv \cdot \dot{Q} \cdot S = Pc/Pv \quad (14.9)$$

If $Pc = P_A$

$$\text{Excretion} = Pc \cdot \dot{V}_A /863 \quad (14.10)$$

then, because mixed venous gas flow = arterial gas flow + amount of gas excreted:

$$Pv \cdot \dot{Q} \cdot S = Pc \cdot \dot{Q} \cdot S + Pc \cdot \dot{V}_A /863$$
$$(14.11)$$

$$Pv = Pc \cdot [1 + \dot{V}_A/\dot{Q}/(S \times 863)] \quad (14.12)$$

$$\text{Fractional retention } Pc/Pv = 1/(1 + \dot{V}_A/\dot{Q} \cdot S') \quad (14.13)$$

$$= S'/(S' + V_a/\dot{Q}) \quad (14.14)$$

Similarly

$$\text{Fractional excretion} = P_E \cdot \dot{V}_E = 1 - \text{retention}$$

$$= \dot{V}_A/\dot{Q}/S' + \dot{V}_A/\dot{Q} \quad (14.15)$$

and by rearrangement

$$\frac{P_E}{P_V} \cdot \frac{S' \cdot \dot{Q}}{\dot{V}_E} \cdot \frac{\dot{V}_A \dot{Q}}{S' + \dot{V}_A / \dot{Q}} \quad (14.16)$$

or

$$\frac{P_E}{P_V} \cdot \frac{\dot{V}_A}{\dot{V}_E} \cdot \frac{S'}{S' + \dot{V}_A / \dot{Q}} \quad (14.17)$$

This is similar to the traditional concept of urinary clearance

$$\text{Clearance} = \frac{P_E \cdot \dot{V}_E}{P_V \cdot S'} = \frac{\dot{Q} \cdot \dot{V}_A / \dot{Q}}{S' \cdot \dot{V}_A / \dot{Q}} \quad (14.18)$$

Note that Eq. 14.17 embodies the concept of dead space, or increase of $\dot{V}_A$ to yield $\dot{V}_E$.

The relationship of total ventilation and total blood flow to those in the individual alveoli or compartments is simply expressed by

$$P_E \cdot \dot{V}_E = \sum_{j=1}^{j=n} P_{Aj} \cdot \dot{V}_{Aj} \quad (14.19)$$

and

$$Pa \cdot \dot{Q}_{tot} = \sum_{j=1}^{j=n} Pc_j \cdot \dot{Q}_j \quad (14.20)$$

that is, the total volume of gas excreted and retained is the sum of the outputs of all the separate compartments, including the completely unventilated shunt compartment (in which $Pc = Pv$) and the ventilated unperfused compartment (in which $P_A = 0$), which contributes air without any tracer gas to the expirate.

These equations embody three concepts:

1. Retention and excretion of inert gases ($Pa/Pv$ and $P_E.\dot{V}_E/Pv.S'$) which may be measured.
2. The blood gas partition coefficient $S'$ (known) for the gas under study.
3. The distribution of ventilation and blood flow, expressed for this purpose as two plots: (a) ventilation to $\dot{V}/\dot{Q}$ ratio and (b) blood flow to $\dot{V}/\dot{Q}$ ratio.

Fig. 14.7 shows an example of retention–solubility and excretion–solubility curves and distribution curves for ventilation and perfusion derived from these. Over a number of years, Wagner and West and other workers have published distribution curves for normal subjects, patients with a variety of moderately severe disease states and a number of experimental animals. Fig. 14.8 shows the narrow range of ventilation–perfusion ratios present in the normal lung. Some abnormalities are illustrated in Fig. 14.9.

The method is sufficiently accurate to discriminate three distinct compartments of high, medium and low ventilation–perfusion ratios, 'dead space' and 'true shunt'. The importance of distinguish-

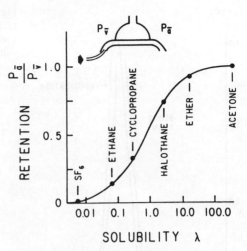

Fig. 14.7. Multiple inert gas exchange (see text). Retention–solubility curve showing typical arterial retentions of inert gases infused into the mixed venous circulation. The most insoluble, sulphur hexafluoride, is excreted instantly unless it passes through very poorly ventilated lung. Acetone is so soluble that it is hardly excreted at all even in well-ventilated alveoli. The measurement of retention for gases of six or more different solubilities can be used to derive a distribution of ventilation–perfusion ratios compatible with the results, using simultaneous equations (see text). (From West, 1981, with permission.)

ing 'dead space' and 'shunt' from areas of very high and very low ventilation–perfusion ratios respectively has already been emphasised.

A further step is to predict, from the model, the arterial blood gases, $Pco_2$ and $Po_2$, knowing the mixed venous gas pressures, the composition of inspired gas and the respiratory exchange ratio. In almost all types of abnormality so far studied, the blood gas pressures predicted from the inert gas results coincided with measured values, the conclusion being that maldistribution of ventilation and perfusion was sufficient to account for abnormalities of $Po_2$ in almost all disease states. The only exception found by Wagner and West was that of patients with diffused lung fibrosis studied during exercise, in whom the degree of arterial hypoxaemia was too great to be explained by the ventilation–perfusion disturbance alone, and it was necessary to postulate a defect of $O_2$ diffusion.

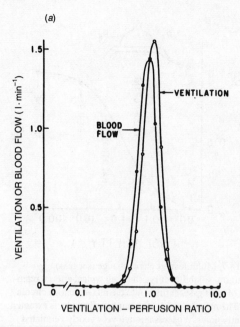

(a)

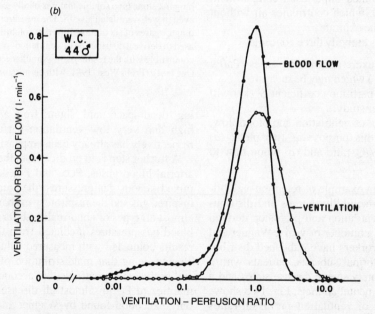

(b)

Fig. 14.8. Distribution of ventilation–perfusion ratios in a young (a) and an older (b) normal subject. Note the increase of poorly ventilated blood flow in the older subject. (From West, 1981, with permission.)

The theoretical limitations of this approach have been studies in great detail. A number of basic assumptions apply to the analysis, notably:

1. Homogeneity within the lung unit.
2. Steady state conditions.
3. Ventilation and blood flow treated as continuous processes.
4. Separate parallel lung units for diffusion.
5. Equilibrium between pulmonary capillary and alveolar gas assumed to be complete for the inert gases.

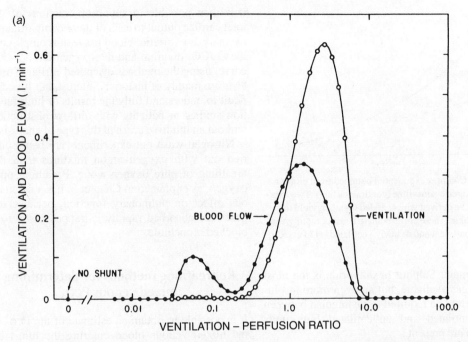

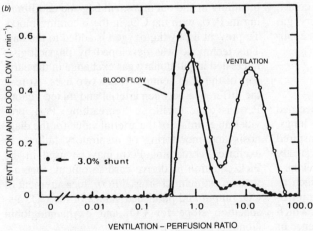

Fig. 14.9. Examples of abnormal ventilation–perfusion distributions in chronic airflow obstruction. (a) Well-preserved blood gases at rest apart from a 3% true shunt: the abnormality is concentrated in the well-ventilated poorly-perfused regions.
(b) Hypoxaemic patient with 'cor pulmonale'. Much of the blood flow is poorly ventilated. (From West, 1981, with permission.)

6. Uniformity of haematocrit.

While none of these assumptions is strictly true, the test appears to work well in practice. Examination of the residual sums of squares after the model has been fitted to data derived from individual patients suggests that departures in real lungs from these approximations have relatively little effect on gas exchange, which can be represented satisfactorily in this way (Evans & Wagner, 1977).

It can be shown mathematically that the resolution of this type of analysis is greatly improved when there is a bi-modal or multi-modal distribution of ventilation–perfusion ratios. Unique solutions are more readily found than when the abnormality consists simply of a splaying of a uni-modal distribution. However, some difficul-

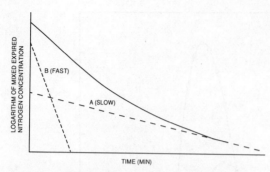

Fig. 14.10. Complex exponential obtained from plotting expired nitrogen against time (continuous line). Two exponentials can be derived which, added together, yield the measured value. These correspond to a fast or rapidly ventilated compartment and a slowly ventilated set of alveoli.

ties do remain. Sulphur hexafluoride is the most insoluble gas available, but an even more insoluble one would be required to distinguish between poorly ventilated and unventilated lung units when both are present.

It would be difficult to over-estimate the contribution to our understanding of pulmonary gas exchange that has followed the meticulous application of this excitingly simple concept.

### Slow and fast compartments

So far the models described have been concerned only with the input and output of the lungs, namely mixed venous and arterial blood, inspired and mixed expired gases, measured in steady state. If patients with airflow obstruction breathe a gas mixture different from inspired air, such as oxygen, or a mixture of argon and oxygen, nitrogen is washed out of the lungs. The rate at which this process occurs is a measure of the presence of slowly ventilated alveoli. Briscoe's two-compartment model is an attempt to measure the delay of alveolar gas mixing by analysing the nitrogen wash-out curve (Fig. 14.10) into exponential decay curves, as if the nitrogen were being excreted from 'fast' and 'slow' compartments. Total ventilation can then be apportioned to the compartments. Having used the time-course of inert gas wash-out to identify the well-ventilated (fast) and poorly ventilated (slow) compartments,

it is then possible to apportion fractions of the total cardiac output to each of these compartments by analysis of arterial blood gas results employing the $O_2/CO_2$ diagram and the oxygen dissociation curve, using the methods discussed earlier. These tests are mainly of historical interest, but it is difficult to understand fully the results of lung function studies in patients with airflow obstruction without an intuitive grasp of this type of analysis.

Nitrogen wash-out experiments are better carried out with oxygen–argon mixtures than the breathing of pure oxygen alone. Breathing pure oxygen, as explained in Chapter 3, has a deleterious effect on pulmonary function, because the gases are absorbed rapidly if trapped distal to a blocked bronchiole.

### Rebreathing methods for determining mixed venous $P_{CO_2}$

It is possible to obtain an estimate of the $P_{CO_2}$ of the mixed venous blood entering the lungs by breathing in and out of a small bag and equilibrating its $P_{CO_2}$ with the $CO_2$ in the incoming blood. To prevent asphyxia, oxygen is added to the bag. This technique was developed by physiologists interested in pulmonary gas exchange in the early part of the 20th century. It has two uses. At rest, the difference between arterial and mixed venous $P_{CO_2}$ is quite small, so 'rebreathing' $P_{CO_2}$ provides an estimate of the arterial value for the diagnosis and monitoring of respiratory failure. In exercise, rebreathing $P_{CO_2}$ may be used in the Fick equation to derive cardiac output, together with an estimate of arterial $P_{CO_2}$, measurement of $CO_2$ output and published values of the $CO_2$ dissociation slope for $CO_2$ and oxyhaemoglobin (Jones *et al.*, 1967).

During breath-holding, gas exchange continues at a progressively falling rate until $P_{O_2}$ and $P_{CO_2}$ approximate to that in the mixed venous blood. Breathing in and out of a small bag enables this process to be studied because it is more comfortable than breath-holding and the tidal gas can be sampled through a rapid continuous analyser.

To avoid hypoxaemia, oxygen is added to the rebreathing bag. Rebreathing $P_{CO_2}$ is strictly speaking an estimate of the $P_{CO_2}$ of the mixed

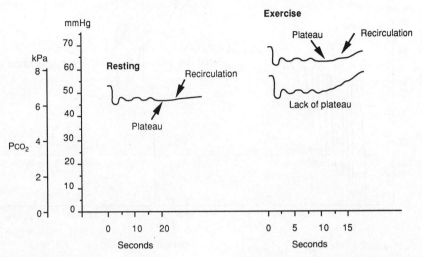

Fig. 14.11. Rebreathing $P_{CO_2}$: the one-stage method. Schematic polygraph trace of the tidal oscillation of $P_{CO_2}$ sampled at the mouth and measured by means of a rapid gas analyser. A plateau, defined as a tidal oscillation of less than 1 mmHg (0.13 kPa), occurs when there is little gas exchange between alveolar and mixed venous blood. This should occur when alveolar $P_{CO_2}$ is equal to the oxygenated mixed venous $P_{CO_2}$, with reservations discussed in the text. In the two examples shown for exercise, the higher is satisfactory, with a plateau occurring 8–10 seconds after the start of rebreathing, before recirculation.

venous blood to which oxygen has been added. This alters the acidity of the haemoglobin and changes the relationship between $P_{CO_2}$ and bicarbonate in the blood (the Christiansen-Douglas-Haldane effect: Chapter 3).

Transient elevations of arterial $P_{CO_2}$ provoke brisk increases in ventilation, but are quite safe if $P_{CO_2}$ does not rise above 60 mmHg (8 kPa).

### One stage measurement of oxygenated mixed venous $P_{CO_2}$ ($P_{\bar{v}}CO_2$)

The principle of this measurement is illustrated in Fig. 14.11. A small bag with a volume of about 1.5 times the tidal volume is primed with a gas containing $CO_2$ at a higher partial pressure than the mixed venous blood. Rebreathing takes place from this bag. If the initial concentration is well chosen, the resulting mixture will be similar to the $P_{CO_2}$ of the oxygenated mixed venous blood

(remembering that this is higher than true mixed venous $P_{CO_2}$ because of the acidifying effect of oxygenating the haemoglobin). As $P_{CO_2}$ is the same in the gas and the blood, no $CO_2$ is absorbed or excreted. Thus, the concentration of $CO_2$ remains the same over several breaths. After 8–15 seconds, depending on cardiac output, blood leaving the lungs at the start of the procedure begins to recirculate, reflecting the rise of $P_{CO_2}$ in the tissues. Thereafter, $P_{CO_2}$ rises in a more or less linear fashion in the rebreathing bag, recording the rise of mixed venous $P_{CO_2}$ as caused by the retention of $CO_2$ produced in the body by metabolism.

When calculating the exact movement of $CO_2$ during this procedure, it is necessary to allow for continued oxygen uptake. This means that during a 'plateau' of constant $P_{CO_2}$ in the bag, there is some $CO_2$ uptake, though not very much. The error produced in the determination of mixed venous $P_{CO_2}$ is unmeasurable at rest (about 1 mmHg (0.7 kPa) at 5 l·min$^{-1}$ cardiac output) and about 3 mmHg (0.4 kPa) when cardiac output is 20 l·min$^{-1}$ (this is calculated from $CO_2$ uptake required to maintain constant bag $P_{CO_2}$ in the presence of oxygen uptake, and from the $CO_2$ dissociation slope of blood).

### Two-stage rebreathing method

This measurement was, for some years, the only simple way of estimating resting $P_{CO_2}$ until blood gas analysers became available. The principle is

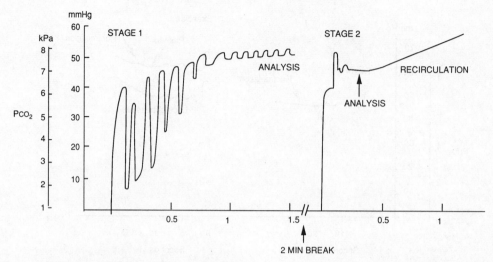

Fig. 14.12. Rebreathing method of measuring resting oxy-genated mixed venous $P_{CO_2}$. Tidal oscillations sampled at the mouth. Stage 1, elevation of bag $P_{CO_2}$ to a value which is nearly in equilibrium with the blood returning to the lungs but higher than the original mixed venous value (because of recirculation of blood during the experiment. The patient is allowed to 'blow off' the remaining excess $CO_2$ for 2 minutes. Stage 2, the bag should now contain gas which, when mixed with patient's alveolar gas yields a value so close to the mixed venous that equilibration takes place within the recirculation time. the subject breathes out fully, rebreathes the gas and is switched out of the bag after 5 breaths. If continuous analysis is not available, analysing the gas at the end of each stage ensures that the procedure is accurate. Stage 1 should not yield a mixture with a lower $P_{CO_2}$ than in the second bag; it may be the same or higher (Campbell & Howell, 1960).

illustrated in Fig. 14.12. The patient first rebreathes into and out of a bag of oxygen. $CO_2$ accumulates until there is equilibrium with the mixed venous blood: this is not achieved until after recirculation has occurred so the $P_{CO_2}$ in the bag is somewhat above the resting mixed venous values. Two minutes is then allowed while the retained $CO_2$ is excreted. Rebreathing for a sec-ond time produces a 'plateau' in 10–15 seconds which represents mixed venous $P_{CO_2}$.

In the original description of this method, $P_{CO_2}$ was described as being on average 6 mmHg (0.9 kPa) less than the rebreathing $P_{CO_2}$: this figure is still widely quoted. In fact, patients in respiratory

failure have a wider veno-arterial $P_{CO_2}$ difference than normal subjects for two reasons:

1. The $CO_2$ dissociation slope is less steep at higher levels than at normal levels of $P_{CO_2}$.
2. Patients in respiratory failure have a low arter-ial, and therefore low mixed venous oxygen saturation. The rebreathing procedure results in full oxygenation, with a correspondingly large Christiansen-Douglas-Haldane effect.

For these reasons, arterial $P_{CO_2}$ is better estimated from the formula

$$P_aCO_2 \approx P_vCO_2 \times 0.8 \qquad (14.21)$$

Rebreathing $P_{CO_2}$ can replace arterial $P_{CO_2}$ in the investigation of stable chronic airflow obstruction and is useful for detecting alveolar hyperventilation.

### Uncertainty regarding the identity of partial pressures of oxygen and carbon dioxide in the alveolar gas and the blood leaving the lungs

Throughout this discussion, it has been assumed that the alveolar membrane acts as a simple dif-fuser for all gases. There are, however, mem-branes which secrete $O_2$. For example, the swim bladder of certain deep-dwelling species of fish contains almost pure $O_2$ secreted by a counter-current mechanism which makes use of the Bohr shift (the effect of pH on the oxyhaemoglobin dis-sociation curve).

Early experimental work from the laboratories of Bohr employing crude analytical methods, later known to be highly inaccurate, suggested that a secretion of $O_2$ might occur in the lungs. There appeared, however, to be $CO_2$ equilibrium. Haldane & Priestly continued to argue the existence of alveolar $O_2$ secretion as late as 1935, while August Krogh (1910), after a series of careful studies, concluded that under steady state conditions no portion of the expired air contained $O_2$ at a lower partial pressure than in the blood. By 1920, most physiology textbooks had accepted Krogh's views. Everyone agreed that the evidence pointed towards perfect alveolar–pulmonary capillary equilibration of $CO_2$.

In about 1967, a few studies were published which suggested that during rebreathing experiments, when alveolar $CO_2$ exchange is minimised, $P_{CO_2}$ in the alveolar gas is higher than in the arterial blood leaving the lungs (Jones *et al.*, 1967; Denison *et al.*, 1971) or in the mixed venous blood entering it (Gurtner, Song & Farhi 1967; Denison *et al.*, 1969), by an amount which may vary from 0 to 30 mmHg (0 to 3.5 kPa). The magnitude of the discrepancy varied with blood flow, pH and other conditions. The difference identified seemed to be too large to be explicable by technical errors, such as a failure to correct the differences in alveolar temperature, which might affect blood gas analysis. Subsequent work showed that the isolated perfused lung worked as a perfect tonometer for $CO_2$. This and other evidence failed to support the idea (which had aroused some interest) that the alveolar membrane and other membranes might sustain a $P_{CO_2}$ gradient (see Gurtner, 1977; Forster, 1977; Piiper, 1986).

Two other possible explanations, apart from experimental error, remain to account for the observations during rebreathing:

1. The long time required for full equilibration of $CO_2$ and bicarbonate ion between the red cells and plasma. Most of the available evidence suggests that this effect is small, perhaps 1–2 mmHg (0.1–0.3 kPa) under extreme conditions.
2. Diffusion of $CO_2$ out of the blood into the myocardium or through the vessels, resulting in a fall of $P_{CO_2}$ between the lungs and the point of sampling after the acute inhalation of $CO_2$. There is no experimental evidence to confirm or refute this.

The best evidence at present indicates that in the steady state, alveolar $P_{CO_2}$ is in equilibrium with the pulmonary capillary blood. There is some doubt as to whether $P_{CO_2}$ in arterial blood is always the same as when it left the lungs.

These findings are important if cardiac output is to be estimated by the indirect Fick method using $CO_2$ as the test gas. A correction factor has to be applied to the plateau value of mixed venous $P_{CO_2}$ which takes this rebreathing $CO_2$ disequilibrium into account (Jones, 1988). Without this correction mixed venous $P_{CO_2}$ is too high, which yields a low value of cardiac output.

## Use of respired gases to measure pulmonary blood flow and tissue volume

### Inert gases

Soluble gases such as nitrous oxide, freon-22, acetylene and a number of anaesthetic gases can be used to measure the transport of gas out of the lung. Pulmonary blood flow is calculated from this, knowing the solubility of the gas in blood. The technique was developed early in the century by Krogh & Lindhard (1912), but refined more recently into the method used today (Fig. 14.13). It is accurate only when gaseous diffusion within the lungs is normal, because it is assumed that the pulmonary perfusion is uniform and that the whole of the measured alveolar volume is accessible to the tracer gas.

The calculation is a modification of the Fick principle for measuring blood flow (Cander & Forster, 1959). By definition, the mixed venous partial pressure of a foreign gas, say nitrous oxide ($N_2O$), is zero when first inspired. Alveolar–arterial equilibration is assumed.

Blood flow = $N_2O$ uptake/(arteriovenous $N_2O$ content difference × solubility)
= $N_2O$ uptake/(alveolar $P_{N_2O}$ × solubility)        (14.22)

This equation is most satisfactorily solved by

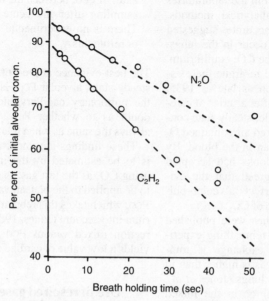

Fig. 14.13. Uptake of the soluble inert gases $N_2O$ and acetylene ($C_2H_2$) from the lungs. In this experiment, refined by Cander & Forster (1959), foreign gas uptake is measured repeatedly during breath-holding. The subject inhales known volumes of gas containing $N_2O$ or $C_2H_2$ from a reservoir, holds the breath for varying lengths of time and exhales into a reservoir; the alveolar concentrations of the foreign gases are measured and plotted as shown. Recently the experiment has been made simpler and more accurate by rebreathing at constant lung volume and measuring end-tidal gas concentrations to determine the uptake of the gas. As shown in this example, the alveolar gas concentrations decrease exponentially until the tracer appears in the mixed venous blood by recirculation. $C_2H_2$ is more soluble than $N_2O$ and can be inhaled in lower concentrations without loss of accuracy.

Uptake of the tracer occurs in three places. Initially, the inspirate is diluted by the alveolar gas which contains no foreign gas. The amount of foreign gas in the lungs after inspiration is calculated from the dilution of helium or another highly insoluble gas and is defined in the figure as a fractional concentration of 1.0. There is immediate uptake of the gas by solution in lung tissue and in the pulmonary blood present in the lung, reducing the alveolar concentration further. The exponential fall of alveolar gas concentration which occurs over the subsequent 10–20 seconds is caused by uptake in the pulmonary blood flowing through the alveoli. Lung tissue uptake can be calculated by backward extrapolation of the alveolar values to zero time. As shown in the figure, the intercept is lower than the value calculated from the dilution of the inspirate by the alveolar gas. From this information it is possible to calculate the blood flow to the ventilated portion of the lung, provided that the solubility of the tracer gas in lung tissue and in blood is known, as explained in the text (Eqs. 14.22–14.33). (From Cander & Forster, 1959, with permission.)

integration as follows: In a single exchanging unit, the uptake of $N_2O$ from alveolar gas in any period of time is:

$$\dot{V}_A \times (F_A N_2 O_{(1)} - F_A N_2 O_{(2)})/t$$
(alveolar vol. × change of alveolar $N_2O$ conc.)/time         (14.23)

In differential form using partial pressures, we get:

$$\dot{V} N_2 O = \frac{-\dot{V}_A}{(P_{BAR} - P_{H_2O})} \cdot \frac{dP N_2 O}{dt}$$
(14.24)

Ignoring for the moment the $N_2O$ dissolved in lung tissue, the test gas is removed in the blood at a rate determined by the blood flow and the amount dissolved in the blood.

$$\dot{V}_{N_2O} = \dot{Q} \cdot P_{N_2O} \cdot \beta$$

Uptake or flux of gas = Blood flow $\times$ (partial pressure) $\times$ solubility in blood per pressure unit             (14.25)

Combining these equations for $\dot{V}_{N_2O}$

$$\dot{Q} = \frac{-\dot{V}_A \, dP_{N_2O}}{(PBAR - P_{H_2O}) \cdot dt} \cdot \frac{1}{P_{N_2O} \cdot \beta}$$

(14.26)

In this equation, alveolar volume, barometric and water vapour pressure and solubility are constants, leaving the variable $[- dP_{N_2O}/dt \div P_{N_2O}]$ which equals

$$\frac{- d\log_e / dt}{P_{N_2O}}$$             (14.27)

the slope of the 'semilog' plot of $P_{N_2O}$ against time.

Combining these equations, but still ignoring the capacity of the pulmonary blood to store gas, permits calculation of cardiac output from the approximate mass equation for transfer of transport of nitrous oxide (or any foreign gas for which there is no diffusion barrier):

$$\dot{Q} = \frac{V_A}{PBAR - P_{H_2O}} \cdot \frac{1}{\beta t_1 - t_2} \cdot \frac{\log_e P_{N_2O}, t_1}{P_{N_2O}, t_2}$$

(14.28)

This equation yields a solution for $\dot{Q}$ which is too low, because after inspiration, some $N_2O$ enters and is dissolved in the lung tissue and pulmonary blood that is already present. The 'pool' from which the incoming blood obtains the $N_2O$ is, in fact, the alveolar gas, the lung tissue and the blood already present. Equation 14.28 has to be modified to take into account the volume of the lung tissue and pulmonary blood ($V_{tis} + V_{blood}$), and the amount of gas removed or added to them for each unit change of $P_{N_2O}$. This is the volume multiplied by the solubility of the gas in tissue and blood respectively ($V_{tis} \cdot \beta_{tis} + V_{blood} \cdot \beta_{blood}$). The flow of blood through the system reduces the $P_{N_2O}$ of the alveolar gas, the lung tissue and the blood within the lung by the same amount: the actual mass of $N_2O$ that is removed from each of these depends

on their capacity (change of content/change of $P_{N_2O}$). Modifying Eq. 14.28, the flux of nitrous oxide into the blood now becomes

$$\frac{- dP_{N_2O}}{dt} \cdot \frac{V_A}{PBAR - P_{H_2O}} + \frac{dP_{N_2O}}{dt} \cdot$$

(14.29)

or

$$\frac{- dP_{N_2O}}{dt} \cdot \frac{V_A}{PBAR - P_{H_2O}} + \frac{dP_{N_2O}}{dt} \cdot$$

$$\frac{dP_{N_2O}}{dt} + (V_{tis} \cdot \beta_{tis} + V_{blood} \cdot \beta_{blood})$$

(14.30)

It is possible to solve for ($V_{tis} \cdot \beta_{tis} + V_{blood} \cdot \beta_{blood}$) from the experimental points (Fig. 14.13). If no foreign gas dissolved in lung tissue, the initial pressure in the rebreathing bag could be calculated from the dilution of the inspired gas by the residual volume; we can call this $P_{N_2O}$ '100%'. Extrapolation of the line through the semilogarithmic plot of $P_{N_2O}$ back to 'zero' time cuts the ordinate at a point lower than 100%, in fact, between 90% and 95%. From these figures we can obtain a factor by which the alveolar volume must be multiplied in order to correct for the capacity of lung tissue. For interest, to complete this account, the calculation is given here.

We assume that the difference between the 100% (diluted inspired) $P_{N_2O}$ and the intercept is all due to the instantaneous passage of gas from the alveoli into the lung tissue and the static pulmonary blood with no removal of $N_2O$ by blood flow. At the start, the alveolar gas is at '100%' $P_{N_2O}$ and the lung liquids contain none. After equalisation, both are at the intercept $P_{N_2O}$. Therefore

$$\frac{V_A \cdot (100\% - \text{intercept} \%)}{PBAR - P_{H_2O}} =$$

Intercept $(V_{tis} \cdot \beta_{tis} + V_{blood} \cdot \beta_{blood})$

(14.31)

and, rearranging

$$(V_{tis} \cdot \beta_{tis} + V_{blood} \cdot \beta_{blood}) =$$

$$\frac{V_A \cdot (100\% - \text{intercept } \%)}{P_{BAR} - P_{H_2O} \text{ intercept } \%} \tag{14.32}$$

Therefore the equation for the flux of gas into the flowing blood becomes

$$\frac{dP_{N_2O}}{dt} \cdot \frac{V_A}{P_{BAR} - P_{H_2O}} \times$$

$$\left[ 1 + \frac{(100\% - \text{intercept } \%)}{\text{intercept } \%} \right] \tag{14.33}$$

In other words, the alveolar volume is multiplied by a number slightly greater than 1 to give an effective volume of the same capacity as the gas. If the inspired breath, and thus alveolar volume is smaller, the factor becomes correspondingly greater.

Nitrous oxide is more or less equally soluble in blood and in lung tissue, so the volume of lung liquids which are in contact with alveolar gas can be calculated from equation 14.32.

The definition of 'zero' time is critical because the intercept is so close to 100%. A finite time is required to breathe in, and it is slightly inaccurate to take the beginning of the test inspirate as the starting point of the exponential fall of gas concentration. The most elegant solution is to combine the procedure with a rebreathing measurement of $TL_{CO}$ (Sackner et al., 1975). CO is very insoluble in water, so to calculate zero time the CO absorption line is extrapolated back to its theoretical '100% after dilution' point to yield the virtual zero time. This requires excellent analytical instruments. Another and even more difficult approach which has been tried experimentally consists of using two gases of differing solubilities and solving the equations for their uptake during rebreathing so that they give the same answer for cardiac output and lung tissue volume (Louderbough, Ozanne & Severinghaus, 1976).

Rebreathing estimates of pulmonary blood flow and lung tissue volume yield consistent and reproducible results in normal subjects, especially during exercise (Winsborough et al. 1980)

In patients with airflow obstruction, the accuracy and usefulness of these techniques is limited in the same way as those of $TL_{CO}$ by the presence of slowly ventilated alveoli. These cause two types of error. Firstly, the portion of the pulmonary blood flow which is poorly ventilated is not measured. Q is an index of the effective (or ventilated) pulmonary blood flow. This problem can only be overcome by injecting tracers into the mixed venous blood, or by traditional measurements involving the Fick principle. Secondly, the slowly ventilated compartment behaves like a sump into which the foreign gases move slowly. This system cannot accurately be analysed as a single exponential, and it is necessary to relate the disappearance of the soluble gas to that of the insoluble gas with each breath.

## References

Campbell, E.J.M. & Howell, J.B.L. (1960). Simple rapid methods of estimating arterial and mixed venous $P_{CO_2}$. British Medical Journal, **i**, 458–462.

Cander, L. & Forster, R.E. (1959). Determination of pulmonary parenchymal tissue volume and pulmonary blood flow in man. Journal of Applied Physiology, **14**, 541–551.

Cherniack, N.S. & Widdicombe, J.G. (1986). Control of breathing. In Handbook of Physiology, section 3, vol. 2, parts I & II. Bethesda: APS.

Clark, T.J.H. (1968). The ventilatory response to $CO_2$ in chronic airways obstruction measured by a rebreathing method. Clinical Science, **34**, 559–568.

Denison, D., Edwards, R.H.T., Jones, G. & Pope, H. (1969). Estimates of the $O_2$ and $CO_2$ pressures in mixed venous blood. Respiration Physiology, **7**, 326–334.

Denison, D., Edwards, R.H.T., Jones, G. & Pope, H. (1971). Estimates of the $CO_2$ pressures in systemic arterial blood during rebreathing in exercise. Respiration Physiology, **11**, 186–196.

Evans, J.W. & Wagner, P.D. (1977). Limits on $\dot{V}_A/\dot{Q}$ distribution from analysis of experimental insert gas elimination. Journal of Applied Physiology, **42**, 889–898.

Farhi, L.E. (1966). Ventilation–perfusion relationship and its role in alveolar gas exchange. In Advances in Respiratory Physiology, ed. C.Y. Caro. London: Edward Arnold.

Farhi, L.E. (1967). Elimination of insert gases by the lung. (1967). Respiration Physiology, **3**, 1–11.

Flenley, D.C. & Millar, J.S. (1967). Ventilatory response to oxygen and carbon dioxide in chronic respiratory failure. *Clinical Science*, **33**, 319–334.

Forster, R.E. (1977). Can alveolar $P_{CO_2}$ exceed pulmonary end-capillary $P_{CO_2}$: No. *Journal of Applied Physiology*, **42**, 323–328.

Fowle, A.S.E. & Campbell, E.J.M. (1964). The immediate carbon dioxide storage capacity of man. *Clinical Science*, **27**, 41–49.

Gribbin, H.R., Gardiner, I.T. & Heinz, G.J. (1983). The role of impaired inspiratory muscle function in limiting the ventilatory response to $CO_2$ in chronic airflow obstruction. *Clinical Science*, **64**, 487–495.

Gurtner, G.H. (1977). Can alveolar $P_{CO_2}$ exceed pulmonary end-capillary $P_{CO_2}$: Yes. *Journal of Applied Physiology*, **42**, 324–326.

Gurtner, G.H., Song, S.H. & Farhi, L.E. (1967). Alveolar and mixed venous $P_{CO_2}$ difference during rebreathing. *Physiologist*, **10**, 190.

Haldane, J.S. & Priestley, J.G. (1935). *Respiration*, 2nd edn. Oxford: Oxford University Press.

Honda, Y., Watanabe, S., Hashizume, I., Satomura, Y., Hata, N. & Sahakibra, Y. (1979). Hypoxic chemosensitivity in asthmatic patients two decades after carotid body resection. *Journal of Applied Physiology*, **46**, 632–638.

Javaheri, F., Lucey, E. & Snider, G.L. (1985). Premorbid ventilatory response to hypercapnia is not related to resting arterial carbon dioxide tension in hamsters with elastase-induced emphysema. *American Review of Respiratory Disease*, **132**, 1055–1059.

Jones, N.L. (1988). *Clinical Exercise Testing*, 3rd edn, p. 193. Philadelphia: Saunders

Jones, N.L., Campbell, E.J.M., McHardy, G.J.M., Higgs, B.E. & Clode, M. (1967). The estimation of carbon dioxide pressure of mixed venous blood during exercise. *Clinical Science*, **32**, 311–327.

Krogh, A. (1910). On the mechanism of gas exchange in the lungs. *Scandinavian Archives of Physiology*, **23**, 248–278.

Krogh, A. & Lindhard, J. (1912). Measurement of blood flow through the lungs of man. *Scandinavian Archives of Physiology*, **27**, 100–125.

Laszlo, G., Clark, T.J.H. & Campbell, E.J.M. (1969). The immediate buffering of $CO_2$ in man. *Clinical Science*, **37**, 299–309.

Linton, R.A.F., Poole-Wilson, P.A., Davies, R.J. & Cameron, I.R. (1973). A comparison of the ventilatory response to carbon dioxide by the steady state and rebreathing methods during metabolic acidosis and alkalosis. *Clinical Science*, **45**, 239–249.

Lloyd, B.B., Jukes, M.G.M. & Cunningham, D.J.C. (1958). The relationship between alveolar oxygen pressure and the respiratory response to carbon dioxide in man. *American Journal of Experimental Physiology*, **43**, 214–227.

Louderbough, H., Ozanne, G. & Severinghaus, J.W. (1976). Lung weight and pulmonary blood flow determination in man and dogs by soluble gas uptake. *Federation Proceedings*, **35**, 729

Lourenço, R.V. (1976). Clinical methods for the study of regulation of breathing. *Chest*, **70** (suppl.), 109–112.

McEvoy, J.D.S., Jones, N.L. & Campbell, E.J.M. (1974). Mixed venous and arterial $P_{CO_2}$. *British Medical Journal*, **iv**, 687–690.

Marazzini, L., Cavestri, R. & Gori, D. (1978). Difference between mouth and oesophageal occlusion pressure during $CO_2$ rebreathing in chronic obstructive pulmonary disease. *American Review of Respiratory Disease*, **118**, 1027–1033.

Matthews, A.W. & Howell, J.B.L. (1975). The rate of isometric inspiratory pressure development as a measure of response to carbon dioxide in man. *Clinical Science*, **49**, 57–68.

Milic-Emili, J. (1982). Recent advances in clinical assessment of control of breathing. *Lung*, **160**, 1–17.

Milic-Emili, J. & Tyler, J.M. (1963). Relation between work output of respiratory muscles and end-tidal $CO_2$ tension. *Journal of Applied Physiology*, **18**, 497–504.

Otis, A.B., & Rahn, H. (1980). Development of concepts in Rochester, New York, in the 1940s. In *Pulmonary Gas Exchange*, vol. 1, ed. J.B. West, pp. 33–66. New York: Academic Press.

Pardy, R.L., Rivington, R.N., Milic-Emili, J. & Mortola, J.P. (1982). Control of breathing in chronic obstructive pulmonary disease. *American Review of Respiratory Disease*, **125**, 6–11.

Piiper, J. (1986). Blood gas equilibrium of carbon dioxide in lungs: a continuing controversy. *Journal of Applied Physiology*, **60**, 1–8.

Plum, F. (1970). Neurological integration of behavioural and metabolic control of breathing. In *Breathing: Hering-Breuer Centenary Symposium*, ed. R. Porter. London: Churchill.

Read, D.J.C. (1967). A clinical method for assessing the ventilatory response to $CO_2$. *Australasian Annals of Medicine*, **16**, 20–32.

Read, D.J.C. & Leigh, J. (1967). Blood:brain:tissue $P_{CO_2}$ relationship and ventilation during rebreathing. *Journal of Applied Physiology*, **23**, 53–70.

Rebuck, A.S. & Campbell, E.J.M. (1974). A clinical method for assessing the ventilatory response to hypoxia. *American Review of Respiratory Disease*, **109**, 345–350.

Riley, R.L. (1980). Development of the three-compartment model for dealing with uneven distribution. In *Pulmonary Gas Exchange*, vol. 1, ed. J.B. West, pp. 67–85. New York: Academic Press.

Riley, R.L. & Permutt, S. (1965). The four quadrant diagram for analyzing the distribution of gas and blood in the lung. In *Handbook of Physiology, Respiration*, vol II, ed. W.O. Fenn & H. Rahn, pp. 1413–1423. Bethesda: APS.

Sackner, M.A., Greeneltch, D., Heiman, M.S., Epstein, L.S. & Atkins, N. (1975). Diffusing capacity, membrane diffusing capacity, capillary blood volume, pulmonary tissue volume and cardiac output measured by a rebreathing technique. *American Review of Respiratory Disease*, **111**, 157–165.

Scheid, P. (1983). Respiratory mass spectrometry. In *Measurement in Clinical Respiratory Physiology*, ed. G. Laszlo & M.F. Sudlow, pp. 131–166. London: Academic Press.

Scheid, P. & Piiper, J. (1980). Intrapulmonary gas mixing and stratification. In *Pulmonary Gas Exchange*, vol. 1, *Ventilation, Blood Flow and Diffusion*, ed. J.B. West. New York: Academic Press.

Shaw, R.A., Schonfield, S.A. & Whitcomb, M.E. (1982). Progressive and transient hypoxic ventilatory drive tests in normal subjects. *American Review of Respiratory Disease*, **126**, 37–40.

von Euler, C. (1986). Brain stem mechanisms for generation and control of breathing pattern. In *Handbook of Physiology*, section 3, vol. 2, part 1, ed. N.S. Cherniack & J.G. Widdicombe. Bethesda: APS.

Wagner, P.D., Naumann, P.F. & Laravuso, R.B. (1974). Simultaneous measurement of eight foreign gases in blood by gas chromatography. *Journal of Applied Physiology*, **36**, 600–605.

Wagner, P.D., Saltzmann, H.A. & West, J.B. (1974). Measurement of continuous distributions of ventilation–perfusion ratios: theory. *Journal of Applied Physiology*, **36**, 588–599.

Wagner, P.D. & West, J.B. (1972). Effects of diffusion impairment on $O_2$ and $CO_2$ time courses in pulmonary capillaries. *Journal of Applied Physiology*, **33**, 62–71.

Wasserman, K.A., Whipp, B.J. & Casaburi, R. (1986). Respiratory control during exercise. In *Handbook of Physiology*, section 3, vol. 2, part 2, ed. N.S. Cherniack & J.G. Widdicombe, pp. 515–619. Bethesda: APS.

Weil, J.V. (1986). Ventilatory control at high altitude. In *Handbook of Physiology*, section 3, vol. 2, part 2, ed. N.S. Cherniack & J.G. Widdicombe, pp. 703–728. Bethesda: APS.

Weil, J.V., Byrne Quinn, E. & Sodal, I.E. (1970). Hypoxic ventilatory drive in normal man. *Journal of Clinical Investigation*, **49**, 1061–1072.

West, J.B. (1980). *Pulmonary Gas Exchange*. Vol. 1, *Ventilation Blood Flow and Diffusion*, pp. 1–339. Vol. 2, *Organism and Environment*, pp. 1–318. New York: Academic Press.

West, J.B. (1981). Ventilation–perfusion relationships. In: *Scientific Foundations of Respiratory Medicine*, pp. 157–158, ed. J.G.Scadding, G. Cumming & W.M. Thurlbeck. London: W. Heinemann.

West, J.B. (1985). *Everest: The Testing Place*, pp. 118–125. New York: McGraw-Hill.

West, J.B., Hackett, K.H., Maret, R.M., Milledge, J.S., Peters, R.M., Pizzo, C.J. & Winslow, R.M. (1983). Pulmonary gas exchange on the summit of Mount Everest. *Journal of Applied Physiology*, **55**, 678–687.

West, J.B., Lahiri, S., Maret, K.H., Peters, R.M. & Pizzo, C.J. (1983). Barometric pressures at extreme altitudes on Mount Everest: physiological significance. *Journal of Applied Physiology*, **54**, 1188–1194.

Whitelaw, W.A., Derenne, J.P. & Milic-Emili, J. (1975). Occlusion pressure as a measure of respiratory centre output in conscious man. *Respiration Physiology*, **23**, 181–199.

Winsborough, M., Miller, J.N., Burgess, D.W. & Laszlo, G. (1980). Estimation of cardiac output from the rate of change of alveolar carbon dioxide pressure during rebreathing. *Clinical Science*, **58**, 263–270.

# 15 Respiratory monitoring during sleep

## Sleep apnoea syndrome

Intermittent cessation or severe reduction of ventilation can occur at night. This is known as sleep apnoea (Guilleminault *et al.*, 1976) or sleep hypopnoea, and may cause a number of manifestations related to the disruption of sleep and to intermittent hypoxaemia in some instances. The commonest type is obstructive sleep apnoea, which is caused by obstruction to respiration due to collapse of the upper airway during inspiration. The condition occurs principally in obese individuals with thick necks and narrow upper airways and is usually accompanied by loud snoring.

### Obstructive apnoea

During the episodes of apnoea, or reduced ventilation, which last several seconds, respiratory movements occur but fail to result in air flow because of obstruction to the upper airway during inspiration. A number of factors combine to cause this phenomenon. The genioglossus and other pharyngeal muscles normally contract during inspiration to maintain normal patency of the upper airways. This mechanism fails to operate satisfactorily in the sleep apnoea syndrome (Mathew & Remmers, 1984; Orem, 1984). In many subjects, there is in addition some organic narrowing by deposition of fat in the upper airway, enlargement of the tongue or some other anatomical abnormality. Enlarged tonsils and adenoids may cause sleep apnoea in children. The common factor is that the effort of inspiration causes the upper airway to collapse by suction so that the entry of air is reduced or altogether impeded (Table 15.1).

## Central apnoea

Central apnoea is caused by damage to the centres in the brain stem which cause breathing to occur automatically in a cyclical fashion even during sleep. Loss of this function is sometimes called 'Ondine's curse'. Respiratory movements cease during this type of apnoea, which is rare. It may occur in infancy. Central and obstructive apnoea may coexist.

### Rapid eye movement sleep

Rapid eye movement (REM) sleep occurs about five times during a normal night's sleep. During REM sleep, dreaming takes place and breathing becomes irregular, often following a behavioural pattern (Chapter 14). This may result in abnormalities of gas exchange including arterial oxygen desaturation, but this is not sleep apnoea.

Sleep apnoea causes daytime sleepiness, by repeatedly waking the patient who achieves very little deep sleep. This can cause poor performance at school in children and a varying amount of disabling hypersomnolence in adults which may have serious consequences, for example, if the patient falls asleep when driving (Findley, Universtadt & Suratt, 1988). Loss of employment and marital disharmony are common. The condition carries a high morbidity and mortality (Partinen, Jamieson & Guilleminault, 1988).

The incidence of obstructive sleep apnoea varies throughout the world. It probably affects about 3 men over the age of 40 per 1000 population in the United Kingdom.

Table 15.1. *Common factors predisposing to the development of obstructive sleep apnoea syndrome*

| Increased nasal resistance | Deviated nasal septum Nasal polyposis Chronic rhinitis |
|---|---|
| Narrow airway | Deposition of fat around neck Enlarged tonsils and adenoids Large tongue (acromegaly, hypothyroidism, amyloid), long uvula, congenital abnormalities |
| Reduced tone of pharyngeal airway | Alcohol Sedation |

## Control of breathing during sleep

In normal subjects, REM sleep occurs after 90 minutes and occupies about 20–25% of the night's sleep. Breathing is irregular and overall ventilation reduced. Behavioural breathing appears to predominate, with sighing, apnoea and periods resembling breathing in speech. There is widespread paralysis. The ventilatory response to $CO_2$ is blunted, although that to hypoxia is preserved. In the early stages of non-REM sleep, there may be periodic breathing of the Cheyne-Stokes type with overall hyperventilation. In deep sleep, the ventilatory response to $CO_2$ may be reduced, but not as much as during REM sleep. $Pco_2$ tends to rise by about 3–4 mmHg (0.5 kPa) in deep sleep (Stradling & Phillipson, 1986).

Central and obstructive sleep apnoea are usually related. Abduction of the pharyngeal wall and larynx is part of the normal inspiratory reflex and is particularly related to the metabolic or chemoreceptor drive to respiration. Airway resistance falls during hypercapnia, but behavioural breathing requires separate control of the pharynx, larynx and the muscles of ventilation. This may account for the coexistence of snoring and obstructive apnoea with central apnoea since, at least in some patients, the underlying mechanism may be reduction of chemoreceptor drive.

## Clinical features of obstructive sleep apnoea

Obstructive sleep apnoea should be suspected when some of the following are present (Whyte *et al.*, 1989):

1. Loud and frequent snoring, especially if apnoea is reported. About a quarter of the patients, or their bed partners, report choking attacks on waking.
2. Daytime hypersomnolence: falling asleep at least once a day when not in bed. About one in twelve seeking advice do this when driving. Restless or unrefreshing sleep is commoner, but not an invariable complaint. Naps taken during the day are refreshing when sleeping in a chair prevents inspiratory obstruction. Severely affected individuals often fall asleep in the waiting room.
3. Severe obesity.
4. Depression and intellectual deterioration.
5. Nocturnal bradycardia, though this is not common.
6. Right ventricular failure out of proportion to any lung disease present.

Heart failure and polycythaemia complicate sleep apnoea only in those who become profoundly hypoxic during episodes of hypoventilation. They are not common findings in patients with sleep apnoea without lung disease (Weitzenblum *et al.*, 1988). They generally occur when daytime arterial $Po_2$ is below normal because of ventilation–perfusion mismatching. In these patients, a minor degree of hypoventilation results in a rapid fall of arterial saturation because of the shape of the dissociation curve for oxygen (Chapter 3). Most of these patients suffer from gross obesity or from one of the lower respiratory disorders most likely to be associated with alveolar hypoventilation: chronic airflow obstruction, kyphoscoliosis, or paresis of the respiratory muscles, notably the muscular dystrophies.

## Investigation of breathing during sleep

Apnoea is defined as cessation of ventilation for longer than 10 seconds. A reduction in respiratory excursions of more than 50% is called hypopnoea and has similar consequences (Whyte *et al.*, 1989). These are abnormal if they occur more

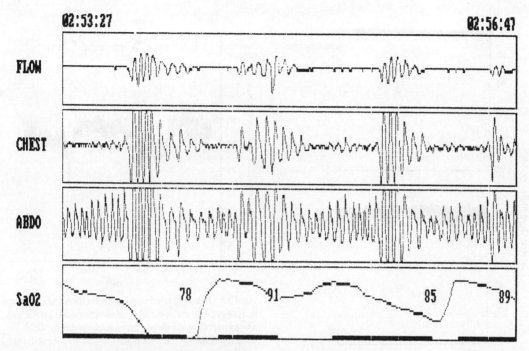

**02:53:27**                                               **02:56:47**

FLOW

CHEST

ABDO

SaO2          78          91          85          89

Fig. 15.1. Records of nasal air flow, chest wall movement, abdominal movement and oxygen saturation in a patient with obstructive sleep apnoea. Note that there is a circulatory delay between changes in pulmonary ventilation and corresponding changes in oxygen saturation recorded from a probe on a finger. In this example, episodes of apnoea and hypopnoea occur regularly, appearing as reduction of nasal airflow. In this instance, abdominal respiratory efforts continue, showing that the apnoea is obstructive. After a while, the patient is aroused and increasing respiratory efforts overcome the obstruction. Three episodes of apnoea are shown in this example. The total time displayed is 3 minutes. (Courtesy of Dr J. R. Catterall and Miss N. Wiltshire.)

than ten times per hour in a 7 hour night during non-REM as well as REM sleep. The frequency of these episodes in healthy subjects increases with age (Berry *et al.*, 1984). Symptoms tend to occur when there are more than 10, or more usually 15 apnoeic episodes per hour. The sleep apnoea syndrome should only be diagnosed if there are significant symptoms accompanied by characteristic sleep recordings, and not simply on the basis of an arbitrary number of apnoeic episodes.

Intermittent apnoea and hypopnoea may be

identified and classified by continuous monitoring of three variables (Fig. 15.1):

1. Respiratory efforts. These are most easily recorded by means of magnetometers attached to the chest and abdomen (impedance pneumography) or by a respiratory jacket. A quite simple pneumograph may suffice. This is a tube containing air which is attached to a transducer; respiratory movements of the chest and abdomen are sensed as pressure changes within the tube.
2. Flow of air through the airways. This may be recorded most simply by means of a thermistor at the nose and mouth recording oscillations of temperature with each breath. Alternatively, a rapid $CO_2$ analyser may be used to sample expired air.
3. Arterial $So_2$. This is most easily measured by means of a pulse oximeter, using a probe on a finger.

Cessation or reduction of airflow are the hallmarks of sleep apnoea and hypopnoea respectively. In central apnoea or hypopnoea, respiratory movements are absent or reduced, while obstructive apnoea is characterised by the

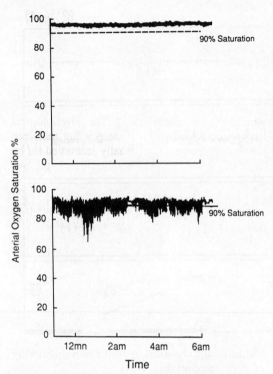

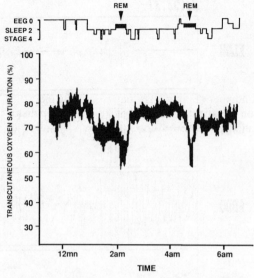

Fig. 15.3. Overnight arterial oxygen saturation and sleep stage in a patient with chronic airflow obstruction and hypoxaemia. The most profound falls of saturation occur during REM sleep (indicated by the thick black lines). This patient did not have obstructive sleep apnoea, as judged by traces of chest wall movement and airflow. (Courtesy of Dr J.R. Catterall.)

Fig. 15.2. Overnight oxygen saturation in a normal subject and a patient with obstructive sleep apnoea. (From Catterall 1992, with permission.)

absence of airflow in the presence of respiratory effort. For simplicity, the term hypopnoea will be used to describe both types of event.

Arterial oxygen desaturation (hypoxaemia) occurs during episodes of hypopnoea in about four fifths of all patients eventually diagnosed as having sleep apnoea syndrome (Douglas *et al.*, 1992). 'Desaturations' are identified from the oximeter trace. Their duration and frequency may readily be assessed. Pulse oximeters capable of storing 8 hours of recordings are inexpensive and easy to apply at home, without the need for skilled operators. They are often used on their own to screen for the presence of nocturnal desaturation, which was previously thought to be the cause of most of the symptoms. Nocturnal traces showing more than 5 desaturations per hour of 4% or more are present in 80% of patients subsequently con-

firmed as having sleep apnoea at polysomnography. These criteria have a specificity of 80%, so are a good basis for more detailed investigation. Stricter criteria are needed for epidemiological surveys. Gross examples of sleep apnoea are easily recognised (Fig. 15.2).

An episode of apnoea will result in arterial oxygen desaturation if it lasts long enough to reduce the $P_{O_2}$ in part of the lung to a level below that required to achieve 95% saturation. Small alveoli store little oxygen and this is rapidly used up if the alveoli are well perfused. Most patients with sleep apnoea are obese. Increased abdominal fat causes FRC to fall, with alveolar underventilation at the bases of the lungs. Very little oxygen is stored in lungs when FRC is low, so arterial $P_{O_2}$ falls rapidly when the breath is held. Other forms of gas exchange impairment cause arterial $P_{O_2}$ to fall during periods of irregular breathing, because of the profound effect of hypoventilation on $O_2$ saturation when alveolar $P_{O_2}$ is close to the steep portion of the oxygen dissociation curve (Fig. 15.3).

Desaturation during REM sleep alone is not the same as the sleep apnoea syndrome, although the effects of prolonged episodes of nocturnal hypoxaemia may perhaps contribute towards the development of 'cor pulmonale' (Catterall *et al.*, 1983).

### Polysomnography

A number of other tests may help in the investigation of patients suspected of having a sleep disturbance.

1. Electrooculography is used to identify REM sleep.
2. The submental muscle relaxes during REM sleep; this is shown by cessation of activity in the electromyogram obtained over the surface of this muscle.
3. Video monitoring by means of an infra-red camera confirms that the patient is asleep, records sleep position and may demonstrate snoring. In some instances, obstructive sleep apnoea is dependent on position, though this finding is not very common in patients who get as far as formal investigation (Anon. 1984).
4. Electromyographic measurement of leg movements helps to diagnose the periodic leg movement syndrome which is fairly common among elderly subjects and may coexist with sleep apnoea. This condition is sometimes called nocturnal myoclonus and is an occasional cause of daytime sleepiness. Rhythmic extension and flexion of the feet and legs occur two or three times a minute in clusters throughout the night.
5. Arterial $PCO_2$. $PCO_2$ rises slowly during hypopnoea because body proteins buffer carbonic acid. $CO_2$ monitoring is therefore used only in patients suspected of nocturnal ventilatory failure with normal daytime $PCO_2$. The majority of these patients have severe thoracic cage or neuromuscular disorders.
6. Electroencephalography. The depth of sleep can be defined (stages I to IV) by means of the electroencephalogram (EEG), combined with the electrooculogram and submental EMG to identify REM sleep (Rechtshaffen & Kales, 1968). In addition to helping to diagnose rare neurological syndromes such as narcolepsy, the EEG shows for how long the patient slept.

These observations are labour intensive but there are a number of good reasons for making them. They furnish proof that the patient has fallen asleep during the investigation. Sleep disruptions can be counted: these are the main cause of hypersomnolence in the sleep apnoea syndrome. They identify the sleep stages during which desaturation occurs: this is important because desaturation which occurs only during the physiological hypopnoea found in REM sleep is not the sleep apnoea syndrome, but is usually accounted for by impaired gas exchange. Finally, narcolepsy and the other rare central nervous system causes of hypersomnolence can be diagnosed by EEG. Narcolepsy is characterised by the rapid onset of REM sleep, usually in less than 15 minutes. The normal value is 90 minutes and this is somewhat reduced in individuals with depression. The classical syndrome of narcolepsy, cataplexy and hypnagogic paralysis occurring at the onset of sleep is easy to diagnose but these associated phenomena do not always occur.

Rigorously, sleep studies performed for research purposes into the effect of intervention in this disorder require a night of acclimatisation to the apparatus. This is not always necessary in clinical studies, especially in patients with hypersomnolence who are capable of falling asleep anywhere. The investigation should, however, be carried out in a room conducive to sleep.

### Daytime studies

It is sometimes necessary to measure the severity of daytime hypersomnolence. For this purpose, the multiple sleep latency test is a useful semi-quantitative measure of how quickly an individual falls asleep in a quiet room during the day (Roehrs *et al.*, 1989). The test is attempted four times during the day at 2 hour intervals, being terminated after 15 minutes of sleep or 20 minutes of wakefulness. Typically, individuals with the sleep apnoea syndrome fall asleep in 6–15 minutes if not sooner. Studies such as this demonstrate that hypersomnolence is caused by arousal rather than by hypoxaemia (Roehrs *et al.*, 1989).

### Limited investigation

The identification of nocturnal hypoxaemia alone does not require a full sleep study (Cooper *et al.*,

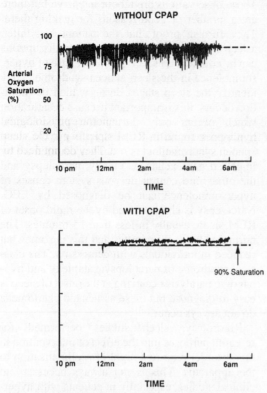

Fig. 15.4. All-night recordings of arterial oxygen saturation before and during the application of continuous positive pressure at the nostrils (CPAP). (From Catterall, 1992,
with permission.)

1991). Oximetry can demonstrate the hypoxaemic
episodes and modern pulse oximeters are capable
of storing observations for several hours. The
investigations may often be carried out without
admission to hospital. In the laboratory, observation of 3 hours of sleep after 12 hours of wakefulness may demonstrate respiratory abnormalities
in many cases, and patients with the grossest form
of hypersomnolence will sleep readily after lunch
in a quiet darkened laboratory (Series et al., 1991;
Sanders et al., 1991).

There are no daytime pulmonary function studies which predict the presence of sleep apnoea
syndrome. Interruption to airflow may occur as a
result of upper airway obstruction during forced
inspiration and expiration. About one fifth of

patients showing this phenomenon during the
measurement of flow volume loops will display
heavy snoring or overt sleep apnoea syndrome.

## Treatment

The identification and treatment of sleep apnoea
syndrome is rewarding. The main benefits are
improved mental performance in children and
loss of daytime sleepiness in adults. The incidence of the condition varies with the amount of
obesity, and is present in about 0.3% of middle-
aged men in the United Kingdom (Stradling &
Crosby, 1991). Treatment is progressive and may
include:

1. Weight reduction.
2. Avoidance of alcohol and sedatives before
   sleep.
3. Surgical correction of remediable nasal and
   nasopharyngeal obstruction such as enlarged
   adenoids in children, (Stradling et al., 1990),
   nasal polyps or grossly deviated nasal septa.
4. Measures to prevent lying on the back when the
   condition is shown to be positional.
5. Continuous positive nasal airway pressure by
   means of a nasal mask to support the upper airway (Sullivan et al., 1981, 1984). This is
   known as nasal CPAP.

Tracheostomy, formerly the mainstay of treatment, is now rarely needed. Protriptyline, an anti-
depressant which causes little sedation, reduces
the time spent in REM sleep but it is rarely found
to be helpful and causes anticholinergic side
effects. Uvulopalatoplasty reduces the sound of
snoring but not the nocturnal desaturations. It is
rarely indicated in hypoxaemic patients, but its
place may need to be re-evaluated.

### Nasal CPAP

To administer nasal CPAP, a quiet pump is used
to blow air continuously past the nose via a well-
fitting nasal mask which is strapped to the
patient's face at night. The flow is adjusted to
achieve a positive pressure of between 5 and 17
cm $H_2O$. It is usually necessary to acclimatise to
the pump for a few hours at low pressure. When a
comfortable level has been reached, and the
patient and the bed partner have become accus-

tomed to the continuous hum of the motor, snoring is abolished and sleep quality is improved. It is necessary to repeat the sleep study for one or two nights to check that the treatment is having the desired effect (Fig. 15.4). Overnight oximetry is sufficient in those instances where this test showed the characteristic abnormalities of obstructive sleep apnoea before treatment.

A few patients appear to lose weight after starting treatment, perhaps because they are able to increase their activity during the day. These are able to discontinue treatment, but the majority of those who benefit symptomatically remain on treatment for life.

This brief summary does not do justice to the large volume of effort expended in this topic since 1970. The study of sleep apnoea and of sleep-disordered breathing is a branch of clinical physiology in its own right. Whether minor degrees of sleep apnoea are important is undecided. The full syndrome of obesity, snoring and daytime hypersomnolence is easily recognisable socially and clinically; such patients are generally grateful for nasal ventilatory support to abolish snoring and reduce the frequency of nocturnal waking.

## Sleep studies in chronic respiratory insufficiency

Muscular dystrophies and neural disorders affecting the respiratory muscles may cause nocturnal hypoventilation, with episodes of profound oxygen desaturation. A weak cough and prolonged reduction of tidal volume make gas exchange worse because they result in basal atelectasis, repeated episodes of infection and ventilation–perfusion mismatching. The end result is chronic respiratory failure. Sleep studies show that nocturnal ventilatory failure may precede abnormalities of daytime blood gases. The techniques employed are similar to those already described in this chapter. In addition, it is helpful to measure arterial $P_{CO_2}$ employing a transcutaneous $CO_2$ analyser applied to the skin. This device responds slowly to changes of $P_{CO_2}$ over about 15 minutes. Prolonged episodes of $CO_2$ retention can be detected with this device. It is not very easy to use, because the skin has to be heated

and the electrode has to be placed on the trunk and moved every few hours (Parker & Delpy, 1983).

The relief of nocturnal hypoventilation may improve well-being in patients with neuromuscular disorders and also with abnormalities of the thoracic wall such as scoliosis. Rather surprisingly, daytime blood gases may sometimes improve as well (Smith, Edwards & Calverley, 1992). Modern ventilators which are able to apply gentle pressure during the inspiratory cycle via a nasal mask are well tolerated. They do not need to be very powerful because if, as is usual, the compliances of the lung and chest wall are normal, an inspiratory pressure rising to 20 cm $H_2O$ is sufficient to generate a tidal volume of over 0.5 litre. The respiratory rate is chosen by the patient and the device can be set to reach a pressure of up to 30 cm $H_2O$ at any frequency, with or without positive end-expired pressure to maintain airway patency.

So far, nocturnal ventilatory assistance appears to have little advantage over the administration of oxygen in patients with chronic airflow obstruction, probably because the gentle positive pressure cannot overcome the inspiratory obstruction and hyperinflation of the lungs and chest wall. About 50% of patients with muscular dystrophy are helped by nocturnal ventilation as are an even greater proportion of those with chronic, stable impairment of respiratory motion. The reason for the improvement is not known; resting the respiratory muscles could be helpful, or it may be that maintaining normal blood gases and normal airway patency at night improves overall lung function or rests the chemoreceptors.

A population of 100 000 may have only 2 or 3 individuals on nocturnal assisted ventilation and a few more using nasal CPAP. Some will try the treatment and not persevere for a variety of reasons. The treatment of those who respond is one of the most rewarding applications of respiratory physiology in clinical practice.

## References

Anonymous (1984). Patient's wife cures his snoring. *Chest*, **85**, 582 (letter).
Berry, D.T.R., West, W.B. & Block, A.J. (1984). Sleep

apnoea syndrome: a critical review of the apnoea index as a diagnostic criterion. *Chest*, **86**, 529–531.

Catterall, J.R. (1992). The sleep apnoea syndromes. In: *Medical Annual: The Year Book of General Practice*, ed. J. Fry & T. Bouchier Hayes. Bristol: Clinical Press.

Catterall, J.R., Douglas, N.R., Calverley, P.M.A., Shapiro, R.M., Brezinova, V., Brash, H.M. & Flenley, D.C. (1983). Transient hypoxaemia during sleep in chronic obstructive pulmonary disease is not sleep apnoea syndrome. *American Review of Respiratory Disease*, **128**, 24–29.

Connaughton, J.J., Catterall, J.R., Elton, R.A., Stradling, J. & Douglas, N.J. (1988). Do sleep studies contribute to the management of patients with severe obstructive pulmonary disease? *American Review of Respiratory Disease*, **138**, 341–344.

Cooper, B.G., Veale, D., Griffiths, C.J. & Gibson G.J. (1991). Value of nocturnal oxygen saturation as a screening test for sleep apnoea. *Thorax*, **46**, 586–588.

Douglas, N.J., Thomas, S. & Jan, M.A. (1992). Clinical value of polysomnography. *Lancet*, **339**, 347–350.

Findley, L., Universtadt, M. & Suratt, P. (1988). Automobile accidents in patients with obstructive sleep apnoea. *American Review of Respiratory Disease*, **138**, 337–340.

Guilleminault, C., Partinen, M., Quera-Jalva, M.A., Hayes, B., Dement, W.C. & Mino-Murcia, G. (1988). Determinants of day time sleepiness in obstructive sleep apnoea. *Chest*, **94**, 32–37.

Guilleminault, C., Tilkian, A. & Dement, W.C. (1976). The sleep apnoea syndromes. *Annual Review of Medicine*, **27**, 465–484.

Leitch, A.G. (1983). Assessment of the control of breathing and monitoring during sleep. In: *Measurement in Clinical Respiratory Physiology*, ed. G. Laszlo & M.F. Sudlow. London: Academic Press.

Letner, M., Young, E. & McGuinty, D. *et al.* (1984). Awake abnormalities of control of breathing and of the upper airway: occurrence in healthy older men with nocturnal disordered breathing. *Chest*, **86**, 573–579.

Mathew, O.P. & Remmers, J.E. (1984). Respiratory functions of the upper airway. In: *Sleep and Breathing*, ed. N.A. Saunders & C.E. Sullivan, pp. 163–200. New York: Marcel Dekker.

Orem, J. (1984). Control of the upper airways during sleep and the hypersomnia–sleep apnea syndrome. In: *Physiology in Sleep*, ed. J. Orem & C.D. Barnes, pp. 273–313. New York: Academic Press.

Parker, D. & Delpy, D.T. (1983). Blood gas analysis by invasive and non-invasive techniques. In: *Measurement in Clinical Respiratory Physiology*, ed. G. Laszlo & M.F. Sudlow, pp. 93–96. London: Academic Press.

Partinen, M., Jamieson, A. & Guilleminault, C. (1988). Long term outcome for obstructive sleep apnea patients: mortality. *Chest*, **94**, 1200–1204.

Rechtschaffen, A. & Kales, A. (1968). A manual of standardized terminology, techniques and scoring system for deep stages of human sleep. NIH Publication 204. Bethesda: National Institutes of Neurological Disease and Blindness.

Roehrs, T., Zorick, F., Wittig, R., Conway, W. & Roth, T. (1989). Predictors of objective level of daytime sleepiness in patients with sleep-related breathing disorders. *Chest*, **95**, 1202–1206.

Sanders, M.H., Black, J., Constantino, J., Kern, N., Studnicki, K. & Coates, J. (1991). Diagnosis of sleep-disordered breathing by half-night polysomnography. *American Review of Respiratory Disease*, **144**, 1256–1261.

Series, F., Cormier, Y. & La Forge, J. (1991). Validity of diurnal sleep recording in the diagnosis of sleep apnea syndrome. *American Review of Respiratory Disease*, **143**, 947–949.

Smith, P.E.M., Edwards, R.H.T. & Calverley, P.M. (1991). Mechanisms of sleep-disordered breathing in chronic neuromuscular disease: implications for management. *Quarterly Journal of Medicine*, 296, 961–973.

Stradling, J.R. & Crosby, J.H. (1991). Predictors and prevalence of obstructive sleep apnoea in 1001 middle-aged men. *Thorax*, **46**, 85–90.

Stradling, J.R. & Phillipson, E.A. (1986). Breathing disorders during sleep. *Quarterly Journal of Medicine*, **225**, 3–18.

Stradling, J.R., Thomas, G., Warley, A.R.H. *et al.* (1990). Effect of adenotonsillectomy on nocturnal hypoxaemia, sleep disturbance and symptoms in snoring children. *Lancet*, **335**, 249–253.

Sullivan, C.E., Berthon-Jones, M., Issa, F.G. & Eves, L. (1981). Perusal of obstructive sleep apnoea by continuous positive airway pressure applied through the nares. *Lancet*, **i**, 841–846.

Sullivan, C.E., Issa, F.G., Berthon-Jones, M., McCauley, V.B. & Costas, L.J.V. (1984). Home treatment of obstructive sleep apnoea with continuous positive airway pressure applied through a nose mask. *Bulletin*, **20**, 49–54.

Weitzenblum, E., Kriegie, J., Apprill, M., Vallee, E., Ratomaharo, J., Oswald, M. & Kurtz, D. (1988). Daytime pulmonary hypertension in patients with obstructive sleep apnoea syndrome. *American Review of Respiratory Disease*, **138**, 345–349.

Whyte, K.F., Allen, M.B., Jeffrey, A.A., Gould, G.A. & Douglas, N.J. (1989). Clinical features of the sleep apnoea/hypopnoea syndrome. *Quarterly Journal of Medicine*, **267**, 659–666.

# APPENDIX

Table A. 1. *Effects of various disorders on the physiology of respiration and the relevance of pulmonary function tests*

| | Pathological change | Physiological consequence | Functional measurements |
|---|---|---|---|
| Airways | Inflammation; scarring; loss of ciliary beat; excessive secretion | Narrowing (variable or fixed obliteration) | Maximal flow; resistance to flow; premature closure; gaseous diffusion; reactivity to constrictors and relaxants |
| Alveoli | Inflammation; mural fibrosis; alveolar filling; alveolar obliteration; disintegration of walls; vascular occlusion | Thickening of walls; reduction of numbers (obliteration or confluence) | Lung size (volume, distensibility, compliance); gas transfer |
| Pulmonary vessels | Constriction; vascular hypertrophy; pulmonary systemic shunts; broncho-pulmonary anastomoses | Pulmonary hypertension; regional variation of blood flow; pulmonary–systemic shunting | Pulmonary arterial pressure; topographical distribution of ventilation and blood flow; measurement of shunt |
| Thoracic cage | Reduced movement of spine and costovertebral joints; pleural air, fluid, obliteration or fibrosis pain; vascular weakness of diaphragm and other muscles | Deformity; impaired excursion | Size and shape of thorax; respiratory muscle power; transdiaphragmatic and intrathoracic pressures |
| Integrated neural control of cyclical action of respiratory muscles | Excessive ventilation; inadequate ventilation; irregular ventilation awake or during sleep | Hyperventilation; $CO_2$ retention; hypoxaemia; nocturnal hypoxaemia | Arterial blood gases, rate, depth and force of breathing at rest, in exercise, in sleep and under abnormal conditions |
| Respiratory sensation | Perception of increased ventilation; perception of increased force | Dyspnoea; respiratory discomfort | Measurement of perceived respiratory and muscular exertion, at rest and under stress |
| Response to environmental change | Altitude (hypobaric); depth (hyperbaric) | Alterations of partial pressures and density of inspired gases | Effects on gas exchange and control of ventilation |

Table A. 2. *Lung function tests in routine use: physiological basis and clinical interpretation*

| Test | Structural implication | Functional implication/clinical usefulness |
| --- | --- | --- |
| Vital capacity | Size of lungs (in the absence of airways disease) | Ventilatory capacity, correlates with dysfunction |
| Derivatives of forced volume–time curve, especially $FEV_1$, $FEV_1/VC\%$, PEF | Airway narrowing | Airflow obstruction (variable or fixed) |
| Static lung volumes: total lung capacity, functional residual capacity, residual volume | Size of lungs | Explains reduced vital capacity: low values indicate small lungs; normal or high values indicate airflow obstruction with premature airway closure |
| Indices of CO uptake: transfer factor (diffusing capacity) and transfer coefficient | An approximate indication of the volume of haemoglobin capable of taking up $O_2$ in the well-ventilated portion of the lungs | In the absence of airflow obstruction, these tests indicate the integrity of alveolar gas exchange |
| Blood gases: arterial $Pco_2$ and arterial $Pco$ (mixed venous $Pco_2$, and transcutaneous capillary $O_2$ saturation may provide estimates) | The respiratory system may fail because of severe disease of the lungs, thorax or respiratory muscles or disturbances of ventilatory control | Blood gases are maintained within close limits at rest and in exercise, given a constant environment |
| Respiratory muscle power: maximal inspiration and expiratory mouth pressures | Damage to efferent innervation of respiratory muscles; acute damage to chest and abdominal wall | Diaphragmatic or global respiratory muscle weakness or fatigue |
| Blood gases, ECG, ventilation and breathing pattern in symptom-limited exercise tests | Tests for coronary artery insufficiency and a wide variety of disorders limiting effort tolerance | Identifies cause of effort intolerance |
| $O_2$ saturation and other measurements during sleep | Upper airway closure or damage to medullary centres governing the cyclical control of respiration | Diagnosis of sleep apnoea syndrome, the common cause of daytime sleepiness |

# INDEX

The index is arranged in word-by-word order. Abbreviations are preferred where appropriate. *Italics* denote illustrations. [ ] denote tables.

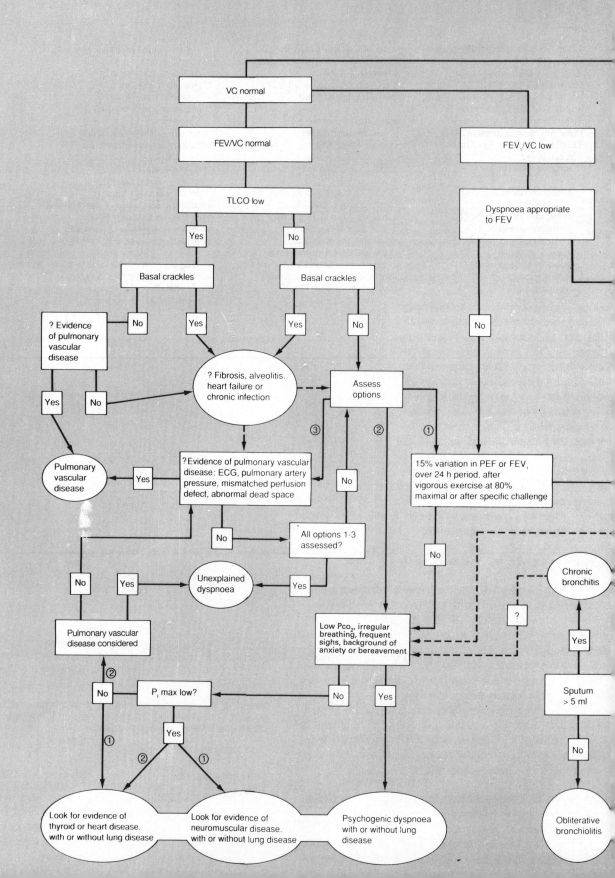

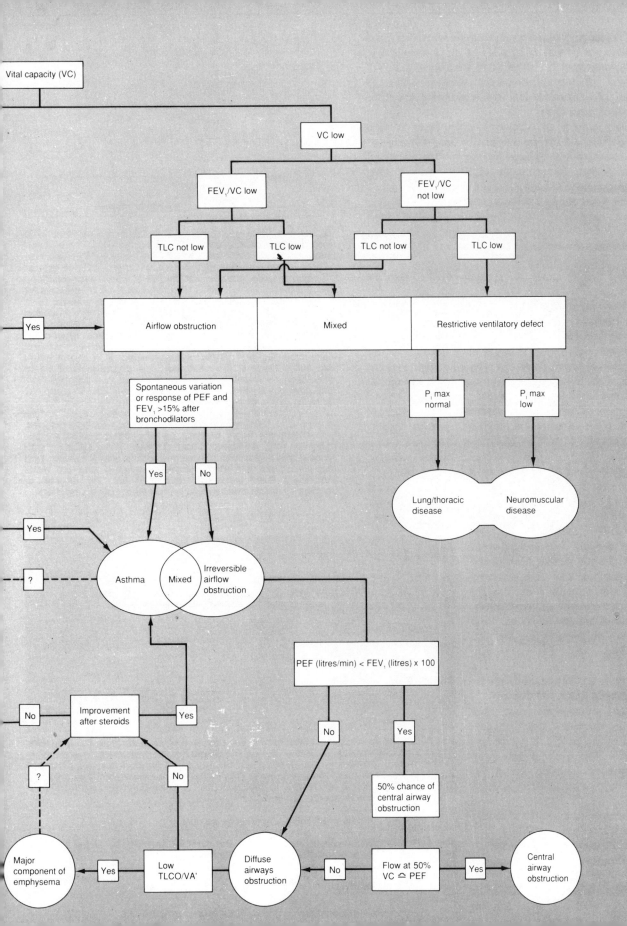